Canine Anatomy

A Systemic Study

Fourth Edition

Canine Anatomy

A Systemic Study

Fourth Edition

Donald R. Adams

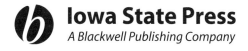

Iowa State Press

A Blackwell Publishing Company

Iowa State Press
2121 State Avenue, Ames, Iowa 50014

Orders:	1-800-862-6657
Office:	1-515-292-0140
Fax:	1-515-292-3348
Web site:	www.iowastatepress.com

⊛Printed on acid-free paper in the United States of America

First edition, 1996
Second edition, 1998
Third Edition, 2001
Fourth Edition, 2004

Library of Congress Cataloging-in-Publication Data

Adams, Donald R. (Donald Robert), 1937–
    Canine anatomy : a systemic study / Donald R. Adams.—4th ed.
        p. cm.
    Includes index.
    ISBN 0-8138-1281-X (alk. paper)
        1. Dogs—Anatomy.   I. Title.

SF767.D6A33 2004
636.7'0891—dc21

                                                    2003049908

The last digit is the print number: 9 8 7 6 5 4 3 2 1

Contents

Preface

This text was written to provide introductory anatomical information on the dog and cat for the first-year veterinary student. Since this text was prepared as an adjunct to the outstanding reference textbook *Miller's Anatomy of the Dog*, specific details and references have been omitted. Terminology generally conforms to that prescribed by *Nomina Anatomica Veterinaria*.

Because this text has been developed to guide students in the systemic dissection of non-embalmed canine carcasses, specific instructions for dissection have been omitted; the diversity in dissection approaches used by student groups provides a variety of learning experiences in the lab, with a periodic replacement of cadavers providing opportunities for repeated dissections of the same anatomical regions.

An effort has been made to present directional and structural terminology gradually and sequentially. Anatomical terms introduced the first time in the text, or emphasized in a particular chapter, are typed in capital letters. Clarification of difficult words has been provided in parentheses the first time the words are used. Such information may include singular and plural spellings, pronunciation, and/or meaning. It is hoped that students will be motivated by this additional information to make regular use of a medical dictionary.

I am indebted to faculty, staff, and administrators of the Iowa State University College of Veterinary Medicine who provided assistance and cooperation in the development of this book. Frank Schneider, one of the student artists, provided numerous detailed illustrations of dissected cadavers and organ systems. This book has been used for over 12 years as a non-required text by veterinary students at Iowa State University.

Unit I

Introduction

In the chapter that follows, you will read about descriptive terms that you will frequently use throughout your academic or professional life.

Contents:

1

Chapter 1
DIRECTIONAL TERMINOLOGY

Objectives: Become familiar with descriptive terms commonly used to describe position of structures within or on the body.

cranial vs. caudal

rostral vs. caudal

dorsal vs. ventral

palmar vs. dorsal

plantar vs. dorsal

anterior vs. posterior

superior vs. inferior

median vs. sagittal planes

dorsal median line vs. ventral medial line

medial vs. intermediate vs. lateral

transverse plane vs. dorsal plane

axial vs. abaxial

superficial vs. deep

A number of adjectives are used to describe the position of structures in the body. Descriptive terms are also used to name many anatomical structures. The terms described in this chapter are utilized throughout the remainder of the text.

An imaginary line through the center of the length of an organ or structure of the body forms the **LONG AXIS** (pl. axes) of that organ or structure (Fig. 1.1). The weight of the organ is almost symmetrically distributed around its long axis. Proximal and distal are used to describe position along the long axis of a structure relative to the main body mass.

PROXIMAL implies a position near or toward the main mass of a structure; **DISTAL** implies a position away from the main mass (Fig. 1.2).

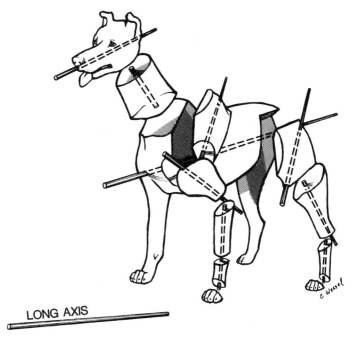

Fig.1.1. Long axis.

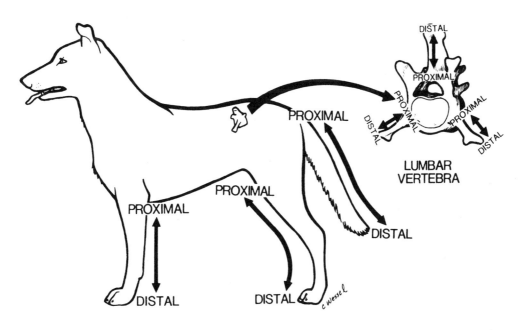

Fig.1.2. Proximal - distal.

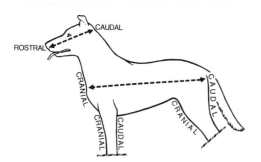

Fig.1.3. Cranial/rostral-caudal.

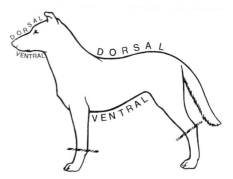

Fig.1.4. Dorsal-ventral.

CRANIAL and **CAUDAL** are directional terms meaning toward or relatively near the cranium (brain case) and tail, respectively (Fig. 1.3). Cranial and caudal, when used in describing structures of the trunk (neck, thorax, abdomen, and pelvis), refer to position along the long axis of the trunk.

Cranial and caudal, when used in reference to forelimb and hind limb structures of a standing dog, refer to the surfaces toward the head and tail, respectively; only the portions of the limbs proximal to the carpus (wrist) and tarsus (ankle) are said to have cranial and caudal surfaces.

ROSTRAL, rather than cranial, is used to describe the positions of most structures along the long axis of the head; the word rostral refers to a position facing the apex of the nose. In the head the opposite direction to rostral is caudal.

DORSAL and **VENTRAL** are directional terms meaning toward or relatively near the back and belly, respectively (Fig. 1.4). Dorsal and ventral, when used in describing structures of the head, trunk, and tail, refer to opposing positions along the long axis.

Distal to the carpus and tarsus, dorsal refers to the surface opposite that of the footpads (Fig. 1.5). The dorsal surfaces of the distal portions of the limbs are continuous proximally with the

cranial surfaces of the respective limb. The surface of the thoracic limb distal to the carpus, which bears footpads, is the **PALMAR** surface; the surface of the pelvic limb distal to the tarsus, which bears footpads, is the **PLANTAR** surface. The palmar and plantar surfaces of the distal portion of the limbs are continuous with the caudal surfaces of the proximal portion of the limbs.

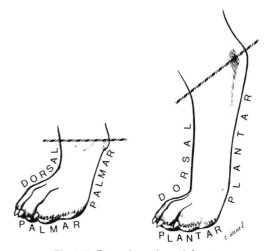

Fig.1.5. Dorsal - palmar/plantar.

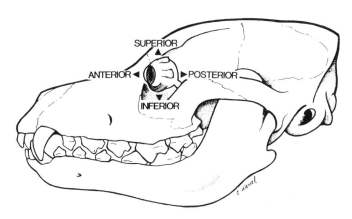

Fig.1.6. Anterior-posterior/superior-inferior.

When describing certain structures of the head (eye, eyelids, lips, inner ear, pituitary gland), the terms cranial, caudal, dorsal, and ventral are replaced by **ANTERIOR, POSTERIOR, SUPERIOR,** and **INFERIOR**, respectively (Fig. 1.6).

An organ or structure may be divided into two nearly identical halves by a **MEDIAN PLANE** (Fig. 1.7). A median plane passing longitudinally through the dog's body divides it into right and left halves. The **DORSAL MEDIAN LINE** and **VENTRAL MEDIAN LINE** are imaginary lines through which the median plane passes on the dorsal and ventral surfaces, respectively, of the dog.

A **SAGITTAL (PARAMEDIAN) PLANE** (Fig. 1.8) is parallel to the median plane.

MEDIAL and **LATERAL** refer to positions toward and away from the median plane, respectively (Fig. 1.9). Some structures, such as blood vessels of the external ear, occur in groups of three and are described as **MEDIAL, INTERMEDIATE,** and **LATERAL**.

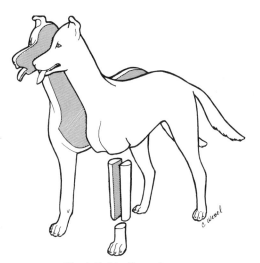

Fig.1.7. Median plane.

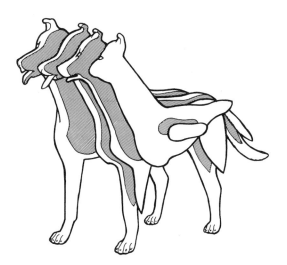

Fig.1.8. Sagittal planes.

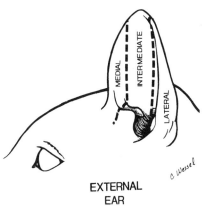

EXTERNAL
EAR

Fig.1.9. Medial-intermediate-lateral.

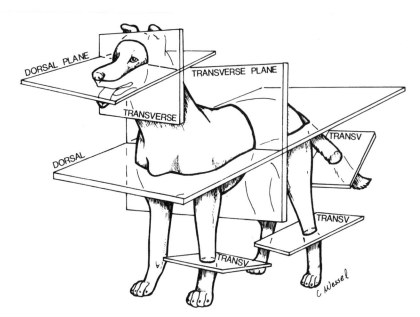

Fig.1.10. Dorsal and transverse planes.

A TRANSVERSE PLANE passes through a structure perpendicular to its long axis; a **DORSAL PLANE**, perpendicular to both the median and transverse planes, divides the body longitudinally into dorsal and ventral portions (Fig. 1.10).

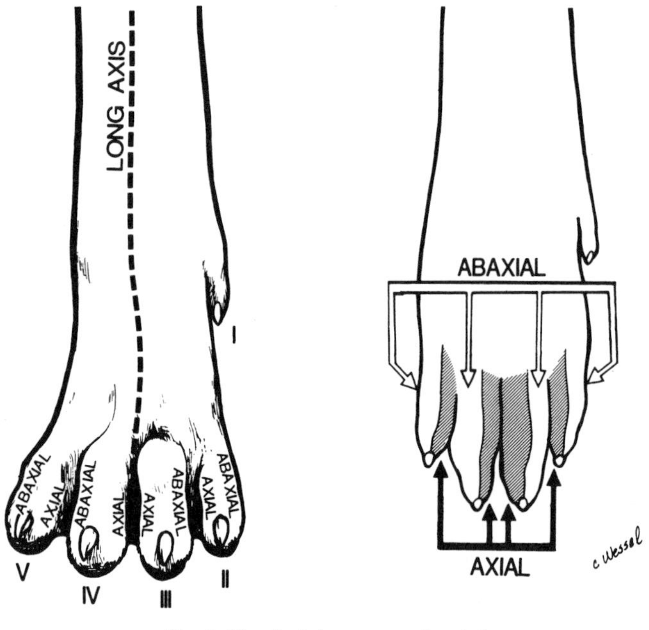

Axial and abaxial are directional terms used in reference to the digits and relate to the long axis of the limb (Fig. 1.11). The long axis of the thoracic and pelvic limbs of the dog passes between the third and fourth digits. Digits are named I, II, III, IV, and V according to position from medial to lateral. If an animal species has less than five digits the remaining digits are usually designated II, III, IV, and V (as in the hind feet of many dogs); II, III, and IV; III and IV; or III.

The **AXIAL** surface of digits I–V is the surface of each digit nearest the axis; the **ABAXIAL** surface of digits I–V is the surface of each digit away from the axis.

Superficial and deep are terms used in reference to position in the body or in a solid organ (Fig. 1.12). **SUPERFICIAL** means near the surface and **DEEP** refers to near the center of the body or solid organ.

Fig.1.11. Axial versus abaxial.

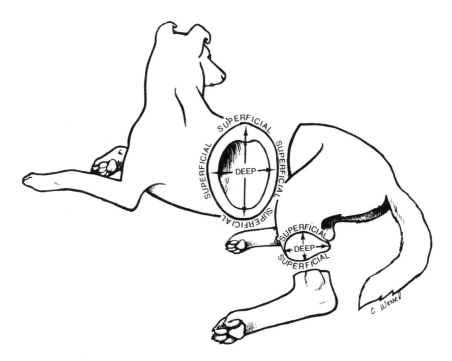

Fig.1.12. Superficial - deep.

Internal and external describe the position of a structure in the body or in a hollow organ (Fig. 1.13). **INTERNAL** implies that a structure is near the lumen of an organ; **EXTERNAL** implies that the structure is away from the center of a hollow organ.

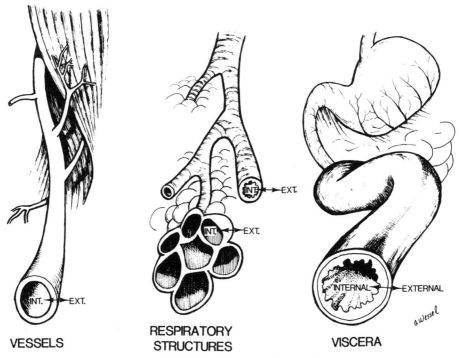

VESSELS   **RESPIRATORY STRUCTURES**   **VISCERA**

Fig.1.13. External - internal.

Unit II

Superficial Morphology

In the two chapters that follow, you will study body structures that are encountered and/or utilized during every clinical examination; dermatology, or the study of the skin, is a major portion of clinical science.

Contents:

Chapter 2
THE COMMON INTEGUMENT

Objectives: Become familiar with structures associated with the skin.

External features of the nose:

Nasal Plane, Nasal Alae, Naris, Nasal Sulci

External features of the eye:

Palpebrae, Superior and Inferior
Cilia
Lateral and Medial Palpebral Commissures
Semilunar Conjunctival Fold (Nictitating Membrane) and Lymph Nodules
Bulbar and Palpebral Conjunctiva
Conjunctival Fornix and Conjunctival Sac
Lacrimal Puncta and Lacrimal Glands
Nasolacrimal Duct
Cornea

External features of the external ear:

External Acoustic Meatus
Tragic and Antitragic Margins
Apex and Scapha
Auricular and Annular Cartilage
Antihelix
Crura
Pretragic Incisure, Tragus, and Intertragic Incisure
Cutaneous Marginal Sac

Other skin structures:

Epidermis and Dermis
Hair Follicle, Primary Hair, Secondary Hairs, and Pore
Cilia, Tragi, Tactile Hairs
Sebaceous, Odoriferous, and Sudoriferous Glands
Ceruminous, Tarsal, and Circumanal Glands

Caudal Gland
Mammary Glands (Mammae) and Mammary Papillae)
Paranala Sinuses (Anal Sacs)
Digital, Metacarpal, Metatarsal, and Carpal Pads
Claw and Dewclaw, Wall and Sole

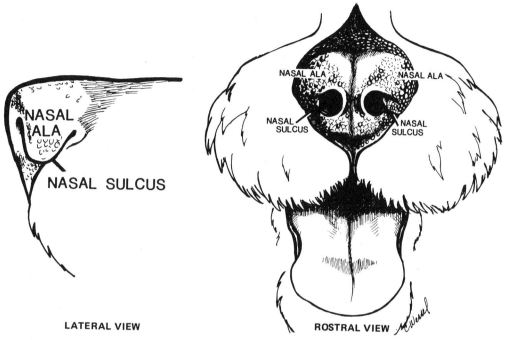

Fig.2.1. Nasal plane.

The term **COMMON INTEGUMENT,** or common covering, includes the skin, hair, skin glands, mammary glands, pads, and claws. The **SKIN,** which covers the external surface of the body, is variously modified over the surface of the external nose, eye, and ear. The **NASAL PLANE** is the nonhaired tip of the nose that is divided by small fissures into numerous polygons (Fig. 2.1). Each external **NARIS** (pl. nares; nostril) is bounded laterally by a movable wing, or **NASAL ALA** (a' lah, pl. alae). The grooves ventral to the nasal alae are the **NASAL SULCI** (sul' kee, sing. sulcus).

The PALPEBRAE (sing. palprebra; eyelids) are modified integumentary structures that protect the anterior surface of the eye (Fig. 2.2).

Both **SUPERIOR** and **INFERIOR PALPEBRAE** have a haired superficial surface, but **CILIA** (sil'e-ah, sing. cilium; eyelashes) are present only on the superior palpebra.

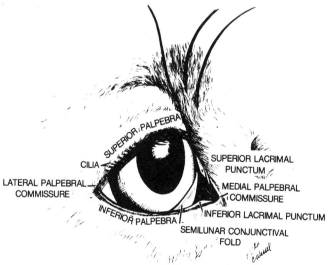

Fig.2.2. Palpebrae.

15

The lateral and medial angles formed by the junctions of the superior and inferior palpebrae are termed **LATERAL** and **MEDIAL PALPEBRAL COMMISSURES (CANTHI)** (can' thie, sing. canthus), respectively. A third eyelid, the **SEMILUNAR CONJUNCTIVAL FOLD (NICTITATING MEMBRANE)**, projects laterally from the medial commissure of the eye.

The skin of the superficial surface of the palpebrae is continuous with the mucous membrane of the deep surface. This mucous membrane is the **CONJUNCTIVA** (Fig. 2.3), a delicate lining that covers the deep surface of the palpebrae (**PALPEBRAL CONJUNCTIVA**) and the anterior surface of the eyeball (**BULBAR CONJUNCTIVA**). The bulbar conjunctiva is continuous with the most superficial layer of the

At the medial palpebral commissure there is a larger fluid–filled space, the **LACRIMAL LAKE** (Fig. 2.4).

A small orifice, difficult to see with the unaided eye, is present in both the superior and inferior palpebrae. These orifices, termed **LACRIMAL PUNCTA** (punk' tah, sing. punctum), are situated near the medial palpebral commissure. **LACRIMAL FLUID** (tears) is produced primarily by **LACRIMAL GLANDS** (70%), located dorsal to the eyeball, and by the superficial gland of the third eyelid (30%).

Fluid collects in the lacrimal lake and passes away from the surface of the eye through the lacrimal puncta; it is then discharged into the rostral part of the nasal cavity by the **NASOLACRIMAL DUCT**.

The posterior (deep) surface of the semilunar conjunctival fold bears prominant **LYMPH NODULES** (Fig. 2.5). These nodules, when inflamed and swollen, may block flow through the secretory ducts of the superficial glands of the third eyelid.

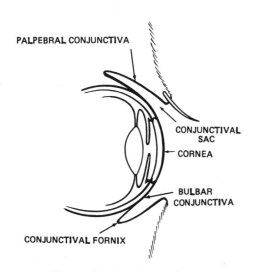

Fig.2.3. Conjunctiva and cornea.

CORNEA, the anterior corneal epithelium. The angle formed by the reflection of the conjunctiva from the palpebral surface to the bulbar surface is termed the **CONJUNCTIVAL FORNIX** (for' niks, pl. fornices). The fluid–filled space between the palpebrae and bulbar conjunctiva is the **CONJUNCTIVAL SAC**.

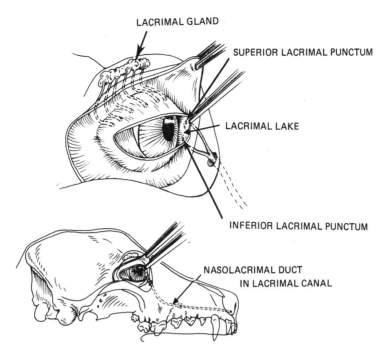

Fig.2.4. Lacrimal apparatus.

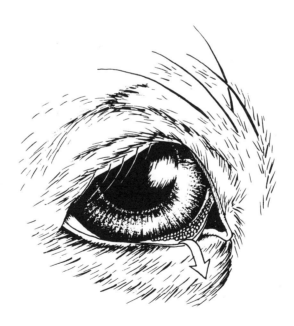

Fig.2.5. Lymph nodules on the deep surface of the semilunar conjunctival fold (third eyelid).

The external ear (Fig. 2.6) consists of a canal, the **EXTERNAL ACOUSTIC MEATUS** (me-a'tus; passage), and the **PINNA** (pin' nah, pl. pinnae). The pinna is that portion of the ear that is readily seen; it is fundamentally the same in the various breeds of dogs. The rostral margin of the pinna is the **TRAGIC MARGIN** and the lateral margin is the **ANTI-TRAGIC MARGIN**.

The tip of the ear is termed the **APEX**. The **SCAPHA** is that portion of the pinna situated between tragic and antitragic margins. The cartilaginous skeleton of the ear is formed by two cartilages: auricular and annular.

The **AURICULAR CARTILAGE**, which provides shape to the external ear, is thin and pliable over most of its distal portion. The proximal portion of the auricular cartilage is rolled, forming a tubelike wall around much of the external acoustic meatus. A number of folds, or wrinkles, formed in the auricular cartilage present structural landmarks for treatment of the ear. The most prominent is a transverse fold on the concave surface of the external ear. The free end of this fold, the **ANTIHELIX** (he' liks, pl. helices; coil), is directed caudolaterally.

At the base of the ear a thickened structure, the **TRAGUS** (tra' gus, pl. tragi), forms the superficial wall of the cartilaginous external acoustic meatus. The tragic margin separates proximally into two **CRURA** (kru' ra, sing. crus) between which is positioned the rostral margin of the tragus. The groove between these crura and the tragus is named the **PRETRAGIC INCISURE**. Caudal to the antihelix on the caudal part of the concave surface of the pinna, several longitudinal ridges may be observed, two of which are the lateral and medial processes of the **ANTITRAGUS**. The fissure between the antitragus and tragus is called the **INTERTRAGIC INCISURE**. The tragus and the pretragic and intertragic incisures are important landmarks for surgery to drain the external acoustic meatus.

A **CUTANEOUS MARGINAL SAC** of unknown significance occurs in the antitragic margin.

The **ANNULAR CARTILAGE** is a short, cartilaginous tube that extends from the osseous external acoustic meatus of the skull to the auricular cartilage; thus it encloses the proximal portion of the membranous external acoustic meatus.

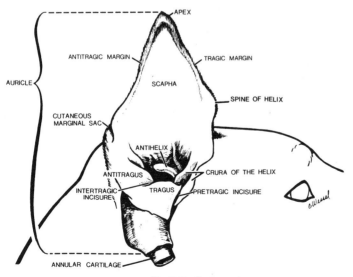

Fig.2.6. External ear.

Microscopically, the skin may be divided into two major parts, the **EPIDERMIS** and **DERMIS** (Fig. 2.7), each of which is subdivided into various layers.

The deepest layer of the epidermis is a layer of living cells, which, by mitosis, produces cells of the more superficial epidermal layers and of hair and claws.

The dermis is a layer of connective tissue deep to the epidermis; it contains blood vessels, nerves, nerve endings, and glands. Macroscopic examination of the dermal layer of the dog reveals the basal portion of hair embedded in it; the layer of living cells of the epidermis folds down into the dermis, forming a sheath or follicle around the base of the hair shaft.

Each hair is a nonliving structure produced by an epidermal **HAIR FOLLICLE**. A number of individual hairs (a larger **PRIMARY HAIR** plus several smaller **SECONDARY HAIRS**), each with its own follicle, project from the surface of the skin through a common opening, or **PORE**. Small muscle fibers attach to the hair follicle deeply and to the dermis superficially. Contraction of these smooth muscle fibers straightens the hair.

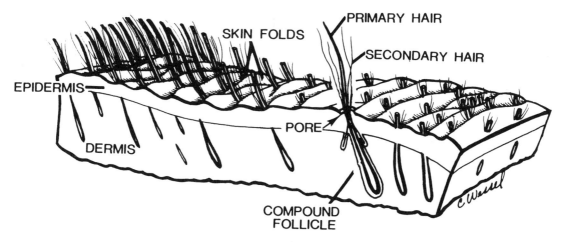

Fig.2.7. Diagram of an excised block of skin.

Some examples of specialized types of hair present over the surface of the body (Fig. 2.8) are: **CILIA, TRAGI** (hair at the opening of the external ear), and the large **TACTILE HAIRS** present over much of the face. Types of tactile hairs include **SUPRAORBITAL, ZYGOMATIC, BUCCAL** (buk'al), **SUPERIOR** and **INFERIOR LABIAL, MENTAL,** and **INTERMANDIBULAR.**

Tactile hairs are termed "vibrissae" by many comparative anatomists. In Veterinary Anatomy the term vibrissae is restricted to specialized hairs present in the nasal vestibule; such vibrissae are not present in the dog.

Tactile hairs are large single hairs, each of which is produced by a large follicle. The tactile hair follicle is surrounded by a blood sinus composed of a superficial ring and a deeper spongy portion. Abundant nerve fiber terminals in the connective tissue walls of the blood sinuses are responsive to tactile sensation. Both the blood pressure in the sinus and the skeletal muscle attaching to the dermal sheath of the follicle may modify the responsiveness of the hair to stimulation.

(*IN THE CAT, Tactile hairs with blood sinuses are also present in the skin of the distal portion of the thoracic limb.*)

Microscopic glands occurring in the dermis are sebaceous, odoriferous, or sudoriferous in character. The SEBACEOUS GLANDS secrete a fatty material and are usually associated with hair follicles. ODORIFEROUS (APOCRINE SUDORIFEROUS) GLANDS, located over most of the dog's surface area, are also associated with hair follicles; these glands, which secrete odorous substances, may function in olfactory communication between animals.

SUDORIFEROUS (MEROCRINE SUDORIFEROUS) GLANDS, or true sweat glands, are restricted in location to the footpads,

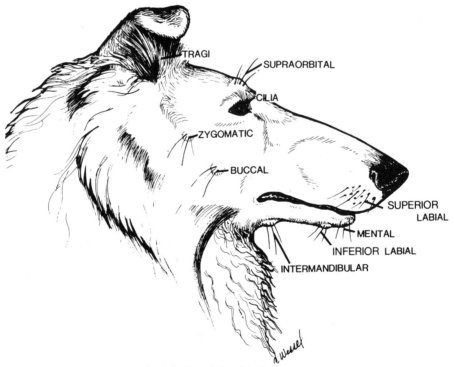

Fig.2.8. Specialized hair types.

where their watery secretions may have a function in gripping the surface. Some larger specialized glands are the **CERUMINOUS GLANDS** of the external auditory meatus, **TARSAL GLANDS** of the palpebrae, **CIRCUMANAL GLANDS** of the anal region, paranal sinus glands (glands of the anal sacs), caudal glands, and mammary glands.

The **PARANAL SINUSES** (anal sacs) are paired cutaneous sacs located one to each side of the anus; a duct from each sinus opens onto the surface of the skin at the lateral margin of the anus (Figs 2.9, 2.10). The paranal sinuses are covered by skeletal muscle that encircles the anal canal.

The **CAUDAL GLAND** is a densely grouped collection of microscopic glands on the dorsal surface of the proximal portion of the tail (Fig. 2.11).

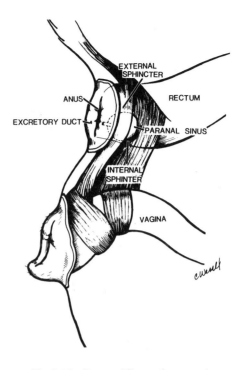

Fig.2.10. Duct orifices of paranal sinuses, anal sphincters relaxed.

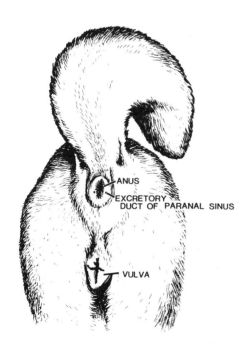

Fig.2.9. Paranal sinusanal sphincter relationship.

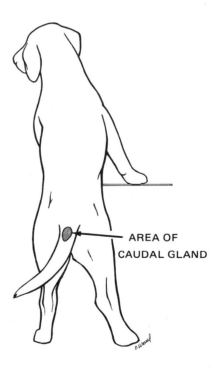

Fig.2.11. Caudal gland.

21

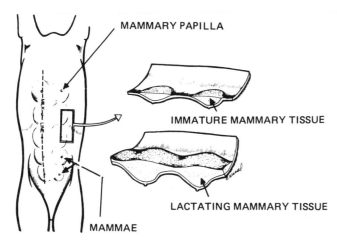

Fig.2.12. Mammary glands.

The **MAMMARY** (milk producing) **GLANDS** – develop in a row on each side of the ventral median line; this row, or line, is termed the "milk line" (Fig. 2.12). Mammary glands (**MAMMAE**) of the bitch are usually present as four to six pairs. Five pairs of mammae are the most common, although there may be four mammae on one side and five on the other.

Each functional mammary gland (**MAMMA**) produces milk, which passes to the surface of the skin via 7–16 ducts in a mammary papilla (pah-pil' ah, pl. papillae), or nipple (Fig. 2.13).

The mammae are described as being thoracic, cranial abdominal, middle abdominal, or caudal abdominal according to their regional placement.

Both male and young female mammae consist of papillae and small primary ducts. Beginning with the onset of the first estrus, the mammary duct system and glandular elements of the bitch develop. After conception, the mammae continue developing until tissue of adjacent glands crowd each other.

PADS, roughened by small projecting papillae, are present on the palmar and plantar surfaces of the limbs. These papillae provide traction as they come into contact with the ground. Each pad consists of thickened epidermal and dermal parts plus a deeper fat pad (Fig. 2.14) that is highly vascular. The pads are named according to their location.

The **DIGITAL PADS** are small pads located in the distal interphalangeal region of digits II–V. The large pads in the metacarpophalangeal and metatarsophalangeal regions are the **METACARPAL** and **METATARSAL** **PADS**, respectively. A small pad on the palmar surface of the carpal region is the **CARPAL PAD**.

A **CLAW** is a cutaneous structure, the proximal portion of which wraps around the distal portion of the digital skeleton (Figs 2.15, 2.16). The dorsal and lateral epidermal portion of the claw (**WALL**) is stronger than the ventral portion (**SOLE**). The proximal portion, or coronary border, of the wall is situated in the osseous depression formed by the ungual crest of the distal phalanx. The dermis of the claw is continuous with connective tissue lining the

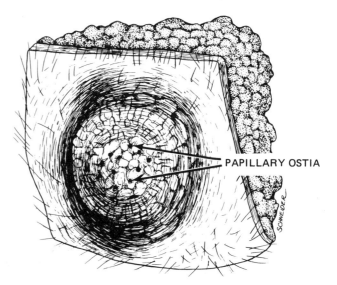

Fig.2.13. Mammary papillae.

22

bone of the distal phalanx. When the claw is
clipped too close, the nerves and blood vessels of
the dermis respond by producing pain and
bleeding.

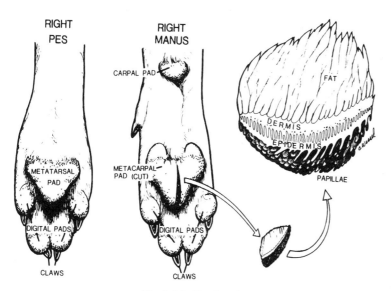

Fig.2.14. Footpads.

A **DEWCLAW** is not a claw but rather a
relatively functionless digit. The dewclaw (first
digit of the hind foot), if present, may possess
one, two, or all three phalanges. For show, the
Briard and Great Pyrenees breeds are required to
have double dewclaws.

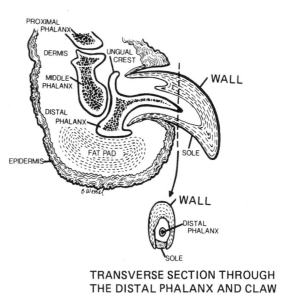

TRANSVERSE SECTION THROUGH
THE DISTAL PHALANX AND CLAW

Fig.2.16. Digit, sectioned sagitally.

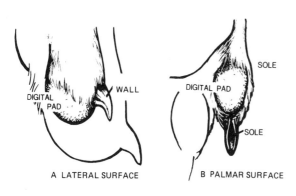

Fig.2.15. Digit.

23

Chapter 3
FASCIA

Objectives: Understand the layering of connective tissue that attaches skin to muscle, interconnects individual muscles, and attaches muscle to bone. Appreciate that nerves and blood and lymph vessels pass through these fascial planes and that when pathogens gain access they may spread within these sheets of fascia.

Superficial Fascia

Cutaneous Trunci, Platysma, Cranial Preputial/Cranial Supramammary Muscle

Panniculus Adiposus

Deep Fascia: Thoracolumbar, Gluteal, Caudal, Antebrachial, Crural Fascia, Fascia Lata, Endothoracic and Transversalis Fascia

Extensor Retinacula: Crural and Tarsal Extensor Retinacula

Flexor Retinaculum

Carotid Sheath

Synovial Bursae and Synovial Tendon Sheaths

Subserous Fascia

FASCIA (fash' e-ah, pl. fasciae; band) is composed of connective tissue bands or sheets that bind skin to deeper structures and ensheath structures deep to the skin.

For descriptive purposes, fascia may be subdivided into three major types: superficial, deep, and subserous (Fig. 3.1); the superficial and deep fascial sheets are named according to the anatomical regions where they are located.

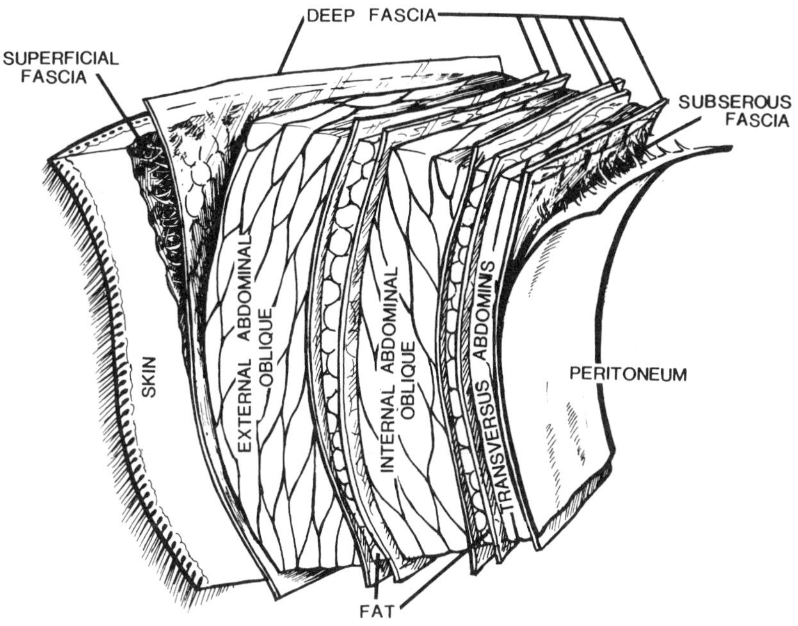

The portion of cutaneous muscle that attaches most of the skin of the trunk to the axillary region is the **CUTANEUS TRUNCI MUSCLE**. Other cutaneous muscles include that of the head (the **PLATYSMA**) and the ventrally situated **CRANIAL PREPUTIAL MUSCLE** of the dog, which, as part of the cutaneus trunci muscle, attaches to the cutaneous sheath of the penis. The mammary glands are located primarily in the superficial fascial layer (the female homolog of the cranial preputial muscle is the **CRANIAL SUPRAMAMMARY MUSCLE**).

In well-fed animals the superficial fascia is often densely infiltrated with fatty deposits; the term **PANNICULUS ADIPOSUS** refers to a fatty superficial fascia. Injections into the superficial fascia are rapidly absorbed by the abundant small blood and lymph vessels present there.

Fig.3.1. Diagram of an excised block of abdominal wall.

The SUPERFICIAL **FASCIA** (**TELA SUBCUTANEA**) (te' lah, pl. telae) is an elastic layer that connects the dermis of the skin to deeper structures. (Many authors consider this layer to be part of the dermis of the skin.) In some locations there is little superficial fascia and the skin is held tightly to underlying structures; in other places the skin is quite loose.

A thin layer of cutaneous muscle, which functions to move or shake the skin, lies within the superficial fascia (Fig. 3.2).

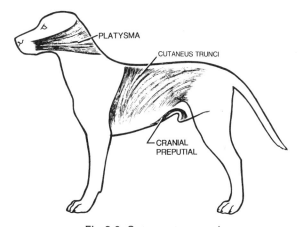

Fig.3.2. Cutaneous muscle.

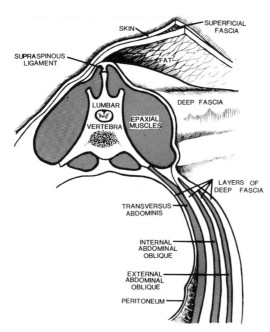

Fig.3.3. Deep lumbar and abdominal fascia.

Some larger veins course near the surface of the body within the superficial fascia.

DEEP FASCIA, a stronger and denser layer than superficial fascia, encases individual muscles and groups of muscles (Fig. 3.3); intermuscular connective tissue **SEPTA** extend between individual muscles, providing a slippery medium in which muscles may shorten during contraction against little resistance. Each layer of fascia splits into other layers that invest muscles, tendons, and bones in a continuous system.

Deep fascia may be arbitrarily described in three levels according to position: (1) a superficial layer that covers the body immediately deep to the superficial fascia; (2) a number of intermediate layers that invest the various muscles and other structures of the body wall; and (3) a deep layer that surfaces the major cavities of the trunk. The intermediate layers interconnect the superficial and deep layers by means of numerous intermuscular septa.

The superficial layer of deep fascia is very well developed in certain anatomical regions (Fig. 3.4) and thus will be given special attention. The **THORACOLUMBAR FASCIA** (1) is present in the thoracic vertebral and lumbar regions; it is continuous caudally with the **GLUTEAL** (2) and **CAUDAL** (3) **FASCIA**. The fascia of the lateral and cranial femoral regions, the **FASCIA LATA** (la'tah; wide) (4), is a very strong connective tissue sheet. The superficial layer of the deep fascia invests the distal portions of the thoracic and pelvic limbs, where it is termed the **ANTEBRACHIAL** (5) and **CRURAL** (6)

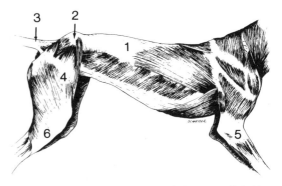

Fig.3.4. Regional thickenings of the superficial layer of deep fascia.

FASCIA. It forms a tight sheath around the limbs that under normal physiological conditions prevents the limbs from accumulating blood and lymph.

The deep fascia forms retaining bands around tendons in the carpal and tarsal regions of the thoracic and pelvic limbs, respectively. The retaining band of dorsal carpal fascia is named the **EXTENSOR RETINACULUM** (ret' i-nak' u-lum, pl. retinacula; rope); it acts to maintain certain tendons in place (Fig. 3.5).

The retaining band of palmar carpal fascia is named the **FLEXOR RETINACULUM.** There

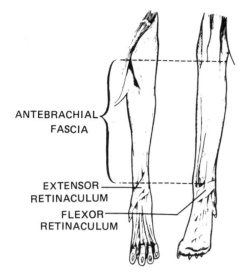

ANTEBRACHIAL
FASCIA

EXTENSOR
RETINACULUM
FLEXOR
RETINACULUM

Fig.3.5. Retinacula of the thoracic limb.

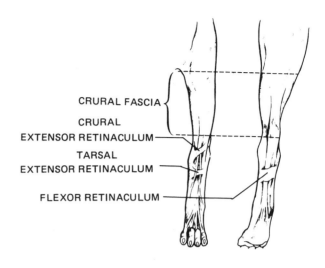

CRURAL FASCIA
CRURAL
EXTENSOR RETINACULUM
TARSAL
EXTENSOR RETINACULUM
FLEXOR RETINACULUM

Fig.3.6. Retinacula of the pelvic limb.

are two dorsal retaining bands of thickened fascia in the pelvic limb, named the **CRURAL** and **TARSAL EXTENSOR RETINACULA,** and one plantar band, the flexor retinaculum (Fig. 3.6).

The deep fascia that forms a sheath around the common carotid artery and vagosympathetic trunk is called the **CAROTID SHEATH** (Fig. 3.7). The compartments between layers of fascia that enclose muscles, vessels, and lymph nodes may contain an infection and delay its spread.

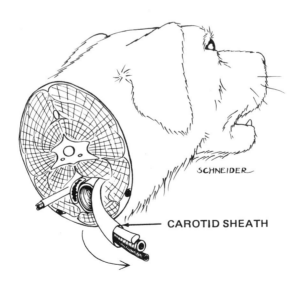

SCHNEIDER

CAROTID SHEATH

Fig.3.7. Carotid sheath.

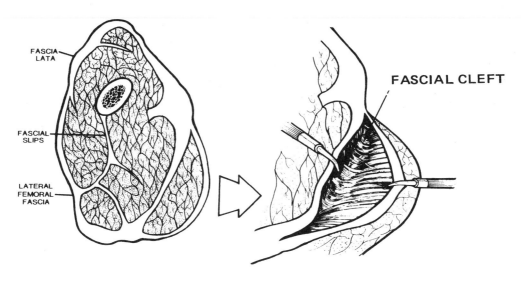

Fig.3.8. Cleavage lines or fascial clefts between muscles.

The greater the freedom needed by muscles for contraction, the greater is the degree of fascial separation from muscle surfaces. As muscles are dissected out, these **FASCIAL CLEFTS** become evident (Fig. 3.8); they are places of cleavage between adjacent muscles.

SYNOVIAL TENDON SHEATHS (Fig. 3.10) occur in the manus and pes as specializations of deep fascia forming elongated sacs that wrap around tendons; the deepest portion of the fascial sac adheres to the tendon. The fluid-filled sheaths permit a degree of movement while reducing friction.

The deep layer of deep fascia that forms part of the deep surface of the thoracic wall is termed

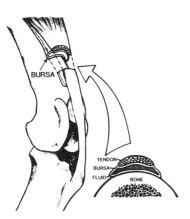

Fig.3.9. Bursa.

Fluid-filled connective tissue sacs, or **SYNOVIAL BURSAE** (ber' sah, pl. bursae), are located in many parts of the body between muscle tendons and underlying bone (Fig. 3.9); bursae reduce friction that otherwise would be produced during muscular activity by tendons sliding on bone.

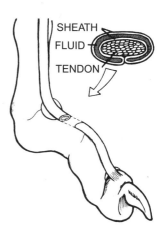

Fig.3.10. Synovial tendon sheath.

ENDOTHORACIC FASCIA (Fig. 3.11). The deep layer of deep fascia in the abdominal and pelvic regions is the **TRANSVERSALIS FASCIA.**

SUBSEROUS FASCIA is situated deep to the deep layer of deep fascia and immediately superficial to the serous membrane that surfaces the body wall of the thoracic, abdominal, and pelvic cavities.

The subserous fascia, grossly indistinguishable from the deep layer of the deep fascia, is continuous from the thoracic and abdominal walls to the various internal organs, where it is internal to the external glistening wet (serous) membrane. The fat deposits around the kidney are located primarily within the subserous fascia.

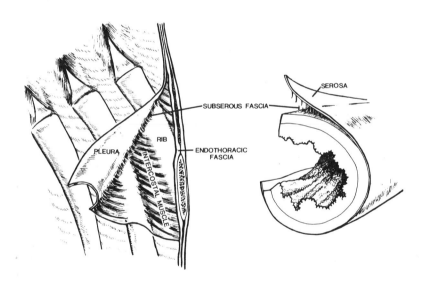

Fig.3.11. Subserous fascia.

Unit III

Musculoskeletal System

The first four chapters of this unit should provide you with an understanding of the muscles and bones that enable the dog to voluntarily move and to reflexly avoid painful or unwanted objects. The fifth chapter of the unit presents some elementary biophysical concepts involved in support and movement of the animal.

Contents:

Chapter 4
THORACIC LIMB

Objectives: Be able to identify structural features of bones, muscles, and joints in radiographs and dissected specimens, and be able to locate their positions in the intact animal.

Regions: Scapular (Supraspinous, Infraspinous), Humeral Articulation, Point of the Shoulder, Axillary, Brachial, Cubital, Point of the Elbow, Olecranon, Antebrachial, Carpal, Metacarpal, and Phalangeal Regions

Manus: Metacarpophalangeal, Proximal Phalangeal, Proximal Interphalangeal, Middle Phalangeal, Distal Interphalangeal, and Claw Regions; Interdigital Space

Bones: Long, Short, Flat, and Pneumatic Bones; Diaphysis, Epiphyses, Metaphyses, Cartilage, Diaphyseal Ossification Centers, Epiphyseal Ossification Centers, and Epiphyseal Plate (Physis); Spongy and Compact Bone

Surfaces, Margins, Prominences, etc., of the Scapula, Humerus, Radius, Ulna, Carpal bones, Metacarpal bones, and Phalanges

Muscles: Insertion and Origin, Muscle Head, Tendons and Aponeuroses; Fixation Muscles; Flexor, Extensor, Abductor, Adductor, Levator, Depressor, Pronator, and Supinator; Antagonistic and Synergistic Muscles; Flat and Pennate Muscles

Extrinsic Muscles: Trapezius, Omotransversarius, Rhomboideus, Serratus Ventralis, Brachiocephalicus, Sternocephalicus, Lattisimus Dorsi, and Superficial and Deep Pectoral Muscles

Intrinsic Muscles: Deltoideus, Infraspinatus, Supraspinatus, Teres Minor, Triceps Brachii, Subscapularis, Teres Major, Biceps Brachii, Coracobrachialis, Tensor Fasciae Antebrachii, Anconeus, Brachialis, Pronator Teres, Extensor Carpi Radialis, Brachioradialis, Common Digital Extensor, Lateral Digital Extensor, Extensor Carpi Ulnaris, Long Abductor Muscle of Digit 1, Flexor Carpi Radialis, Superficial Digital Flexor, Flexor Carpi Ulnaris, Deep Digital Flexor, and Pronator Quadratus

Sesamoid bones, Jugular Fossa, and Carpal Canal

Joints: Cartilaginous and Synovial Joints; Synchondroses and Symphyses; Articular Cavity, Articular Capsule, and Synovia; Extracapsular Ligaments, Collateral Ligaments; Simple and Composite Articulation; Ginglymus; Plane, Spheroidal, Ellipsoidal, Condylar, Trochoid, and Saddle Articulations

Structures, Ligaments, and Joints of the Proximal Humeral, Cubital, Carpal, and Interphalangeal Articulations

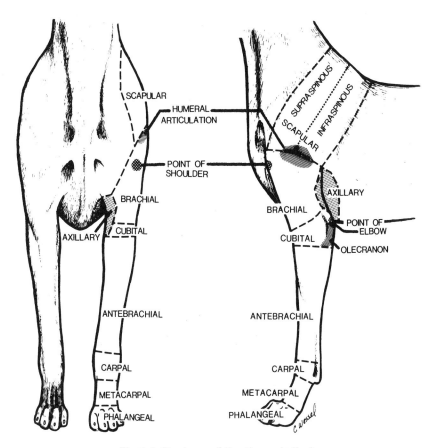

Fig.4.1. Regions of the thoracic limb.

The thoracic limb has scapular, humeral articulation, axillary, brachial, cubital, antebrachial, carpal, metacarpal and phalangeal regions (Fig. 4.1). The **SCAPULAR REGION** is subdivided longitudinally by the spine of the scapula into the **SUPRASPINOUS REGION** (craniodorsally) and the **INFRASPINOUS REGION** (caudoventrally).

The region of the **HUMERAL ARTICULATION** is superficial to the shoulder joint; the POINT OF THE SHOULDER is the most cranial osseous prominence of the bones forming the shoulder joint. The AXILLARY REGION is the area superficial to the AXILLA, a space or tissue compartment medial to the proximal portion of the arm and lateral to the cranial portion of the thorax.

The BRACHIAL REGION is superficial to the arm to which it refers. The CUBITAL REGION is superficial to the elbow joint.

The POINT OF THE ELBOW is the most caudal osseous projection at the elbow joint; the specific area of the cubital region over the point of the elbow is the OLECRANON (o-lek'rah—non) REGION.

The ANTEBRACHIAL REGION is the surface of the forearm. The area of the wrist is the CARPAL REGION. The METACARPAL REGION is distal to the carpal region and proximal to the digits. The area superficial to the digits is the PHALANGEAL REGION.

The MANUS (ma' nus, pl. manus) isthe portion of the thoracic limb that includes the carpal, meta-carpal, and phalangeal regions (Fig. 4.2).

The area superficial to the junction of the digits with the remainder of the foot of the thoracic limb is the METACARPOPHALANGEAL REGION. The regions superficial to the bones of the proximal and middle segments of the digits are termed PROXIMAL and MIDDLE PHALANGEAL; the distal area of each digit is termed the CLAW REGION.

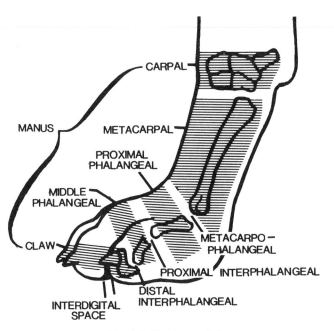

Fig.4.2. Regions of the manus.

Regions superficial to the joints between osseous elements of the digit are termed PROXIMAL and DISTAL INTERPHALANGEAL. The area between individual digits is the INTERDIGITAL SPACE.

The bones and muscles of the major appendages of the body, the thoracic and pelvic limbs, form the APPENDICULAR SKELETON and MUSCLES (Fig. 4.3).

The thoracic limb is arbitrarily divided into a number of anatomical segments, which correspond to the names of regions that overlay then (Fig. 4.4).

Bones are classified according to their shape as long, short, flat, or pneumatic (Fig. 4.5). LONG BONES generally are longer than they are wide or thick. SHORT BONES are of various shapes and are usually nearly as wide as they are long. FLAT BONES are those laterally compressed bones that provide protection for soft structures. PNEUMATIC

BONES are those with air—filled cavities or sinuses. The various bones of the thoracic limb are long, short, or flat.

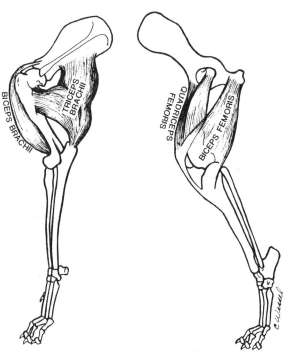

Fig.4.3. Appendicular structures.

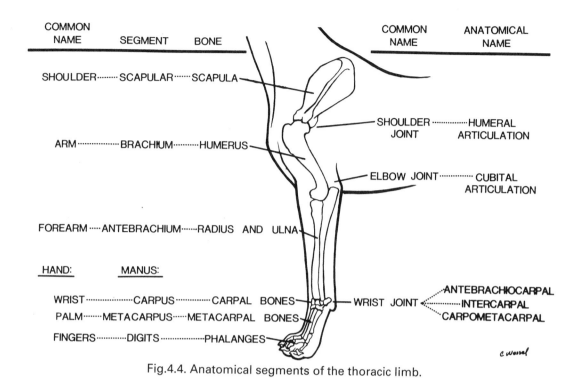

Fig.4.4. Anatomical segments of the thoracic limb.

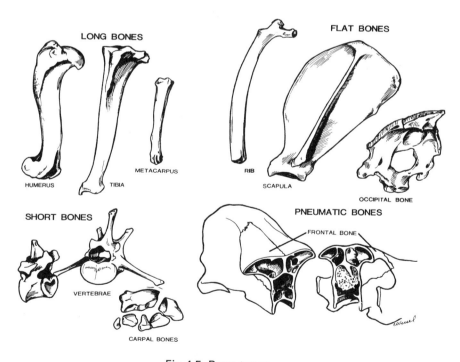

Fig.4.5. Bone types.

A long bone (Fig. 4.6) is composed of a shaft (DIAPHYSIS) and two extremities (EPIPHYSES). The epiphyses usually have larger diameters than does the diaphysis. The thickened portions of the diaphysis adjacent to the epiphyses are termed METAPHYSES.

of long bones possess epiphyseal (secondary) centers of ossification at 4 months. Many long bones have accessory centers of ossification.

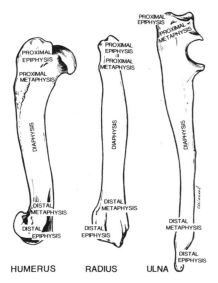

Fig.4.6. Portions of long bone.

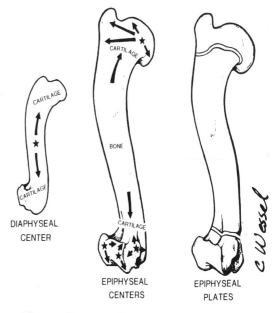

Fig.4.7. Centers of ossification in long bone.

With few exceptions, all bones of the neck, trunk, and appendages develop from CARTILAGE. Cartilaginous models of long bone undergo ossification in DIAPHYSEAL CENTERS present in the middle of the models and in EPIPHYSEAL CENTERS at the extremities (Fig. 4.7); in addition, ossification occurs in tissue around the perimeter of the model.

The first appearance of ossification centers occurs in the dog embryo about half way through the gestation period. The diaphyseal (primary) ossification centers are present in the diaphyses prior to birth; short bones and the epiphyses of long bones are without ossification centers at the time of birth. In the dog, short bones develop centers of ossification between the ages of 2 weeks and 10 months; all epiphyses

Prior to a dog achieving full growth, cartilage is present in long bones over the surface of the epiphyses and as a plate between the diaphysis and the epiphyses (Fig. 4.8). Bone growth is achieved by proliferation of cartilaginous cells concurrent with ossification of some of the cartilage tissue.

The EPIPHYSEAL PLATE (PHYSIS) (fi' sis, pl. physes; growth) consists of a zone of resting cartilage adjacent to the epiphysis, a zone of proliferating cartilage, a zone of hypertrophy and maturation, and a zone of calcification adjacent to the metaphysis. When cartilaginous cells of the physis (which are under the influence of growth hormone) cease to proliferate, the plate becomes ossified and growth in length of the long bone ceases. Growth in diameter occurs by deposition of calcium around the outside of the diaphysis coincident with reabsorption of bone from the inside of the diaphysis.

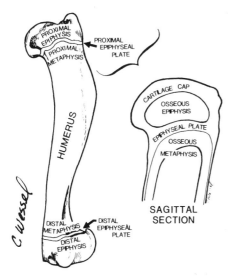

Fig.4.8. Physes of long bones.

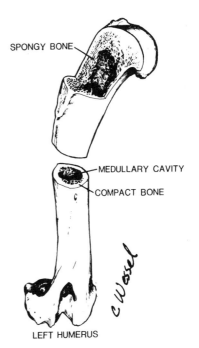

Fig.4.9. Spongy and compact bone.

Bones of the skeleton are described as being spongy or compact (Fig. 4.9) depending upon the ratio of osseous to nonosseous material present.

SPONGY BONE is composed of numerous interlacing OSSEOUS TRABECULAE (trah-bek' u-lee, sing. trabecula) or fibers, the direction of which indicates the various lines of stress imposed on the bone. COMPACT BONE appears visually as a solid substance. Compact bone, with a compressive strength four times that of concrete and a tensile strength half that of steel, forms the superficial layer of the entire osseous skeleton, the diaphysis of long bones, and much of the pectoral and pelvic girdles. Spongy bone is present in the deeper portions of short and flat bones and in the epiphyses and metaphyses of long bones.

Bones of the Thoracic Limb

The SCAPULA (pl. scapulae) (Fig. 4.10) is the most proximal bone of the thoracic limb. Its borders are the DORSAL (1), CRANIAL (2), and CAUDAL (3) MARGINS and the CRANIAL (4), CAUDAL (5), and VENTRAL (6) ANGLES.

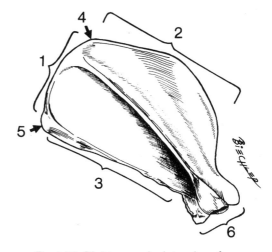

Fig.4.10. Right scapula, lateral surface.

The ventral angle of the scapula (Fig. 4.11) is that portion articulating with the humerus; it is characterized by a shallow concavity, the GLENOID (socket shape) CAVITY (1), and a cranial enlargement, the SUPRAGLENOID TUBERCLE (2).

The CORACOID PROCESS (3) is a small medial projection from the supraglenoid tubercle. Located near the caudal edge of the

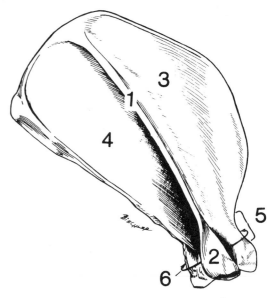

Fig.4.12. Right scapula, lateral surface.

The deep surface of the scapula (Fig. 4.13) is divided into a proximal SERRATED FACE (1) and a distal SUBSCAPULAR FOSSA (2).

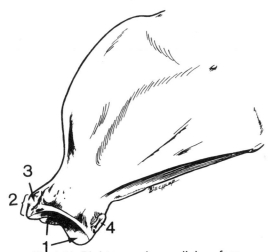

Fig.4.11. Right scapula, medial surface.

ventral angle is another enlargement, the INFRAGLENOID TUBERCLE (4).

On the lateral surface of the scapula (Fig. 4.12), an elongated projection, the SCAPULAR SPINE (1), protrudes distally as the ACROMION (2). Two spaces, one on either side of the scapular spine, are termed from cranial to caudal, SUPRASPINOUS (3) and INFRASPINOUS (4) FOSSAE (fos' ee, sing. fossa; channel).

The cranial margin forms the SCAPULAR NOTCH (5) just proximal to the supraglenoid tubercle. The NECK OF the SCAPULA (6) is the constricted portion of the scapula at the transverse plane of the acromion and scapular notch.

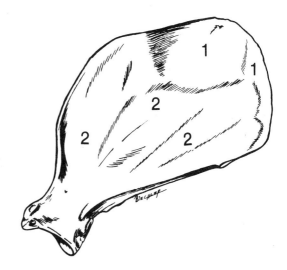

Fig.4.13. Right scapula, medial surface.

(DIFFERENCES TO BE NOTED IN THE CAT: The cat possesses an osseous CLAVICLE. This radiographically observable one, embedded in the brachiocephalicus muscle, does not articulate with other bones.

The feline acromion is composed of HAMATE (ham'ate; hooked) and SUPRAHAMATE PROCESSES. The suprahamate process is a caudally projecting prominence near the distal end of the scapular spine; the hamate process is a distal extension of the acromion that reaches the level of the humeral articulation.)

tubercles on the proximal craniomedial surface of the humerus is the INTERTUBERCULAR GROOVE (4). The major tubercle of the humerus forms the point of the shoulder.

The linear elevation on the lateral surface of the proximal part of the humerus (Fig. 4.15) is termed the TRICIPITAL MUSCLE LINE (1). It terminates distally at a roughened prominence, the DELTOID TUBEROSITY (2).

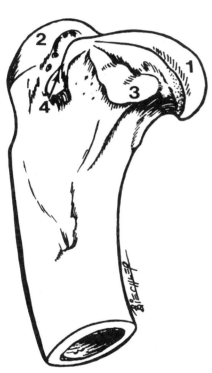

Fig.4.14. Right humerus, medial.

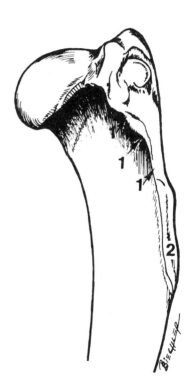

Fig.4.15. Right humerus, lateral surface.

The scapula articulates with the HUMERUS (pl. humeri). The proximal portion of the humerus (Fig. 4.14) consists of a caudal articular projection, or HEAD (1); a large semicircular prominence, or MAJOR TUBERCLE (2), cranial to the head; and a smaller MINOR TUBERCLE (3), located medial to the head. The depression between the minor and major

43

The TERES (te' reez; round and long) MAJOR TUBEROSITY (1, Fig. 4.16) is a small, roughened eminence on the medial surface of the humerus opposite and just proximal to the deltoid tuberosity (2). The NUTRIENT FORAMEN (pl. foramina) (3) of the diaphysis is on the caudal surface of the distal half of the humerus. There are a number of nutrient foramina on the medial and lateral surfaces of the major and minor tubercles.

The distal end of the humerus is composed of a CONDYLE (kon' dil; knuckle) (4) and LATERAL and MEDIAL EPICONDYLES (5). (Many clinicians consider the distal end of the humerus to be composed of both medial and lateral condyles.)

The HUMERAL CONDYLE includes the HUMERAL TROCHLEA (trok' le-ah; pulley)

(1, Fig. 4.17) and several depressions formed proximal to the trochlea by the radius and ulna. The trochlea forms most of the humeral surface that articulates with the ulna. The OLECRANON FOSSA (2) is the large depression on the distal caudal surface of the humerus. It is continuous with a depression on the cranial surface of the humerus via the SUPRATROCHLEAR FORAMEN. The depression on the distal cranial surface of the humerus (RADIAL FOSSA) is formed by articulations with the radius.

The epicondyles are the laterally and medially projecting prominences on the distal end of the humerus. The medial epicondyle (3) is larger than the lateral epicondyle (4). The ridge of bone proximal to the lateral epicondyle on the caudolateral surface of the humerus is the LATERAL EPICONDYLAR CREST (5).

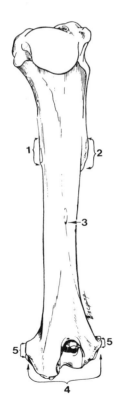

Fig.4.16. Right humerus, caudal surface.

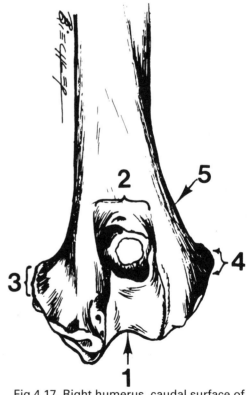

Fig.4.17. Right humerus, caudal surface of distal portion.

(DIFFERENCES TO BE NOTED IN THE CAT: The supratrochlear foramen is usually absent; however, a SUPRACONDYLAR FORAMEN is present in the distal medial portion of the feline humerus, forming an osseous passageway for the median nerve and brachial artery.)

The ULNA (pl. ulnae) (Fig. 4.18), the longest bone of the dog's body, extends from the point of the elbow to the carpus.

The OLECRANON (1), or proximal extremity of the ulna, projects caudally past the cubital articulation forming the point of the elbow. A relatively long olecranon provides strength in extending the cubital articulation, whereas a relatively short olecranon provides for rapid extension.

A large TROCHLEAR NOTCH (2), present on the proximal cranial surface of the ulna, articulates with the humeral trochlea. The two projections forming the proximal and distal margins of the trochlear notch are the ANCONEAL (ang-ko' ne-al) (3) and CORONOID (crownlike) (4) PROCESSES, respectively.

When the cubital articulation is extended, the anconeal process is positioned within the olecranon fossa of the humerus. There are two coronoid processes; the RADIAL NOTCH (5) of the ulna is present between the large medial and small lateral coronoid processes. When rotator muscles contract, the proximal portion of the radius rotates against the radial notch of the ulna.

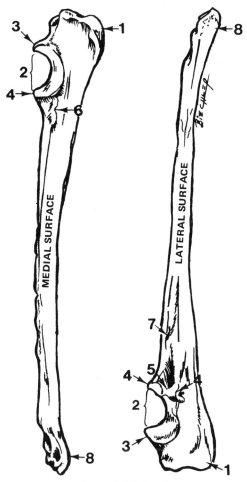

Fig.4.18. Right ulna.

The ULNAR TUBEROSITY (6) is a small prominence just distal to the medial coronoid process. The roughened cranial surface of the body of the ulna is the border facing the radius. Note the nutrient foramen (7) in the proximal portion of this rough surface. The distal pointed portion of the ulna is termed the LATERAL STYLOID (pillarlike) PROCESS (8).

In the prone position, the RADIUS (pl. radii) (Fig. 4.19) is positioned craniolaterally to the ulna at the cubital articulation and craniomedially at the carpal articulation.

The concave FOVEA (fo' ve-ah, pl. foveae) CAPITIS (1) of the head of the radius articulates with the lateral portion of the condyle of the humerus.

The RADIAL TUBEROSITY (2) is a small eminence on the medial surface of the radius near the transverse level of the ulnar tuberosity. The tendons of insertion of the brachialis and biceps brachii muscles, which attach to the ulna, also attach to the radial tuberosity.

The RADIAL TROCHLEA (3) is the distal articular surface by which the radius articulates with carpal bones. The elongated medial projection of the distal end of the radius is the MEDIAL STYLOID PROCESS (4). The rough caudal surface of the radius is the border facing the ulna; this interosseous surface has a nutrient foramen (5) near the proximal end of the radius.

Seven bones form the skeleton of the dog CARPUS; the carpal bones are arranged in two rows, a proximal row of three bones and a distal row of four bones (Fig. 4.20). The medial bone of the proximal row articulates with the radius; it is the largest of the carpal bones and is termed the INTER-MEDIORADIAL CARPAL BONE (1). The lateral bone of the proximal row, which articulates with both ulna and radius, is the ULNAR CARPAL BONE (2).

The ACCESSORY CARPAL BONE (3) is caudal to the ulnar carpal bone on the lateral surface of the carpus. The distal row of four carpal bones is named from medial to lateral as CARPAL BONES I, II, III, and IV.

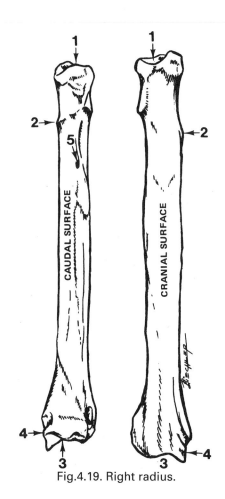

Fig.4.19. Right radius.

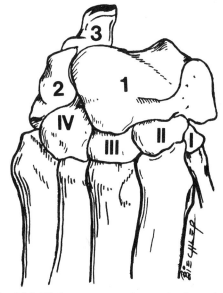

Fig.4.20. Right carpus and prominal portion of the metacarpus dorsal surface.

The METACARPUS, which is distal to the carpus and proximal to the digits, contains five METACARPAL BONES numbered I through V (Fig. 4.21).

Each metacarpal bone has a proximal BASE (1), a BODY (2), and a distal HEAD (3). Metacarpus I is quite small.

DIGITS II, III, IV, and V (Fig. 4.22) have three PHALANGES (fa' lan-jez, sing. phalanx) each; digit I usually has two. The proximal phalanx of digit I and the proximal and middle phalanges of digits II, III, IV, and V have a proximal base (I), a body (2), and a distal head (3).

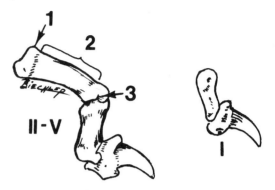

Fig.4.22. Digits, lateral surface.

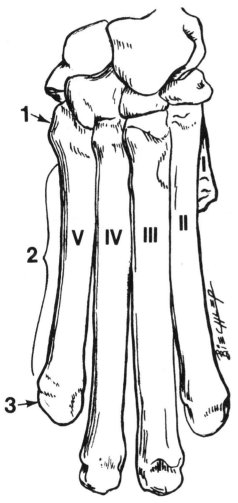

Fig.4.21. Right carpus and metacarpus, dorsal surface.

The distal phalanx (Fig. 4.23) of digits I through V has a dorsal prominence, the EXTENSOR PROCESS (I); a palmar FLEXOR TUBERCLE (2); a distal CREST OF THE CLAW (3); and a PROCESS OF THE CLAW (4). The crest of the distal phalanx projects distally superficial to the dorsal and lateral proximal surfaces of the cutaneous claw; the base of the crest of the distal phalanx is the extensor process.

A pair of elastic ligaments attach the crest of the distal phalanx to the middle phalanx, resulting in overextension of the distal interphalangeal joint (see p. 94). The process of the claw is the bony extension of the distal phalanx into the cutaneous claw.

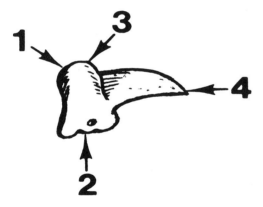

Fig.4.23. Distal phalanx, lateral surface.

MUSCLES

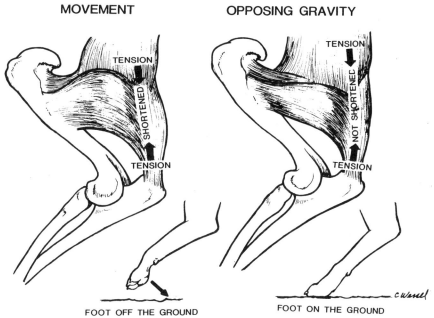

Fig.4.24. Results of tension in appendicular muscle.

Microscopically, skeletal muscle is composed of fibers (cells) that function by creating tension along their long axes. This tension may result in shortening of a muscle, which effects movement of osseous structures to which the muscle is attached, or it may prevent movement by either acting against opposing gravitational forces or countering contraction of other muscles (Fig. 4.24).

A skeletal muscle (Fig. 4.25) is composed of a main portion and two extremities; the major portion, or **BELLY,** of a muscle contains the greatest number of muscle fibers. The muscle extremities attach to bone or fascia. If contraction of a muscle results in movement, the most mobile end of the muscle is termed the **INSERTION** (TERMINATION); the extremity with least movement is called the **ORIGIN.** The portion of a muscle adjacent to the origin is the **HEAD.**

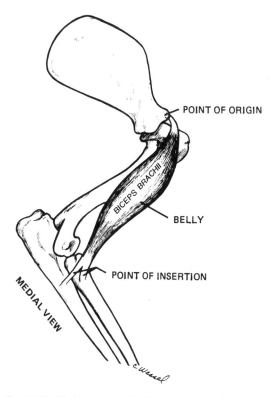

Fig.4.25. Skeletal muscle, its regions and points of attachment.

Usually the origin of an appendicular muscle is the attachment closest to the body. Many muscles produce movement at both points of attachment, while other muscles produce movement at one end one time and at the other end another time, depending on the position of the body and its functional state. In these cases it is not necessary to describe points of origin and insertion, only points of attachment.

Among the muscle fibers in the belly of a muscle are numerous connective tissue fibers; these fibers coalesce at the extremities of most muscles, forming tough cords called **TENDONS** or flat sheets termed **APONEUROSES** (ap" o-nuro' ses, sing. aponeurosis) (Fig. 4.26).

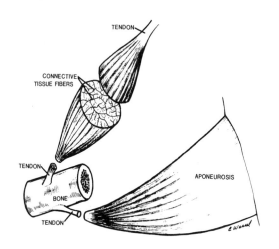

Fig.4.26. Skeletal muscle, types of attachment.

Aponeuroses are often continuous with deep fascia. Some muscles attach directly to bone by means of their investing fascia and by connective tissue fibers within the muscle rather than by means of tendons or aponeuroses. Connective tissue fibers of tendons, by merging into the intercellular substance of bone, are strongly attached. Muscle fibers are more likely to tear under stress than are the tendons of attachment.

Descriptive terms indicate the action of groups of muscles on the structures to which they attach. **FIXATION MUSCLES** are those that fix or stabilize bones of a joint against movement in one direction, while other muscles act to effect movement of the joint in another direction. Muscles that span a joint, attaching to two different bones, may either increase the angle of the joint, **EXTENSION,** or decrease it, **FLEXION** (Fig. 4.27).

Muscles that move a structure toward the median plane are said to be **ADDUCTORS;** those that move the limbs away from the median plane are **ABDUCTORS** (Fig. 4.28).

A muscle that raises a structure dorsally is a **LEVATOR.** The antagonistic muscle to a levator is a **DEPRESSOR** (Fig. 4.29).

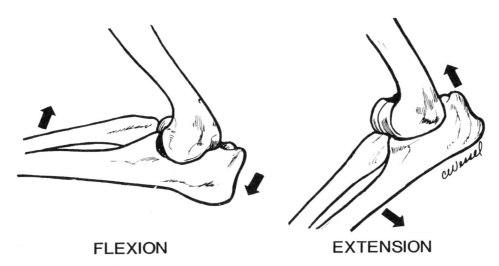

FLEXION   **EXTENSION**

Fig.4.27. Action of muscles, flexion versus extension.

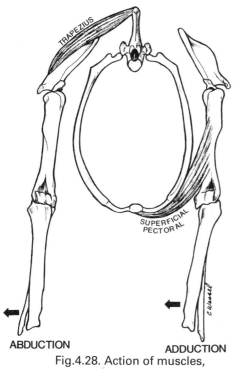

ABDUCTION   ADDUCTION
Fig.4.28. Action of muscles,
abduction versus adduction.

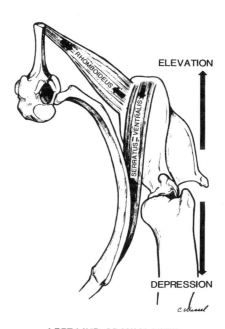

LEFT LIMB, CRANIAL VIEW

Fig.4.29. Action of muscles, elevation
versus depression.

A muscle responsible for rotating the cranial surface of a limb medially is a **PRONATOR**, while the opposing muscle, which rotates the cranial surface of the limb laterally, is a **SUPINATOR** (su " pi- na' tor) (Fig. 4.30).

The function of one muscle is usually opposed by another; e.g., if a muscle functions to straighten a joint, another one, an **ANTAGONISTIC MUSCLE**, will have the function of bending the joint. If two or more muscles work together to perform a function, they are said to be **SYNERGISTIC** (Fig. 4.31).

The pattern of muscle fibers within a muscle and the number of motor units activated (a motor unit is one motor nerve fiber and all the muscle fibers it activates) determine the amount of change in length and the force that a contracting muscle may produce (Fig. 4.32).

The longer a muscle is and the more parallel its fibers are to the long axis, the greater will be the length of contraction. **FLAT (STRAPLIKE) MUSCLES** have long fibers parallel to the long axis of the muscle.

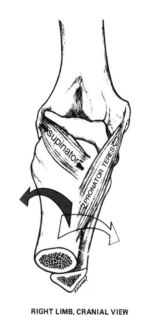

RIGHT LIMB, CRANIAL VIEW

Fig.4.30. Action of muscles, supination versus pronation.

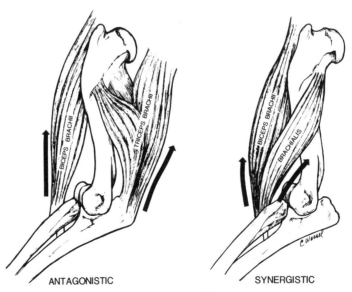

ANTAGONISTIC   SYNERGISTIC

Fig.4.31. Action of muscles, antagonistic versus synergistic.

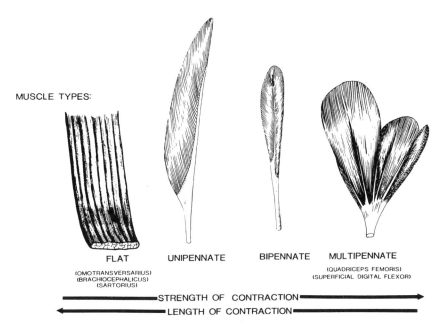

MUSCLE TYPES:

FLAT
(OMOTRANSVERSARIUS)
(BRACHIOCEPHALICUS)
(SARTORIUS)

UNIPENNATE

BIPENNATE

MULTIPENNATE
(QUADRICEPS FEMORIS)
(SUPERFICIAL DIGITAL FLEXOR)

STRENGTH OF CONTRACTION

LENGTH OF CONTRACTION

Fig.4.32. Skeletal muscle, muscle fiber arrangement.

PENNATE MUSCLES have fibers that are oriented at an angle to the long axis of the muscle; the fibers are shorter and more numerous in pennate than in straplike muscles. Various types of pennate muscles are classified by the complexity of fiber arrangement: unipennate, bipennate, and multipennate.

A **UNIPENNATE MUSCLE** has a row of fibers parallel to each other but at an angle to the long axis of the muscle.

A **BIPENNATE MUSCLE** has two rows of fibers converging on the long axis of the muscle. The most powerful is the **MULTIPENNATE MUSCLE**, which is characterized by more than two rows of parallel fibers, each attaching to longitudinally oriented tendinous tissue within the muscle itself.

Muscles are usually named according to their action, shape, or attachment. A muscle with the name common digital extensor produces extension of the digits. The pronator teres muscle is a round muscle that produces pronation. The trapezius muscle is shaped like a trapezoid.

However, the name of a muscle may be misleading for a particular species; e.g., the triceps brachii muscle has three heads in the human and four in the dog. The names of some muscles provide information on both origin and insertion; e.g., the spinodeltoideus arises on the spinous process of the scapula and inserts on the deltoid tuberosity of the humerus.

Muscles of the Thoracic Limb

More than 53 muscles act upon the thoracic limb. The actions of individual muscles or muscle groups may be readily estimated by mentally visualizing relative positions of bone, muscle, and muscle attachments. By shortening the length of a muscle or part of a muscle, the function or action of that muscle (whether a flexor, extensor, abductor, adductor, levator, depressor, pronator, supinator, sphincter, dilatator, or other) is determined. However, a muscle acts in conjunction with a number of other muscles, and the direction of pull on the skeletal part is due to the sum of the forces applied by individual muscles.

Eight of the thoracic limb muscles are **EXTRINSIC**, i.e., these muscles are related or attach to bones that are not a part of the thoracic limb skeleton. Extrinsic muscles of the limbs produce differential movement of axial and appendicular structures. The extrinsic muscles of the thoracic limb are responsible for movement of the shoulder and upper arm; a small movement of the limb proximally may result in a much larger displacement of the distal end of the limb (Fig. 4.33).

Four extrinsic muscles of the thoracic limb that attach the scapula to the axial skeleton are the trapezius (trah-pe' ze-us), rhomboideus, omotransversarius (omo; shoulder), and serratus ventralis. Three of these may be observed from a lateral view (Figs. 4.34, 4.35): two superficially, the trapezius (1) and omotransversarius muscles (2), and one more deeply, the rhomboideus muscle (3). The fourth extrinsic muscle of the scapular region, the serratus ventralis (4), requires considerable dissection for visualization.

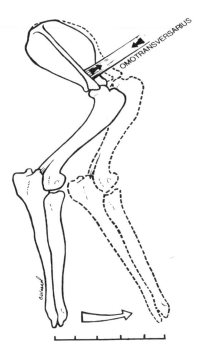

Fig.4.33. Magnification of limb displacement.

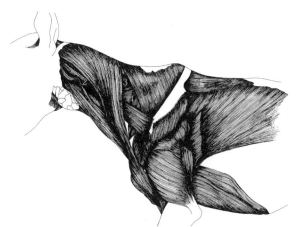

Fig.4.34. Extrinsic muscles of the thoracic limb that attach to the scapula.

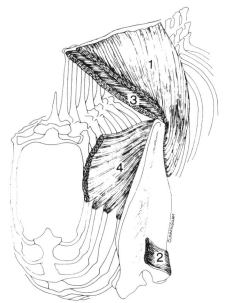

Fig.4.35. Schematic: Craniolateral view of muscles that attach to the scapula.

The **TRAPEZIUS MUSCLE** of each side attaches the spine of a scapula to a ligament positioned longitudinally along the dorsal median line of the body (Fig. 4.36). Each trapezius is divided cranially into a cervical portion (1) and caudally into a thoracic portion (2), named according to region of origin. The two trapezii span the interscapular region, forming the shape for which they are named.

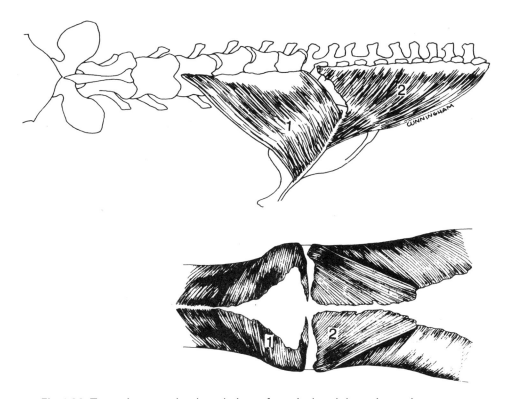

Fig.4.36. Trapezius muscle, dorsal view of cervical and thoracic portions.

The **OMOTRANSVERSARIUS** (1, Fig. 4.37) is a strap-shaped muscle that connects the distal end of the scapular spine (acromion) to the transverse process of the 1st (most cranial) cervical vertebra. Another extrinsic muscle of the thoracic limb, the brachiocephalicus, is superficial to the omotransversarius muscle in the lateral cervical region.

Deep to the trapezius muscles, a pair of muscles arise from the dorsal median line and insert on the proximal end of each scapula near the dorsal border (Fig. 4.38). This paired muscle has a rhomboid (diamond) shape, hence its name, **RHOMBOIDEUS.** The rhomboideus muscle is divided into a capital portion (1), a cervical portion (2), and a thoracic portion (3). The **RHOMBOIDEUS CAPITIS MUSCLE** is a slender straplike portion that separates proximally from the **RHOMBOIDEUS CERVICIS MUSCLE** to attach to the skull.

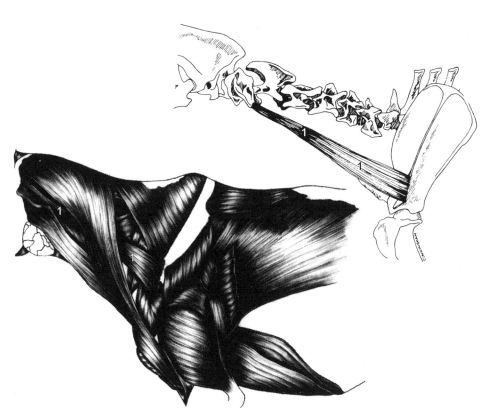

Fig.4.37. Omotransversarius muscle.

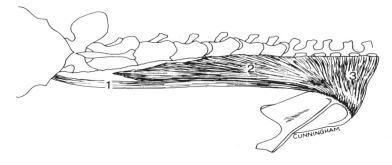

Fig.4.38. Left rhomboideus muscle, dorsal view of three subdivisions.

The remaining extrinsic muscle that inserts on the scapula, the **SERRATUS VENTRALIS**, is situated deep to the scapula (Figs. 4.39, 4.40).

The long axis of the serratus ventralis muscle is in a dorsolateral direction from the trunk to the scapula. The serratus ventralis muscles suspend the thorax from the deep proximal surfaces (serrated faces) of the scapulae. Each serratus

ventralis arises from the neck and from the thorax; the serrated origins give the muscle its name.

The **SERRATUS VENTRALIS CERVICIS MUSCLE** (1) arises from the transverse processes of the caudal five cervical vertebrae (note that at the base of the neck the cervical vertebrae are situated quite far ventrally). The muscular slips of the **SERRATUS VENTRALIS THORACIS MUSCLE** (2) arise ventral to the midlength of the first seven or eight ribs.

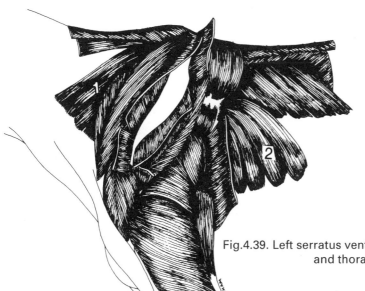

Fig.4.39. Left serratus ventralis muscle, lateral view of cervical and thoracic portions.

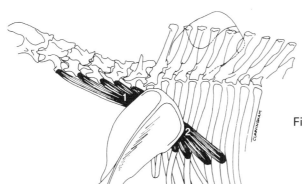

Fig.4.40. Schematic of the left serratus ventralis muscle, dorsolateral view.

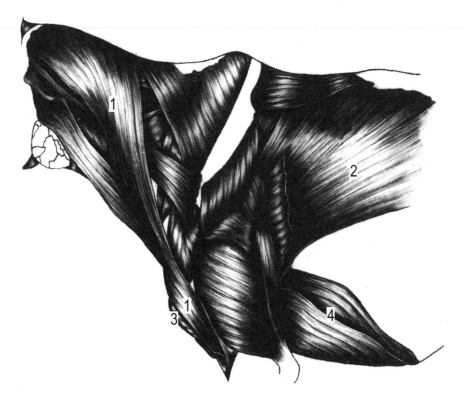

Fig.4.41. Extrinsic muscles of the thoracic limb, humeral attachment.

Four extrinsic muscles of the thoracic limb that attach the humerus to the axial skeleton (Fig. 4.41) are the brachiocephalicus (1), latissimus dorsi (2), superficial pectoral (3), and deep pectoral (4).

The **BRACHIOCEPHALICUS** (brak " e-o-se-fal' i-kus; arm and head) **MUSCLE** attaches by one end to the skull and median dorsal line of the neck and by the other to the distal cranial surface of the humerus (Fig. 4.42). A transverse tendinous line is present in the brachiocephalicus dorsal to the level of the point of the shoulder. The vestige of the clavicle may be palpable at this **CLAVICULAR INTERSECTION** (arrow) as a small piece of cartilage or bone. Considering the clavicular intersection as the least movable point within this muscle (which is several separate muscles in animals with functional clavicles), the part of the brachiocephalicus that inserts on the humerus is the **CLEIDO-BRACHIALIS MUSCLE** (1); the other two

portions, which insert on the neck and skull, are the cervical (2) and mastoid (3) parts of the **CLEIDOCEPHALICUS MUSCLE**, respectively. The **STERNOCEPHALICUS** (4), a trunk muscle (see p. 141), is located immediately cranioventral to the cleidocephalicus and adjacent to the external jugular vein.

The **LATISSIMUS** (lah-tis' i-mus) **DORSI** (1, Fig. 4.43) is a broad, flat muscle caudal to the thoracic limb region and deep to the cutaneus trunci muscle. It is wide at its aponeurotic origin from the dorsal median line and relatively narrow and thick near its insertion on the proximal medial surface of the humerus (teres major tuberosity). The caudal portion of the trapezius muscle is superficial to the craniodorsal portion of the latissimus dorsi muscle.

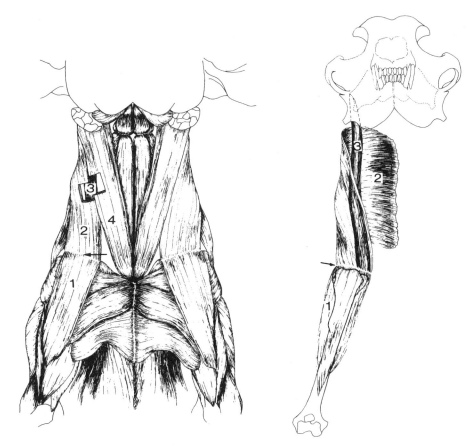

Fig.4.42. Right brachiocephalicus muscle, ventral view.

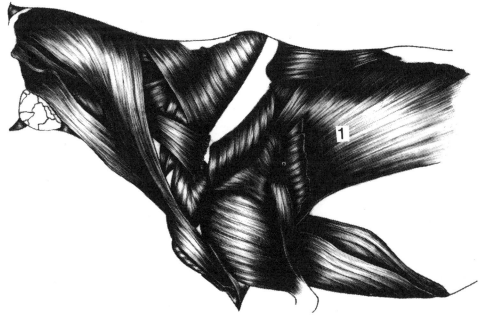

Fig.4.43. Left latissimus dorsi muscle, lateral view.

The **SUPERFICIAL PECTORAL MUSCLE** (Fig. 4.44) arises from the ventral median line and

inserts on the cranial proximal surface of the humerus. It is subdivided into two parts, a smaller, superficial descending portion and a deeper, broader transverse portion.

The fibers of the **DESCENDING PECTORAL** (1) are oriented in a caudolateral direction; those of the **TRANSVERSE PECTORAL** (2) are oriented transversely. The **DEEP (ASCENDING) PECTORAL** (3) arises from the ventral median line and inserts on the proximal medial surface of the humerus. It may be divided by fascial clefts into several smaller muscles. The muscle fibers of the cranial portion of the deep pectoral are deep to the superficial pectoral and are oriented transversely. The caudal portion of the deep pectoral is superficial and is oriented craniolaterally.

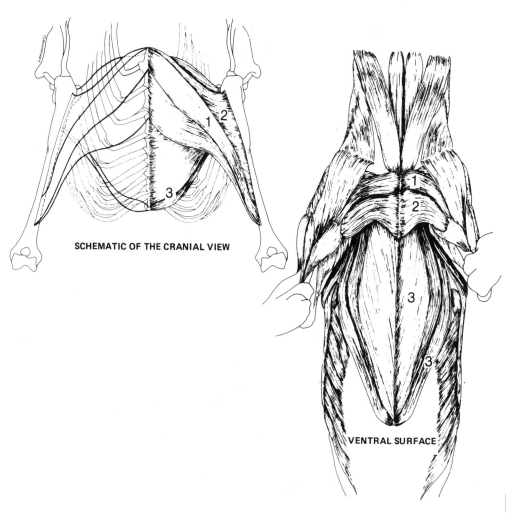

SCHEMATIC OF THE CRANIAL VIEW

VENTRAL SURFACE

Fig. 4.44. Pectoral muscles.

A depression, the **JUGULAR** (jug' u-lar; neck) **FOSSA** (arrow, Fig. 4.45), is present on each side of the ventral median line, cranial to the superficial pectoral (1, 2), medial to the cleidobrachialis (3) and the clavicular intersection (4), and lateral to the straplike sternocephalicus (5), which attaches the sternum to the skull. The superficially situated external jugular vein passes deeply from the neck at the jugular fossa into the thoracic cavity.

(DIFFERENCES TO BE NOTED IN THE CAT: The descending portion of the superficial pectoral muscle arises more caudally on the sternum and is thus more transversely oriented than that of the dog. Extrinsic muscles such as the brachiocephalicus andsuperficial pectoral insert distally on the proximal portion of the antebrachium.)

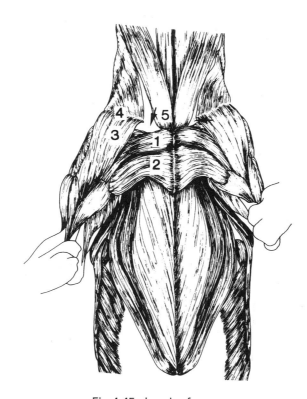

Fig.4.45. Jugular fossae.

INTRINSIC muscles of the thoracic limb are those that both arise from and insert upon bone or fascia of the thoracic limb. Nine intrinsic muscles of the thoracic limb that span the surfaces of the humeral articulation are: laterally —the deltoideus, infraspinatus, teres minor, and supraspinatus; caudally—the teres major and triceps brachii; cranially—the biceps brachii; and medially—the subscapularis and coracobrachialis.

The **DELTOIDEUS MUSCLE** (1, 2, Fig. 4.46) is the most superficial of four intrinsic muscles that cross the lateral surface of the shoulder joint. It has two origins, two bellies, and one insertion. The most distal portion of the deltoideus (1), which arises from the acromion, is situated across the humeral articulation, caudal to the major tubercle. Both the acromial portion and a second more proximal portion (2), which arises by an aponeurosis from the scapular spine, insert in common on the deltoid tuberosity, deep to the cleidobrachialis muscle.

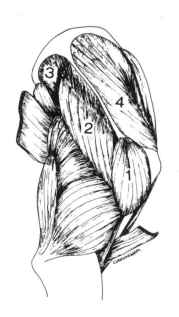

Figure 4.46 Instrinsic muscles of the right shoulder, lateral view.

The portion of the deltoideus that arises from the scapular spine is easily confused with a deeper muscle, the **INFRASPINATUS** (3), which arises from the infraspinous fossa. The tendon of the infraspinatus muscle is situated lengthwise across the lateral surface of the humeral articulation and inserts on the lateral surface of the major tubercle.

The **SUPRASPINATUS MUSCLE** (4) arises from the supraspinous fossa of the scapula, deep to the trapezius and omotransversarius muscles, and inserts on the major tubercle of the humerus.

The small **TERES MINOR MUSCLE** (1, Fig. 4.47) arises from the caudal border of the scapula and inserts distally on the lateral surface of the proximal portion of the humerus. The teres minor is deep to the deltoideus muscle and caudal to the distal portion of the infraspinatus muscle.

The **TRICEPS** (three heads) **BRACHII MUSCLE** has four heads of origin, three of which are from the proximal portion of the humerus and one is from the caudal border of the scapula. The head of the triceps brachii, which has a muscular origin from the caudal margin of the scapula, appears to have two or three bellies; these muscle masses are the **LONG HEAD OF THE TRICEPS BRACHII** (2, 3, 4), which forms the major portion of the muscle. The other three heads of the triceps brachii muscle are named lateral, medial, and accessory according to their positions around the caudal surface of the humerus.

The common point of insertion of the triceps brachii muscle is on the olecranon of the ulna (point of the elbow); the caudal margin of the triceps brachii muscle mass along the caudal surface of the arm, formed mostly by the long head, is termed the **TRICIPITAL MARGIN** (5).

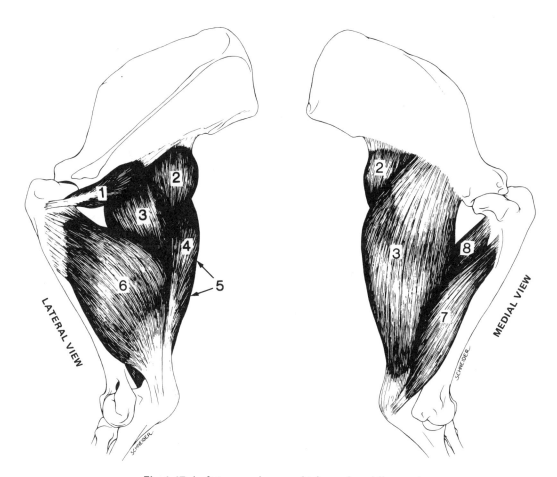

Fig.4.47. Left teres minor and triceps brachii muscles.

The **LATERAL HEAD** (6) arises from the tricipital line of the humerus; this part of the triceps brachii forms the major muscular mass on the lateral surface of the arm. The **MEDIAL HEAD** (7) arises from the proximal medial surface of the humeral diaphysis and by position forms the medial portion of the four-part triceps. The **ACCESSORY HEAD** (8), which is positioned between the medial, lateral, and long heads, arises from the proximal surface of the humerus.

The **SUBSCAPULARIS** (1, Fig. 4.48) is a muscle situated on the deep surface or subscapular fossa of the scapula from which it arises. It crosses the medial surface of the humeral articulation and inserts on the minor tubercle of the humerus. A portion of the belly of the supraspinatus muscle (2), which overlaps the cranial border of the scapula onto its medial surface, is often mistaken for the subscapularis muscle.

On the medial surface of the thoracic limb the proximal portion of the **TERES MAJOR MUSCLE** (3) may be observed between the more craniodorsally located subscapularis muscle and the more caudally positioned latissimus dorsi muscle (4). The teres major muscle arises from the caudal angle of the scapula and inserts, in common with the latissimus dorsi and cutaneus trunci muscles, on the teres major tuberosity of the humerus.

The **BICEPS** (two heads) **BRACHII MUSCLE** (1, Fig. 4.49) arises from the supraglenoid tubercle of the scapula and inserts on the proximal cranial surface of the radius and ulna in the **ANTEBRACHIUM**. The tendon of origin of the biceps brachii muscle passes through the intertubercular groove of the craniomedial surface of the humerus, where the tendon is held in place by the **TRANSVERSE HUMERAL LIGAMENT** (2). The transverse humeral ligament attaches to the major and minor tubercles of the humerus.

The **CORACOBRACHIALIS MUSCLE** (3) arises from the coracoid process of the scapula, crosses the minor tubercle, and inserts on the medial surface of the proximal half of the humerus.

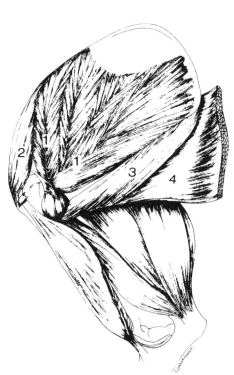

Fig.4.48. Intrinsic muscles of the right shoulder, medial view.

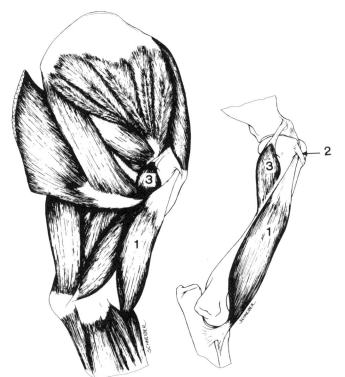

Fig.4.49. Left biceps brachii and coracobrachialis muscles, medial view.

Fifteen intrinsic muscles of the thoracic limb span the cubital articulation; seven of these directly effect movement of the antebrachium. The other muscles arise from the humerus and effect movement of the carpus and/or digits.

The intrinsic muscles of the **BRACHIUM** that act upon the antebrachium may be grouped into muscles that are caudal to the long axis of the limb—the triceps brachii, tensor fasciae antebrachii, and anconeus; craniolateral to the cubital articulation—the brachialis and supinator; and craniomedial to the cubital articulation—the biceps brachii and pronator teres.

The **TENSOR FASCIAE ANTEBRACHII** (1, Fig. 4.50) is a thin, strap-shaped muscle located on the caudomedial surface of the arm, superficial to the long head of the triceps (2). It arises from the latissimus dorsi muscle (3), near its attachment on the teres major tuberosity, and inserts on fascia of the olecranon.

The **ANCONEUS** (4) is a short muscle that arises on the distal caudal surface of the humerus and inserts on the proximal lateral surface of the ulna.

(DIFFERENCES TO BE NOTED IN THE CAT: Both the cleidobrachialis and the superficial pectoral muscles of the cat insert on the proximal portion of the antebrachium. A small EPITROCHLEOANCONEUS MUSCLE, present on the proximomedial surface of the feline cubital articulation, arises from the medial epicondylar crest and inserts on the olecranon.)

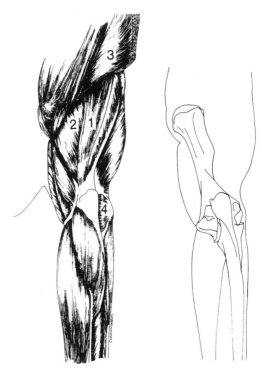

Fig.4.50. Right tensor fasciae antebrachii and anconeus muscles, caudal view.

The **BRACHIALIS MUSCLE** (1, Fig. 4.51) arises from the proximal caudolateral surface of the humerus and inserts craniomedially on the ulna and radius, just distal to the cubital articulation. It forms a half spiral around the humerus in its course from origin to insertion.

The **SUPINATOR** (2) is a short muscle that arises from the lateral epicondyle of the humerus and inserts on the cranial surface of the radius. This rotator muscle of the antebrachium is situated craniolateral to the cubital articulation, deep to other antebrachial muscles. The biceps brachii muscle (3) stretches from the scapula (proximally) through the intertubercular groove of the humerus to its dual insertion on the radius

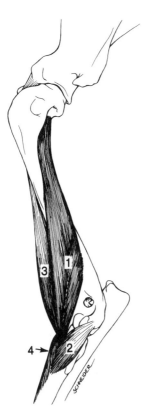

Fig.4.51. Muscles adjacent to the cranial surface of the cubital articulation.

and ulna, distal to the cubital articulation (see Fig. 4.49). The biceps brachii muscle is situated along the craniomedial surface of the humerus, superficial and cranial to the medial head of the triceps muscle. Much of the proximal portion of the biceps brachii muscle is covered by the superficial and deep pectoral muscles. The **PRONATOR TERES** (4) is a small muscle that arises from the medial humeral epicondyle and inserts on the medial border of the radius.

The intrinsic muscles of the thoracic limb that arise, at least in part, from the humerus and insert on bones of the manus may be grouped into extensors of the carpus, extensors of the carpus and digits, flexors of the carpus, and flexors of the carpus and digits. They arise, at least in part, from an epicondyle of the humerus and cross two or more joints. Those muscles originating from the lateral epicondyle are **EXTENSOR MUSCLES OF THE MANUS;** those arising from the medial epicondyle are **FLEXOR MUSCLES OF THE MANUS.** The extensor group of muscles, located on the craniolateral surface of the antebrachium, includes the extensor carpi radialis, common digital extensor, lateral digital extensor, and extensor carpi ulnaris (ulnaris lateralis).

The **EXTENSOR CARPI RADIALIS** (1, Fig. 4.52) is the large muscle palpable through the skin on the cranial surface of the radius. The craniomedial border of the extensor carpi radialis muscle is a commonly used site for injections into the cephalic vein. A rudimentary thin strip of muscle, the **BRACHIORADIALIS,** may be present medial to and parallel with the cephalic vein. The extensor carpi radialis muscle originates from the lateral epicondylar crest and inserts on the proximal dorsal surface of metacarpal bones II and III. A transversely oriented thick band of carpal fascia, the **EXTENSOR RETINACULUM** (2), binds the two extensor carpi radialis tendons in place against the carpus (dorsally).

(DIFFERENCE TO BE NOTED IN THE CAT: The brachioradialis muscle is well developed.)

The **COMMON DIGITAL EXTENSOR MUSCLE** (3) is lateral and partially deep to the extensor carpi radialis. It arises from the lateral epicondyle and inserts by four tendons on the proximal surface (extensor process) of the distal phalanx of digits II, III, IV, and V. The extensor retinaculum (2) on the dorsal surface of the carpus also retains the four common digital extensor tendons in position.

The **LATERAL DIGITAL EXTENSOR MUSCLE** (4) is caudolateral and partially deep to the common digital extensor muscle. It arises from the lateral epicondyle of the humerus and inserts by three tendons, which join with tendons of the common digital extensor muscle on the proximal dorsal surface of the distal phalanx of digits III, IV, and V. The three tendons of insertion of the lateral digital extensor are also held in place on the dorsal surface of the carpus by the extensor retinaculum (2).

The **EXTENSOR CARPI ULNARIS** (5), which is considered to be a flexor muscle in the dog, is situated along the lateral surface of the antebrachium, where it arises from the lateral epicondyle of the humerus and inserts via two tendons on the accessory carpal bone and proximal lateral surface of metacarpal V.

The **LONG ABDUCTOR MUSCLE OF DIGIT I** (6), which is oriented distomedially, arises from the craniolateral surface of the ulna and inserts on the proximal end of metacarpus I. A **SESAMOID** (ses' ah-moid; sesame-seed-like) **BONE**, frequently observed in radiographs of the carpal joint, is present in the tendon of insertion.

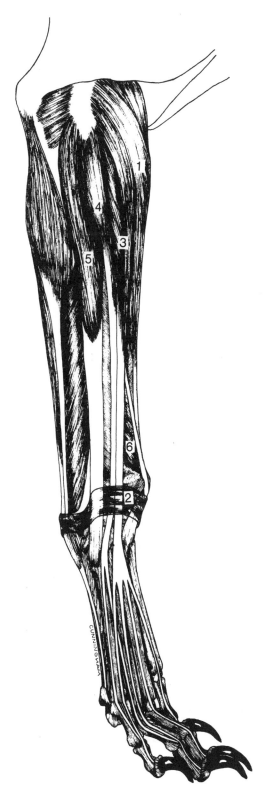

Fig.4.52. Extensor muscles of the right manus, lateral view.

The flexor group of muscles (Fig. 4.53), located on the caudomedial surface of the antebrachium, includes the flexor carpi radialis, superficial digital flexor, flexor carpi ulnaris, and deep digital flexor. The short belly of the **FLEXOR CARPI RADIALIS MUSCLE** (1), present on the medial surface of the proximal portion of the antebrachium, is caudal and partially deep to the pronator teres.

The flexor carpi radialis muscle arises from the medial epicondyle of the humerus and inserts on the proximal palmar surface of metacarpals II and III. The **SUPERFICIAL DIGITAL FLEXOR MUSCLE** (2) is caudal to the flexor carpi radialis and forms the caudomedial surface of the antebrachium. It arises from the medial epicondyle of the humerus and inserts by means of four tendons on the proximal palmar surfaces of the middle phalanx of digits II, III, IV, and V.

A thickening of deep fascia, the **FLEXOR RETINACULUM**, binds the insertion tendon of the superficial digital flexor into a hollow in the palmar surface of the carpus. The **CARPAL CANAL** is a space formed by the flexor retinaculum and the accessory, ulnar, and radial carpal bones. The flexor retinaculum is divided into two parts, one superficial and the other deep to the superficial digital flexor tendon.

The **FLEXOR CARPI ULNARIS** (3) consists of two parts that appear as separate muscles, an ulnar (3a) and a humeral (3b) head. The short bellied ulnar head arises from the caudal surface of the olecranon and inserts distally as a tendon on the accessory carpal bone. The humeral head originates proximally from the medial epicondyle, deep to the ulnar head, and also inserts on the accessory carpal bone.

The **DEEP DIGITAL FLEXOR MUSCLE** (4) has three points of origin: the medial epicondyle of the humerus, the proximal caudal border of the ulna, and the medial border of the radius. The two portions that arise from the ulna and radius are small and combine with the tendon of the humeral head at the level of the carpus.

All three heads of the deep digital flexor have one common tendon of insertion, which, after passing through the carpal canal, divides into five tendons. The five tendons insert on the proximal palmar surface (flexor tubercle) of the distal phalanx of digits I, II, III, IV, and V. The flexor retinaculum maintains the deep digital flexor tendon in the carpal canal.

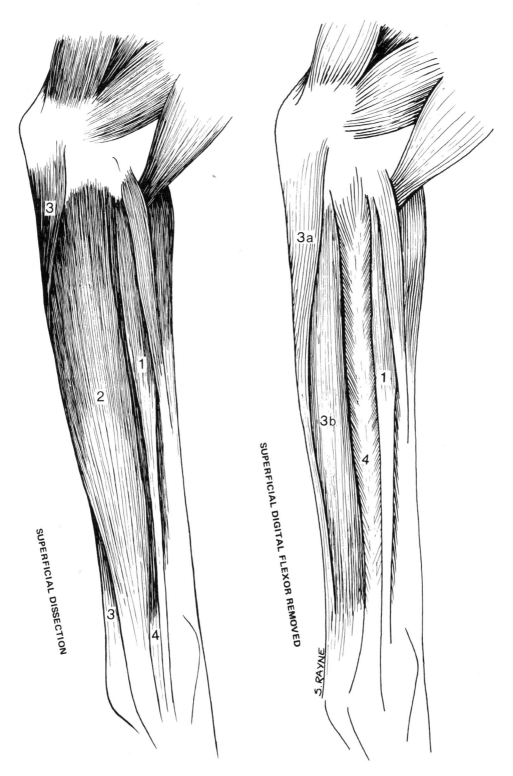

Fig.4.53. Flexor muscles of the left manus, medical view.

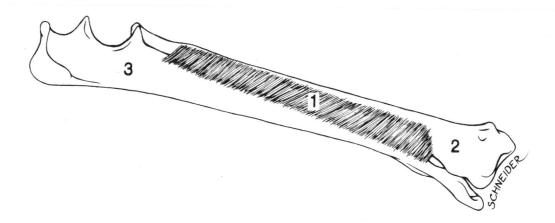

Fig.4.54. Left pronator quadratus muscle, caudomedial view.

A muscle in the interosseous space between the ulna and radius (Fig. 4.54), deep to the deep digital flexor, is the **PRONATOR QUADRATUS** (four sided) (1). This muscle attaches to the rough surfaces of the radius (2) and ulna (3).

JOINTS

There are a number of osseous joint types in the body (Table 4.1), but the articulations of greatest importance in veterinary medicine are the cartilaginous and synovial joints.

CARTILAGINOUS JOINTS permit limited movement; **SYNOVIAL JOINTS**, with lubricating fluid between opposing bones, are characterized by greater freedom in movement.

Table 4.1 Classification of articulations.

General Type	Class of Joint
Synarthroses (little movement)	
A. One bone directly fused to another bone	Synostosis
B. Bone attached to bone by cartilage (cartilaginous articulations)	
1. Hyaline cartilage	Synchondrosis
2. Fibrocartilage	Symphysis
C. Bone attached to bone by dense connective tissue (fibrous articulations)	
1. Broad zone of dense connective tissue	Syndesmosis
2. Narrow zone of dense connective tissue between flat bones	Suture
3. Tooth anchored in an alveolus of the jaw by dense connective tissue	Gomphosis
Synovial Articulations (movable)	
A. Shape (of opposing articular surfaces)	
1. Flat surface with a flat surface	Plane
2. Convex surface with a concave surface	Spheroidal
3. Elongated convex surface with an elongated concave surface	Ellipsoidal
4. Knuckle-shaped surface fitting into a reciprocal depression	Condylar
5. Circular surface rotating in a concave or ring-shaped surface	Trochoid
6. Concavoconvex surface with a reciprocal convexoconcave surface	Saddle (sellar)
B. Plane of movement—one plane only	Ginglymus
C. Number of bones involved	
1. Two opposing surfaces	Simple
2. More than two articular surfaces	Composite

Cartilaginous joints are composed of two bones united by either hyaline cartilage or fibrocartilage; these two types of joints are termed **SYNCHONDROSES** and **SYMPHYSES** (sim' fi-ses, sing. symphysis). An osseous epiphysis joined to the diaphysis of a long bone by epiphyseal cartilage is an example of a synchondrosis (Fig. 4.55); most synchondroses are lost through ossification during the maturation process. Junctions between right and left pelvic bones and between individual vertebrae are examples of symphyses.

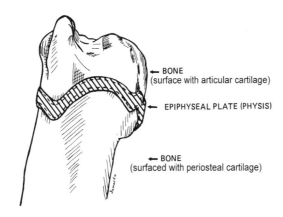

Fig.4.55. A synchondrosis.

Synovial joints are characterized by the presence of an **ARTICULAR CAVITY** between the articular cartilages surfacing opposing bones (Fig. 4.56).

The **ARTICULAR CAPSULE** of a synovial joint passes from the superficial layer of one bone to the superficial layer of the opposing bone, forming a sheath around the articular cavity; thus the articular cavity is completed by walls of articular cartilage and the articular capsule.

The articular capsule is composed of two connective tissue layers: a deep **SYNOVIAL STRATUM** and superficial **FIBROUS STRATUM.**

The thin synovial membrane produces the lubricating fluid, **SYNOVIA,** which fills the articular cavity. Fat deposits are often present between the synovial and fibrous membranes. Such deposits may protrude into the space between the opposing bones of a joint; however, the synovial membrane folds around the deep surface of the fat.

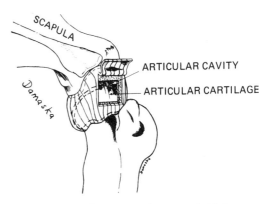

Fig.4.56. Contents of a synovial joint.

Thickenings of the fibrons membrane, called EXTRACAPSULAR LIGAMENTS, aid in maintaining the integrity of synovial joints. A pair of extracapsular ligaments, termed **COLLATERAL LIGAMENTS** (Fig. 4.57) are associated with the fibrous membrane of the articular capsule of a number of articulations; these articulations are characterized by bending in only one plane. Collateral ligaments that cross the joint to each side of the plane of movement help prevent lateral movement and overextension.

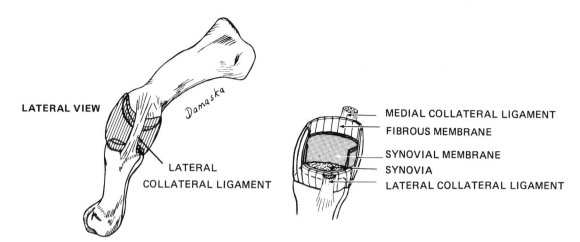

LATERAL VIEW

Damaska

LATERAL
COLLATERAL LIGAMENT

MEDIAL COLLATERAL LIGAMENT
FIBROUS MEMBRANE
SYNOVIAL MEMBRANE
SYNOVIA
LATERAL COLLATERAL LIGAMENT

Fig.4.57. Collateral ligaments of a synovial joint.

Synovial joints are described in subtypes according to the shape of their articular surfaces, the direction of movement they permit, and the number of articular surfaces within the same capsule.

A SIMPLE ARTICULATION (Fig. 4.58) is a synovial joint formed by only two opposing articular surfaces within the same connective tissue sheath or joint capsule; many of the synovial joints classed according to shape are also simple articulations.

A COMPOSITE ARTICULATION (Fig. 4.59) is a synovial joint having more than one pair of opposing articular surfaces within the same articular capsule. The **GINGLYMUS** (jing' glimus; hinge) **ARTICULATION** is a type of synovial joint that permits movement in one plane only.

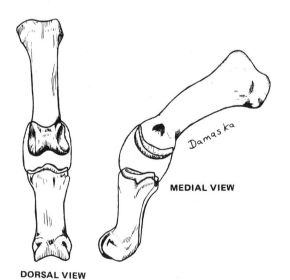

MEDIAL VIEW

Damaska

DORSAL VIEW

Fig.4.58. Synovial joint, simple articulation.

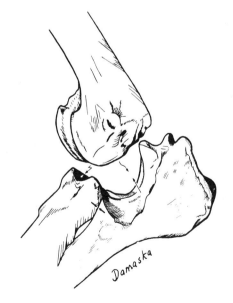

Damaska

Fig.4.59. Synovial joint, composite articulation.

Synovial joints are described according to shape (Fig. 4.60) as: **PLANE ARTICULATIONS** (A), opposing bones with flat surfaces; **SPHEROIDAL ARTICULATIONS** (B), opposing convex surface fitting into a reciprocally concave surface; **ELLIPSOIDAL ARTICULATIONS** (C), similar to spheroidal but elongated; **CONDYLAR ARTICULATIONS** (D), surface with knuckle-shaped prominences fitting into opposing surface with reciprocal depressions; **TROCHOID ARTICULATIONS** (E), shaped like a wheel, with a circular surface turning or pivoting within an opposing ring-shaped surface or on an opposing circular surface; and **SADDLE ARTICULATIONS** (F), opposing bones with concavoconvex surfaces.

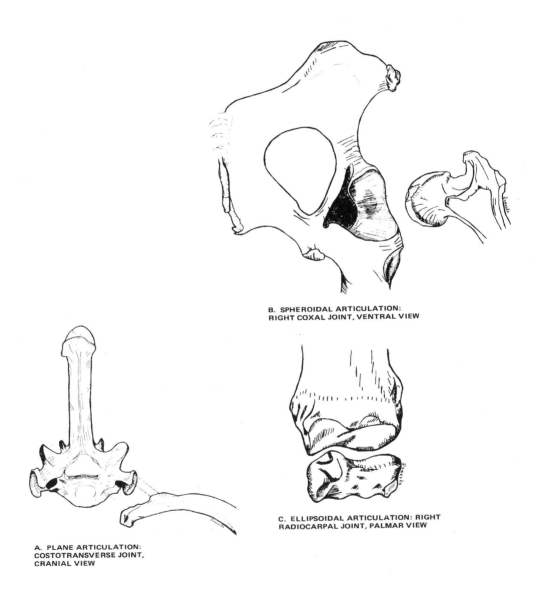

B. SPHEROIDAL ARTICULATION:
RIGHT COXAL JOINT, VENTRAL VIEW

C. ELLIPSOIDAL ARTICULATION: RIGHT
RADIOCARPAL JOINT, PALMAR VIEW

A. PLANE ARTICULATION:
COSTOTRANSVERSE JOINT,
CRANIAL VIEW

Fig.4.60 (A). Synovial joints, classed according to the shape of the articular surface.

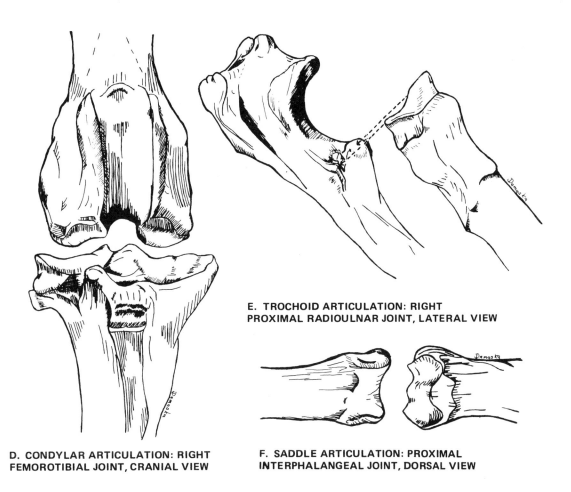

E. TROCHOID ARTICULATION: RIGHT PROXIMAL RADIOULNAR JOINT, LATERAL VIEW

D. CONDYLAR ARTICULATION: RIGHT FEMOROTIBIAL JOINT, CRANIAL VIEW

F. SADDLE ARTICULATION: PROXIMAL INTERPHALANGEAL JOINT, DORSAL VIEW

Fig.4.60 (B). Synovial joints, classed according to the shape of the articular surfaces.

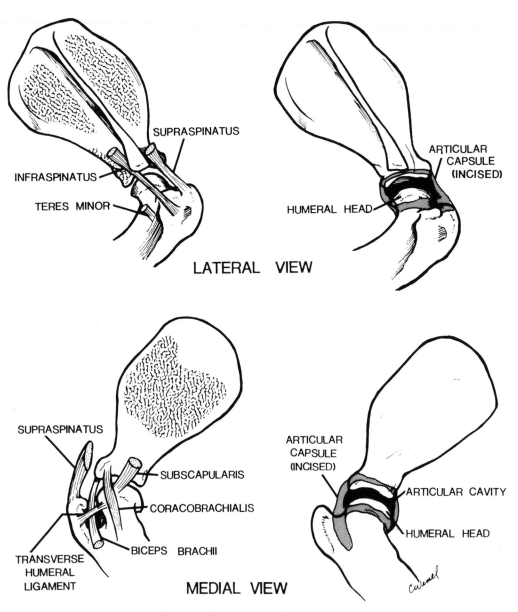

SUPRASPINATUS

INFRASPINATUS

TERES MINOR

LATERAL VIEW

ARTICULAR CAPSULE (INCISED)

HUMERAL HEAD

SUPRASPINATUS

SUBSCAPULARIS

CORACOBRACHIALIS

BICEPS BRACHII

TRANSVERSE HUMERAL LIGAMENT

MEDIAL VIEW

ARTICULAR CAPSULE (INCISED)

ARTICULAR CAVITY

HUMERAL HEAD

Fig.4.61. Right humeral articulation.

Joints of the Thoracic Limb

The **HUMERAL ARTICULATION** (Fig. 4.61) is a spheroidal type of synovial joint. It is characterized by a small amount of movement in any direction. The fibrous membrane of the articular capsule blends with the transverse humeral ligament and the tendons of insertion of the subscapularis, infraspinatus, and supraspinatus muscles. The articular capsule, with synovial fluid, extends distally through the intertubercular groove between the humerus and tendon of the biceps brachii.

The tendons of the subscapularis, infraspinatus, and supraspinatus, which act as muscular (active) collateral ligaments, are quite efficient; dislocations of the humeral articulation are rare. The tendons of the biceps brachii and coracobrachialis muscles also strengthen the humeral articulation.

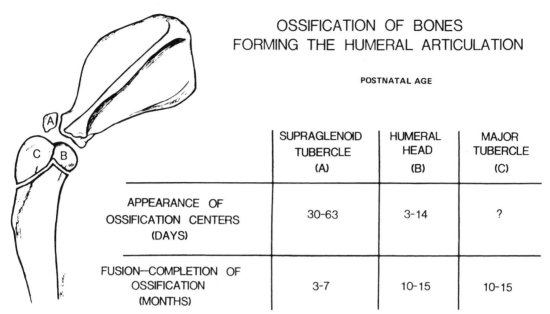

OSSIFICATION OF BONES FORMING THE HUMERAL ARTICULATION

POSTNATAL AGE

	SUPRAGLENOID TUBERCLE (A)	HUMERAL HEAD (B)	MAJOR TUBERCLE (C)
APPEARANCE OF OSSIFICATION CENTERS (DAYS)	30-63	3-14	?
FUSION—COMPLETION OF OSSIFICATION (MONTHS)	3-7	10-15	10-15

Fig.4.62. Ossification of bones forming the left humeral articulation.

When radiographing the humeral articulation of dogs younger than 7 months, a separate accessory epiphyseal center of ossification may be noted in the region of the supraglenoid tubercle, which has not yet undergone fusion to the remainder of the scapula (Fig. 4.62). The proximal epiphysis of the humerus may be separated from the diaphysis by a cartilaginous plate in dogs younger than 1 year.

The **CUBITAL ARTICULATION** (Fig. 4.63), an example of a ginglymus, is composed of three articulations: **HUMEROULNAR** (1), **HUMERORADIAL** (2), and **PROXIMAL RADIOULNAR** (3).

A single articular capsule and articular cavity filled with synovial fluid serve all three articulations of the cubital region (Fig. 4.64). Thus the cubital articulation is a composite articulation.

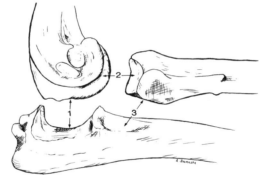

Fig.4.63. Right cubital articulation, lateral view.

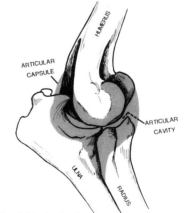

Fig.4.64. Articular capsule of the right cubital articulation, lateral view.

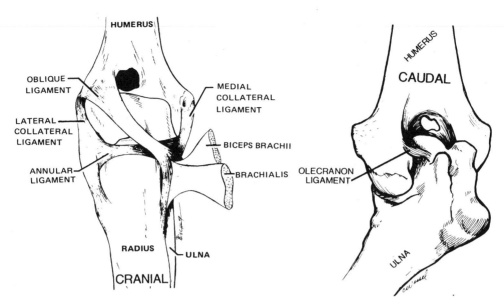

Fig.4.65. Extracapsular ligaments of the right cubital articulation.

All ligaments associated with the cubital articulation are extracapsular (Fig. 4.65). Thickenings of the fibrous membrane of the articular capsule form the **LATERAL** and **MEDIAL COLLATERAL LIGAMENTS,** which attach the lateral and medial epicondyles of the humerus, respectively, to the radius and ulna.

The **ANNULAR LIGAMENT OF THE RADIUS** is a connective tissue band, deep to the collateral ligaments, that partially encircles the head of the radius; the annular ligament and radial notch of the ulna form a ring in which the radius rotates. The **OBLIQUE LIGAMENT** crosses the flexor angle of the cubital articulation; attaching to the humerus and ulna, it aids in preventing overextension. The **OLECRANON LIGAMENT** attaches the anconeal process of the ulna to the caudal surface of the medial epicondylar crest.

Dislocations (luxations) of the cubital articulation are infrequent; however, the condyle is prone to fracture because of the presence of the olecranon fossa and

supratrochlear foramen. These fractures result in a separation of either one or both of the medial and lateral portions of the condyle from the diaphysis. The main axis of stress in the thoracic limb during locomotion is through radial carpal bone, radius, and lateral portion of the humeral condyle.

The distal portion of the humerus develops three ossification centers by 9 weeks of age; the distal centers fuse with the diaphysis and each other by 9 months (Fig. 4.66).

The radius and ulna each have one proximal ossification center, which is present by 7 weeks and is fused by 10 months of age; in addition, a center of ossification may be present in the anconeal process of the ulna. Elbow dysplasia, which is characterized by the partial or complete failure of the anconeal process to fuse with the olecranon, is most frequent in large dogs such as the German Shepherd.

The **CARPAL ARTICULATION** (Fig. 4.67) includes the **ANTEBRACHIOCARPAL** (1), b (2), other **INTERCARPAL** (3), and

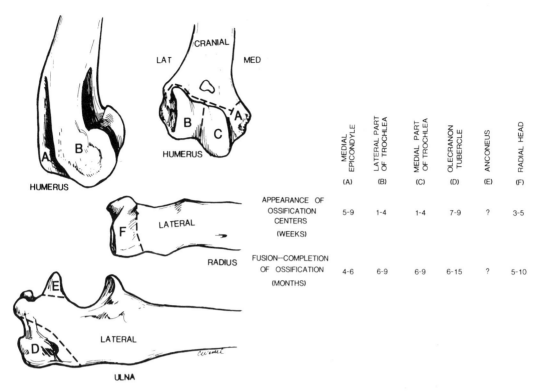

	MEDIAL EPICONDYLE	LATERAL PART OF TROCHLEA	MEDIAL PART OF TROCHLEA	OLECRANON TUBERCLE	ANCONEUS	RADIAL HEAD
	(A)	(B)	(C)	(D)	(E)	(F)
APPEARANCE OF OSSIFICATION CENTERS (WEEKS)	5-9	1-4	1-4	7-9	?	3-5
FUSION—COMPLETION OF OSSIFICATION (MONTHS)	4-6	6-9	6-9	6-15	?	5-10

Fig.4.66. Ossification of bones forming the right cubital articulation.

CARPOMETACARPAL (4) ARTICULATIONS.

Opposing articular surfaces of individual carpal bones constitute the various intercarpal articulations. The middle carpal articulation, a joint between proximal and distal rows of carpal bones, includes several intercarpal articulations. The combined action of individual portions of the carpal articulation is described as a ginglymus.

The fibrous membrane portion of the carpal articulation capsule extends as a sleeve from the distal end of the radius and ulna, over the carpal bones, to the proximal end of the metacarpal bones. The synovial membrane is present as two separate entities, forming two articular cavities, each containing synovia: one between the antebrachium and the proximal row of carpal bones, the other between the proximal and distal rows of carpal bones and between the distal carpal and metacarpal bones. The antebrachiocarpal articulation is a composite articulation since a common articular cavity extends between the **DISTAL RADIOULNAR ARTICULATION** and the **RADIOCARPAL** and **ULNOCARPAL ARTICULATIONS**.

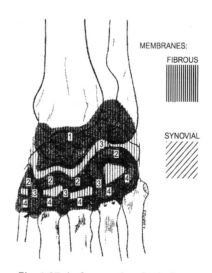

MEMBRANES:

FIBROUS

SYNOVIAL

Fig.4.67. Left carpal articulation.

79

Ossification centers appear in the carpal bones and in the distal epiphyses of the radius and ulna postnatally; ossification is completed with loss of cartilaginous epiphyseal plates by the age of 12 months (Fig. 4.68).

Fracture of the accessory carpal bone occurs frequently in Greyhounds. The sesamoid bone of the long abductor of digit I is present on the medial surface of the carpus.

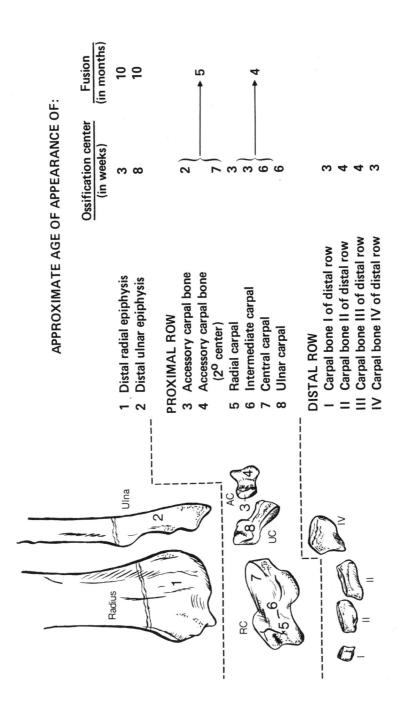

APPROXIMATE AGE OF APPEARANCE OF:

	Ossification center (in weeks)	Fusion (in months)
1 Distal radial epiphysis	3	10
2 Distal ulnar epiphysis	8	10
PROXIMAL ROW		
3 Accessory carpal bone	2	5
4 Accessory carpal bone (2° center)	7	
5 Radial carpal	3	
6 Intermediate carpal	3	4
7 Central carpal	6	
8 Ulnar carpal	6	
DISTAL ROW		
I Carpal bone I of distal row	3	
II Carpal bone II of distal row	4	
III Carpal bone III of distal row	4	
IV Carpal bone IV of distal row	3	

Fig. 4.68. Ossification of bones forming the left carpal articulation.

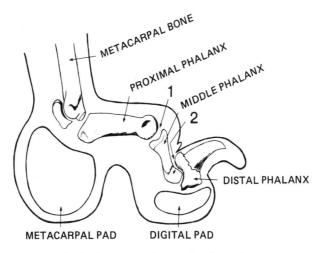

Fig.4.69. Interphalangeal articulation.

The articulations between proximal and middle phalanges and between the middle and distal phalanges are termed the **PROXIMAL** (1) and **DISTAL** (2) **INTERPHALANGEAL ARTICULATIONS**, respectively (Fig. 4.69).

The digital pads are located on the palmar surfaces of the distal interphalangeal articulations.

A small sesamoid bone, present dorsally in the joint capsule of each metacarpophalangeal joint, is positioned between the common digital extensor tendon and joint. Larger, paired sesamoid bones on the palmar surface of each metacarpophalangeal joint are positioned between superficial digital flexor tendons and each joint.

Chapter 5

PELVIC LIMB

Objectives: Be able to identify structural features of bones, muscles, and joints in radiographs and dissected specimens, and be able to locate their positions in the intact animal.

Regions: Coxal Articulation, Femoral, Genual, Patellar, Popliteal, Crural, Tarsal, Metatarsal, and Phalangeal Regions

Pes: Tarsal, Metatarsal, Metatarsophalangeal and Phalangeal Regions

Surfaces, Margins, Prominences, etc., of the Pelvis, Femoral Bone, Patella, Tibia, Fibula, Tarsus, Metatarsus, Phalanges

Muscles: Gluteal Muscles, Biceps Femoris, Semitendinosus, Semimembranosus, Caudal Crural Abductor, Sartorius, Pectineus, Gracilis, Adductor, Tensor Fasciae Latae, Quadriceps Femoris, Iliopsoas, Articularis Coxae, Internal Obturator, Gemelli, Quadratus Femoris, External Obturator, Cranial Tibial, Long Digital Extensor, Fibularis Longus, Lateral Digital Extensor, Fibularis Brevis, Long Digital Extensor of Digit 1, Gastrocnemius, Superficial Digital Flexor, Deep Digital Flexor, Popliteus, and Caudal Tibial Muscle

Sesamoid bones, Symphyseal Tendon, Cranial Pubic Ligament, Prepubic Tendon, Fascia Lata, Crural and Tarsal Extensor Retinacula, Tarsal Canal, and Common Calcanean Tendon

Structures and Ligaments of the Coxal, Stifle, and Tarsal Joints; Menisci and Cruciate Ligaments

The pelvic limb is divided into coxal articulation, femoral, genual, crural, tarsal, metatarsal, and phalangeal regions (Fig. 5.1). **COXAL ARTICULATION** refers to the hip joint, **FEMORAL** to the thigh, **GENUAL** to the knee, **CRURAL** to the leg, and **TARSAL** to the ankle. The **PATELLAR REGION** is the subregion of the genual region that overlies the patella (knee cap). The **POPLITEAL** (pop-lit'e-al) **REGION** is the area caudal to the knee.

superficial to the joint between the skeleton of the metatarsus and the proximal segment of the digit is the **METATARSOPHALANGEAL REGION**. The other regions distal to the metatarsus are named the same as corresponding areas of the thoracic limb (see Fig. 4.2).

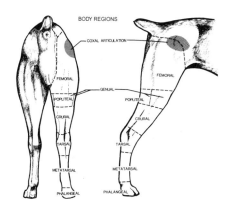

Fig.5.1. Subregions of pelvic limb.

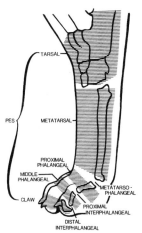

Fig.5.2. Regions of the pes.

BONES OF THE PELVIC LIMB

The **METATARSUS** is that portion of the foot (**PES**) (pes, pl. pedes) between the ankle and the digits (Fig. 5.2). The term pes signifies the **TARSAL, METATARSAL, and PHALANGEAL REGIONS**. The surface area

The bones of the pelvic limb include those of the pelvic girdle and the femoral, genual, crural, tarsal, metatarsal, and phalangeal regions (Fig. 5.3).

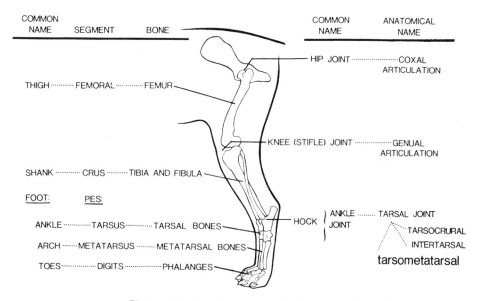

Fig.5.3. Anatomical segments of the pelvic limb.

The **PELVIS** (Fig. 5.4) consists of the **PELVIC GIRDLE** (1) and the **SACRUM** (2). The pelvic girdle (**OSSA COXARUM**) consists of right and left **OS** (pl. **ossa**) **COXAE** (kok' see, sing. coxa).

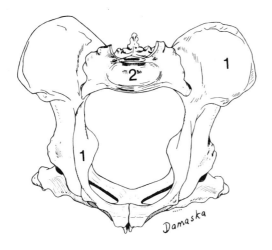

Fig.5.4. Bony pelvis, cranial view.

The three bones forming the mature os coxae (Fig. 5.5)—**ILIUM** (1), **ISCHIUM** (is' ke-um, pl. ischia) (2), and **PUBIS** (3)—are united to each other around the **ACETABULUM** (4), a concave articular surface. The ilium forms the craniodorsal portion, the pubis the cranioventral portion, and the ischium the caudoventral portion of the os coxae. Dogs younger than 7 months have a separate acetabular bone, which may be apparent on radiographs.

The dorsocranial marginal ridge of the ilium is the **ILIAC CREST** (1, Fig. 5.6), which includes a cranioventral prominence, the **TUBER COXAE** (2), and a long dorsal prominence, the **TUBER SACRAL** (3).

The **MAJOR ISCHIATIC NOTCH** (4) is the elongated concavity on the dorsal surface of the ilium, caudal to the tuber sacral. The smooth, shallow depression in the lateral surface of the thin wing of the ilium is named the **GLUTEAL** (gloo' te-al) **SURFACE** (5). A smooth prominence on the lateral surface of the body of the ilium, cranial to the acetabulum, is the **RECTUS FEMORIS AREA** (6), the point of origin of a muscle of similar name.

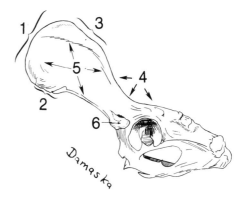

Fig.5.6. Left ilium, lateral view.

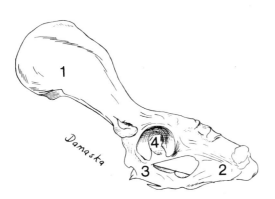

Fig.5.5. Bones forming the left os coxae lateral view.

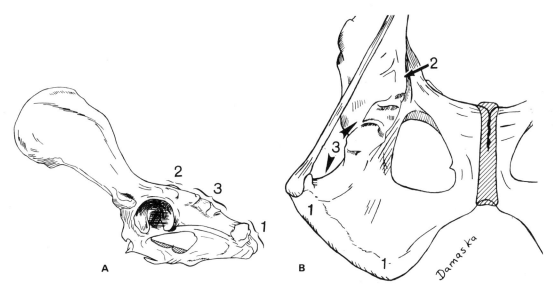

Fig.5.7. Left ischium: lateral view (A); caudodorsal view (B).

The **TUBER ISCHIADICUM** (1, Fig. 5.7) is the broad, caudally projecting margin of the ischium and its lateral projection. A space present on the dorsal margin of the ischium between the **ISCHIATIC SPINE** (2) and the tuber ischiadicum is termed the **MINOR ISCHIATIC NOTCH** (3).

The **ILIOPUBIC EMINENCE** (1, Fig. 5.8) is a small prominence on the cranial margin of the pubic bone, lateral to the **PELVIC SYMPHYSIS** (2).

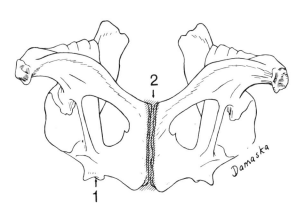

Fig.5.8. Ossa coxarum, caudoventral view.

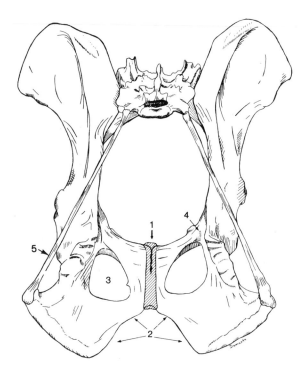

Fig.5.9. Bony pelvis and sacrotuberous
ligament, caudodorsal view.

The two halves of the ossa coxarum articulate
ventrally at the pelvic symphysis (1, Fig. 5.9);
this articulation is composed of two parts, the
PUBIC and **ISCHIATIC SYMPHYSES.** The
pelvic symphysis becomes ossified in dogs older
than 5 years.

The **ISCHIATIC ARCH** (2), on the
caudoventral margin of the two ischia, extends
from one tuber ischiadicum to the other.

The two large **OBTURATOR FORAMINA** (3),
one on each side, are enclosed by the ischiatic
and pubic bones. A smooth surface on the
craniodorsal margin of the obturator foramen is
the **OBTURATOR GROOVE** (4).

A cordlike structure, the **SACROTUBEROUS
LIGAMENT** (5), attaches the lateral portion of
the tuber ischiadicum to the sacrum and 1st
caudal vertebra

*(DIFFERENCES TO BE NOTED IN THE
CAT: A sacrotuberous ligament is not present in
the cat.)*

The **ACETABULAR FOSSA** (1, Fig. 5.10) is
incomplete ventromedially due to the presence
of the **ACETABULAR NOTCH** (2).

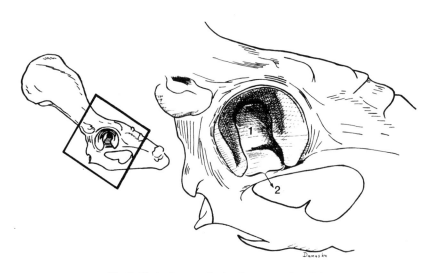

Fig.5.10. Left acetabular fossa and notch.

The proximal portion of the **FEMORAL BONE** (Fig. 5.11) bears an articular **HEAD** (1), which is directed medially; a small **FOVEA** (fo'veah, pl. foveae) of **THE FEMORAL HEAD** (2) is present on the caudomedial surface. A distinct constriction, the **NECK OF THE FEMORAL BONE** (3), is present between the head and the remainder of the proximal extremity.

The large, dorsally projecting **MAJOR TROCHANTER** (4) is separated from the head and neck by the large, cavernous **TROCHANTERIC FOSSA** (5) on the caudal surface of the proximal extremity.

The **MINOR TROCHANTER** (6) is present on the caudomedial surface of the femoral bone, distal to the neck.

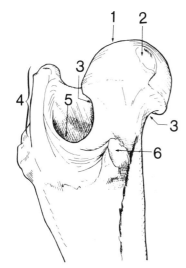

Fig.5.11. Proximal portion of the left femoral bone, caudal view.

The ridge of bone that extends from the minor to the major trochanter is the **INTERTROCHANTERIC CREST** (1, Fig. 5.12). The area of the **THIRD TROCHANTER** (2) occurs on the caudolateral surface of the femoral bone, near the same transverse plane as the minor trochanter.

A ROUGH SURFACE extends longitudinally along the caudal surface of the femoral bone; the edges of the rough surface are termed the **MEDIAL** (3) and **LATERAL** (4) **LIPS** of the rough surface. The **NUTRIENT FORAMEN** is present in the rough surface (5).

The distal caudal surface of the femoral diaphysis is named the **POPLITEAL SURFACE** (6).

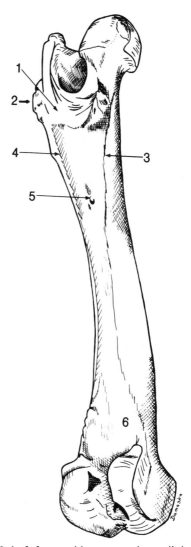

Fig.5.12. Left femoral bone, caudomedial view.

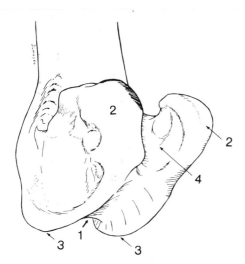

Fig.5.13. Distal portion of the left femoral bone, caudolateral view.

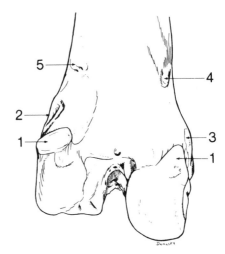

Fig.5.14. Distal portion of the left femoral bone, caudal view.

The distal end of the femoral bone (Fig. 5.13) is characterized by a **TROCHLEA** (1) and two caudally projecting **CONDYLES** (2). The trochlea is a smoothly grooved surface with lateral and medial lips (3); each lip is continuous distally with a condyle. The trochlear groove of the femoral bone is continuous distally with the **INTERCONDYLAR FOSSA** (4), a large concavity between the condyles.

Smooth, circular, articular surfaces (1, Fig. 5.14) are present proximally on the caudally projecting condyles. These are the articular surfaces of the medial and lateral sesamoid bones of the gastrocnemius muscle. Two small prominences, the **LATERAL** (2) and **MEDIAL** (3) **EPICONDYLES**, are on the caudolateral and caudomedial surfaces, respectively, of the distal extremity; each epicondyle is adjacent to a particular surface of a sesamoid bone. Proximal to the epicondyles are two large prominences on the caudal surface of the diaphysis; these **SUPRACONDYLAR TUBEROSITIES, MEDIAL** (4) and **LATERAL** (5), are continuous with the lips of the rough surface of the femoral bone.

A small concave depression, the **EXTENSOR FOSSA** (1, Fig. 5.15), is present on the distal end of the femoral bone at the junction of the lateral lip of the trochlea and the lateral condyle. Between the articular surface (2) of the lateral sesamoid bone and the extensor fossa, a third smooth articular surface may be noted, the **FOSSA OF THE POPLITEAL MUSCLE** (3).

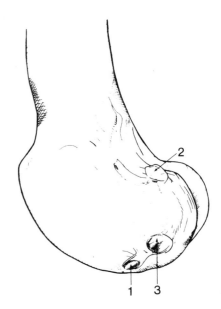

Fig.5.15. Distal portion of the right femoral bone, lateral view.

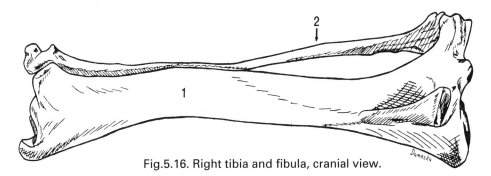

Fig.5.16. Right tibia and fibula, cranial view.

The crural region is nearly the same length as the femoral region; two bones (Fig. 5.16), a large **TIBIA** (1) and a slender **FIBULA** (2) are present in the **CRUS** (krus, pl. crura; leg).

The proximal end of the tibia (Fig. 5.17) bears three large prominences: a caudomedial prominence, the **MEDIAL CONDYLE** (1); a caudolateral prominence, the **LATERAL CONDYLE** (2); and a cranial longitudinal crest, the **CRANIAL MARGIN** (3). The proximal portion of the cranial margin, the **TIBIAL TUBEROSITY** (4), provides for insertion of the primary extensor muscle mass of the knee joint.

Two small eminences on the proximal tibial articular surface project proximally into the intercondylar fossa of the femoral bone; these medial and lateral intercondylar tubercles are collectively termed the **INTERCONDYLAR EMINENCE** (5). Depressions cranial and caudal to the intercondylar eminence are the **CRANIAL** (6) and **CAUDAL** (7) **INTERCONDYLAR AREAS**, respectively.

The groove in the caudal surface of the tibial epiphysis, distal to the caudal intercondylar area, is the **POPLITEAL NOTCH** (8). The **EXTENSOR GROOVE** (9) is a furrow in the proximolateral surface between the lateral tibial condyle and the tibial tuberosity.

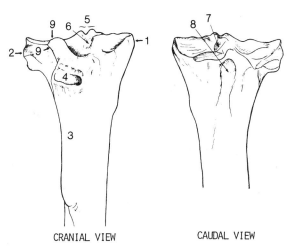

CRANIAL VIEW   CAUDAL VIEW

Fig.5.17. Proximal portion of the right tibia.

The medial portion of the distal end of the tibia (Fig. 5.18) projects distally as the **MEDIAL MALLEOLUS** (mal-le' o-lus, pl. malleoli) (1). The distal articular surface of the tibia is the **TIBIAL COCHLEA** (2).

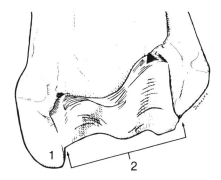

Fig.5.18. Distal portion of the right tibia, caudal view.

91

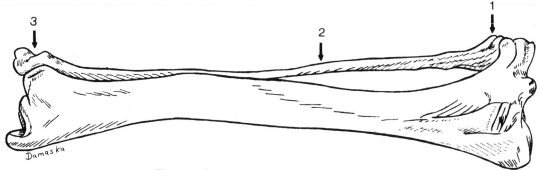

Fig.5.19. Right tibia and fibula, cranial view.

The fibula (Fig. 5.19), which is lateral to the tibia, is characterized by a proximally enlarged **HEAD** (1), a long, slender **BODY** (2), and an enlarged distal extremity, the **LATERAL MALLEOLUS** (3).

The bones of the **TARSUS** (Fig. 5.20) are arranged in three rows: a proximal row of two bones, the **CALCANEUS** (kal- ka'ne-us) (1) and **TALUS** (2); a middle row formed by a single bone, the **CENTRAL TARSAL BONE** (3); and a distal row of four bones, **TARSAL BONES I, II, III**, and **IV**. The laterally positioned calcaneus is the largest bone of the tarsus.

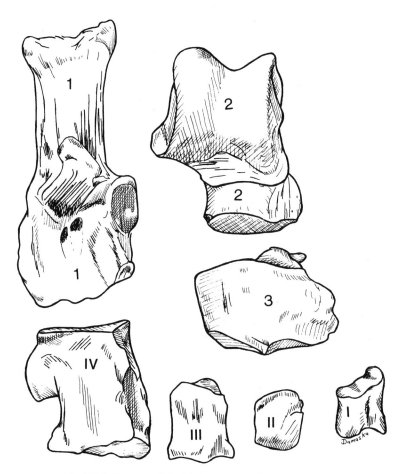

Fig.5.20. Bones of the right tarsus, dorsal view.

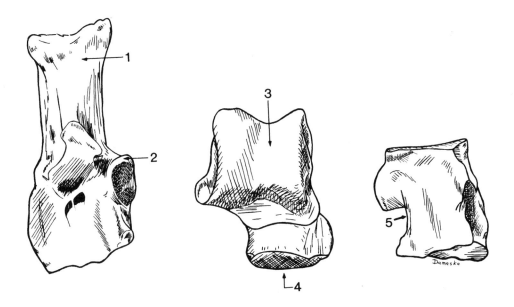

Fig.5.21. Right calcaneus, talus, and fourth tarsal bones, dorsal view.

The **TUBER CALCANEI** (1, Fig. 5.21) is the large, proximally projecting prominence of the calcaneus on which the common calcanean tendon inserts. A medial projection near the distal end of the calcaneus, the **SUSTENTACULUM** (sus " ten-tak' u-lum; support) **TALI** (2), articulates with the medial plantar surface of the talus.

The talus articulates with the dorsal surface of the calcaneus and with the distal extremity of the tibia. The proximal dorsal surface of the talus is in the form of a trochlea (3), which matches, in a reciprocal manner, the cochlear surface of the tibia. The head (4), or distal end, of the talus articulates with the central tarsal bone, which in turn articulates with tarsal bones I, II, and III.The distal articular surface of the calcaneus contacts the proximal articular surface of tarsal bone IV. A groove (5) in the lateral surface of tarsal bone IV indicates the site where the fibularis longus tendon crosses to the plantar surface of the pes.

There are four main **METATARSAL BONES, II–V** (Fig. 5.22); in most breeds a small

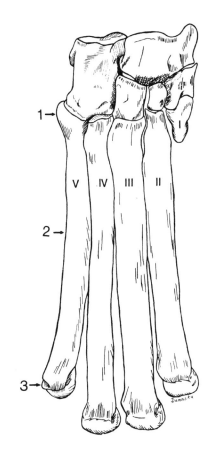

Fig.5.22. Right metatarsal bones and distal two rows of tarsal bones, dorsal view.

93

metatarsal I is also present. Each metatarsal bone has a proximal **BASE** (1), a **BODY** (2), and a distal **HEAD** (3). The metatarsus is longer than the metacarpus of the same dog.

DIGITS II–V have **PROXIMAL** (1), **MIDDLE** (2), and **DISTAL** (3) **PHALANGES** (Fig. 5.23). Digit I may be absent; if present, it will usually contain one or two phalanges.

(DIFFERENCES TO BE NOTED IN THE CAT: Retractile claws (Fig. 5.24) are characteristic of the Felidae (cat family). The articular surfaces of the distal interphalangeal articulation are shaped such that during hyperextension, the distal phalanx (1) swivels past the lateral surface of the middle phalanx (2).

Two elastic ligaments (3), tautly stretched between the middle and distal phalanges, maintain the claw in retraction. Protrusion of

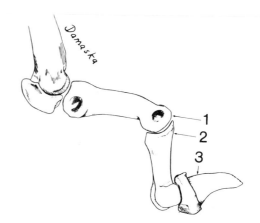

Fig.5.23. Bones of a digit (II–V) lateral view.

the claw requires contraction of the digital extensors (4) for fixation of the proximal interphalangeal articulation and of the deep digital flexor muscle (5) for flexion of the distal interphalangeal articulation.)

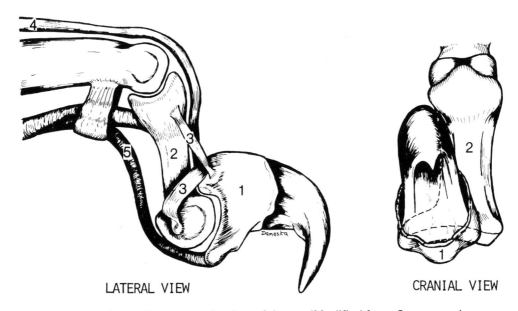

LATERAL VIEW

CRANIAL VIEW

Fig.5.24. Retractile claw mechanism of the cat (Modified from Gonyea and Ashworth 1975 *J.Morphol* 145(2): 229–38).

MUSCLES OF THE PELVIC LIMB

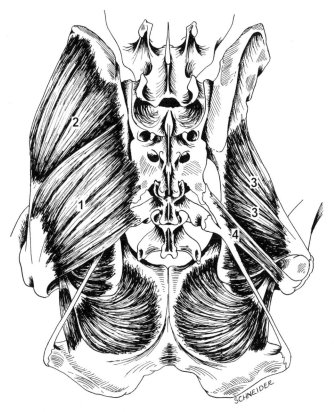

Fig.5.25. Gluteal muscles, dorsal view.

The proximal portion of the pelvic limb contains gluteal, caudal femoral, medial femoral, cranial femoral, and coxal articulation muscles.

The **GLUTEAL MUSCLES** (Fig. 5.25) include the small, caudal superficial gluteus (1), the large middle gluteus (2), and the deeply situated deep gluteus (3). The **SUPERFICIAL GLUTEUS** (1), which arises from gluteal fascia (the sacrum) and the sacrotuberous ligament, inserts on the third trochanter of the proximal caudolateral surface of the femoral bone.

The **MIDDLE GLUTEUS** (2), the fibers of which are oriented caudodistally, is the major superficial muscle of the gluteal region. It arises from the iliac crest and the gluteal surface of the ilium; its tendon inserts on the major trochanter of the proximal surface of the femoral bone. A caudal portion of the middle gluteus, the **PIRIFORMIS** (pear shape) **MUSCLE,** situated deep to the superficial gluteus, arises from the caudal vertebrae and is easily confused with a small deep slip (4) of the superficial gluteus.

Fibers of the **DEEP GLUTEUS MUSCLE** (3) are oriented caudodistally from the ilium to the major trochanter on the proximal lateral surface of the femoral bone. The origin of the deep gluteus muscle is from the ilium at the dorsal level of the major ischiatic notch.

Caudal femoral muscles (Fig. 5.26) are the biceps femoris (1), semitendinosus (2), semimembranosus (3), and the slender caudal crural abductor (4). The **BICEPS FEMORIS** (1) forms the major muscle mass on the caudolateral surface of the femoral region; it arises from the tuber ischiadicum and the sacrotuberous ligament, passes over the insertion of the superficial gluteus muscle (5), and inserts by means of aponeuroses at various points distally.

The **SEMITENDINOSUS** (sem˝ e-tend˝ i-no′ sus) **MUSCLE** (2) arises from the tuber ischiadicum and inserts distally on the medial surface of the tibia; it also inserts by means of a fascial attachment on the tuber calcanei. The **SEMIMEMBRANOSUS MUSCLE** (3) arises from the tuber ischiadicum, at which level it is visible superficially. Distally, the muscle fibers are covered laterally by the semitendinosus muscle and medially by the gracilis muscle (6).

The semimembranosus muscle attaches by means of two tendons of insertion, one to the distal medial lip of the femoral rough surface and one to the proximal medial surface of the tibia (medial tibial condyle).

The long, thin, straplike **CAUDAL CRURAL ABDUCTOR MUSCLE** (4) is situated along the caudal deep margin of the biceps femoris; it arises from the sacrotuberous ligament and inserts by a fascial attachment on the lateral surface of the crus.

(DIFFERENCES TO BE NOTED IN THE CAT: The GLUTEOFEMORALIS, an elongate muscle adjacent to the cranial margin of the biceps femoris muscle, arises from the 2nd and 3rd caudal vertebrae and inserts on the patella.)

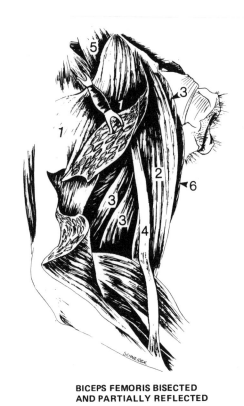

BICEPS FEMORIS BISECTED AND PARTIALLY REFLECTED

Fig.5.26. Caudal femoral muscles, lateral view.

Medial femoral muscles (Fig. 5.27) are the sartorius (1), pectineus (pek-tin′ e-us) (2), gracilis (gras′il-is; slender) (3), and adductor (4). The **SARTORIUS MUSCLE** (1) forms the craniomedial surface of the femoral region. This muscle is divided longitudinally into two straplike muscles, one caudal to the other. The cranial part of the sartorius muscle arises from the iliac crest and inserts on the patella; the caudal part arises from the tuber coxae and inserts on the cranial margin of the tibia. The **PECTINEUS** (2) is a spindle-shaped muscle that is palpable in the abducted limb on the proximal medial surface of the femoral region. It arises from the iliopubic eminence and inserts deep to the sartorius muscle on the distal rough surface of the femoral bone (caudomedially). A triangular "space," formed by the converging

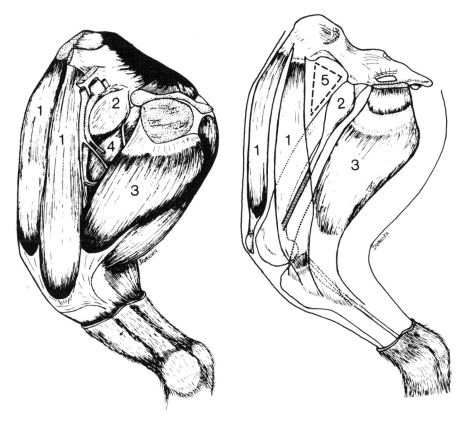

SUPERFICIAL DISSECTION   **SCHEMATIC, DEEP MUSCLES REMOVED**

Fig.5.27. Medial femoral muscles, medial view.

sartorius and pectineus muscles, is termed the
FEMORAL TRIANGLE (5). The **GRACILIS** (3)
is a broad, flat muscle that forms the
caudomedial surface of the femoral region. The
fibers of the **ADDUCTOR MUSCLE** (4), deep
to the gracilis muscle and caudal to the femur,
are directed distolaterally from the pelvic
symphysis to the caudal surface of the
femoral bone.

Viewed from the caudal aspect (Fig. 5.28), the
gracilis is the most medial of the four superficial
muscles observed: biceps femoris (1),
semitendinosus (2), semimembranosus (3), and
gracilis (4). The gracilis muscle arises from the
pelvic symphysis and inserts by an aponeurosis
on the proximal craniomedial surface of the
tibia; a caudal portion of the aponeurosis inserts
on the tuber calcanei.

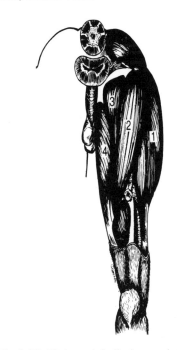

Fig.5.28. Right pelvic limb, caudal view.

The adductor muscle (Fig. 5.29) may be subdivided into two parts: adductor magnus et brevis (1) and adductor longus (2). The adductor muscle is deep and caudal to the pectineus muscle (3) and cranial to the semimembranosus muscle (4).

The **ADDUCTOR MAGNUS ET BREVIS** (large and short) **MUSCLE** (1) arises from the pelvic symphysis and inserts on the lateral lip of the rough surface of the femoral bone.

The **ADDUCTOR LONGUS MUSCLE** (2) arises from the pubic bone and inserts on the caudal surface of the femoral bone near the intertrochanteric crest.

Both the gracilis and adductor muscles arise from the pelvic symphysis via strong connective tissue termed the symphyseal tendon.

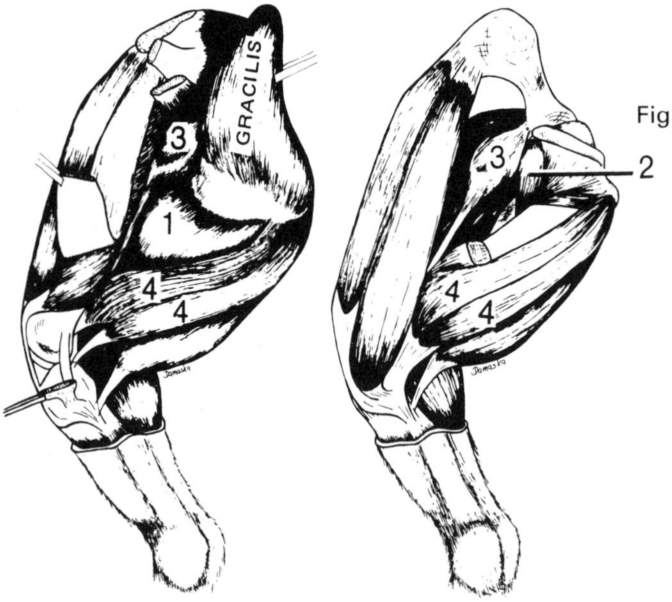

Fig.5.29. Medial femoral muscles, medial view.

The **SYMPHYSEAL TENDON** (1, Fig. 5.30) is situated along the ventral median line superficial to the pelvic symphysis. The transversely oriented **CRANIAL PUBIC LIGAMENT** (2)

attaches one iliopubic eminence to the other at right angles to the symphyseal tendon. Abdominal muscles attach to the cranial pubic ligament via a strong **PREPUBIC TENDON** (3).

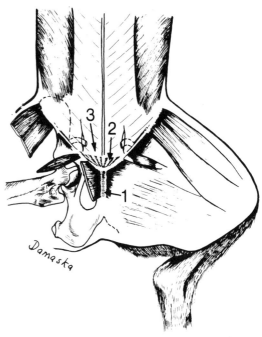

Fig.5.30. Schematic of prepubic and symphyseal tendons, ventral view.

The cranial femoral muscles (Fig. 5.31) include the tensor fasciae latae and quadriceps femoris. The **TENSOR FASCIAE LATAE** (1) is a short, double-bellied muscle situated on the proximal lateral surface of the femoral region between the sartorius muscle (2) craniomedially, the middle gluteus muscle (3) proximally, and the biceps femoris muscle (4) caudally. The tensor fasciae latae muscle arises from the tuber coxae and inserts on the **FASCIA LATA** (5).

The large **QUADRICEPS** (four heads) **FEMORIS MUSCLE** (Fig. 5.32) arises from four points, three from the proximal end of the

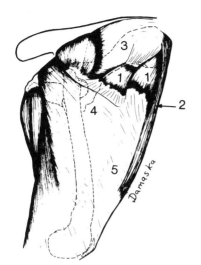

Fig.5.31. Schematic of cranial femoral muscles,
lateral view.

femoral diaphysis and one from the ilium. The three heads, which arise from the femoral bone, are partially separable and are named according to their position as **VASTUS LATERALIS** (1), **VASTUS MEDIALIS** (2), and **VASTUS INTERMEDIUS** (3) **MUSCLES**. The vastus intermedius muscle is positioned directly against the cranial surface of the femoral bone.

The **RECTUS** (straight) **FEMORIS MUSCLE** (4), the fourth and most cranial portion of the quadriceps femoris, arises from an attachment area on the lateral surface of the ilium, cranial to the acetabulum. All four bellies of the quadriceps muscle form one common tendon of insertion that extends distally around the patella to insert on the tibial tuberosity.

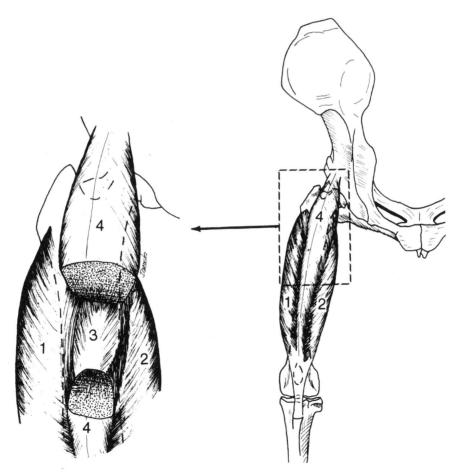

Fig.5.32. Schematic of quadriceps femoris muscle, cranial view.

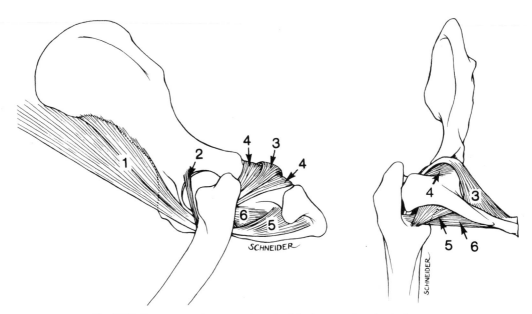

Fig.5.33. Deep muscles associated with the coxal articulation.

Deep muscles closely associated with the coxal articulation (Fig. 5.33) are the iliopsoas (il " e-o-so' as) (1), articularis coxae (2), internal obturator (3), gemelli (jem'el-li) (4), quadratus femoris (5), and external obturator (6).

The **ILIOPSOAS MUSCLE** (1, Fig. 5.34), which will be described later with the trunk (see p. 157), is formed by two muscles, the **PSOAS** (so as) **MAJOR** (2) and **ILIACUS** (3). The iliacus muscle arises from the ventral concave surface of

the ilium, caudal to the tuber coxae, and extends caudally past the proximal medial surface of the femoral bone to attach to the minor trochanter.

The **ARTICULARIS COXAE** (4) is a short, straplike muscle that arises from the ilium caudal to the origin of the rectus femoris and inserts on the proximal cranial surface of the femoral diaphysis. The articularis coxae muscle is in contact with the more deeply situated articular capsule.

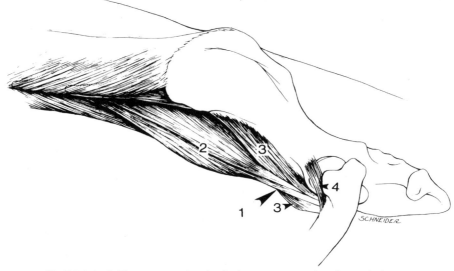

Fig.5.34. Left iliopsoas and articularis coxae muscles, lateral view.

The **INTERNAL OBTURATOR MUSCLE** (1, Fig. 5.35) arises from the dorsal marginal surface of the obturator foramen. This obturator muscle is considered internal since it arises from within the canal formed by the pelvic bones. The tendon of the internal obturator muscle crosses the dorsal surface of the minor ischiatic notch, ventral to the sacrotuberous ligament, and inserts on the trochanteric fossa of the femoral bone.

The **GEMELLI** (2) are small muscular masses arising from the dorsolateral surface of the minor ischiatic notch, deep to the tendon of the internal obturator muscle.

The tendon of the gemelli muscles inserts on the trochanteric fossa. The **QUADRATUS FEMORIS** (3) is a short, strong muscle arising from the ventral surface of the ischium, medial to the tuber ischiadicum, and inserting on the intertrochanteric crest of the femoral bone.

The quadratus femoris (1, Fig. 5.36) and adductor longus (2) muscles together form a V shape; they have a common area of insertion and one arises from the ischium (caudally) and the other from the pelvic symphysis (cranially).

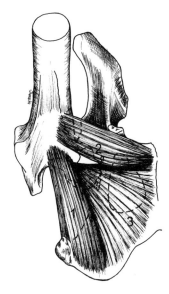

Fig.5.36. Deep muscles of the right coxal articulation, ventral view.

The broad, flat **EXTERNAL OBTURATOR MUSCLE** (3) arises from the ventral surface of bones forming the obturator foramen and inserts on the proximal caudal surface of the femoral bone in the trochanteric fossa.

The external obturator muscle is covered cranially by the more superficial long adductor muscle and caudally by the quadratus femoris muscle.

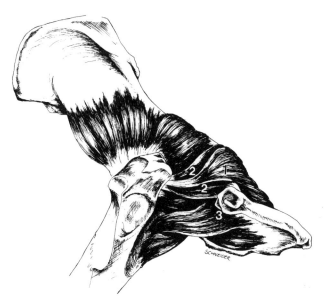

Fig.5.35. Deep muscles of the left coxal articulation, ventral view.

101

The muscles that arise from the femoral bone or proximal portion of the crus and insert on bones of the pes (Fig. 5.37) may be grouped into flexors of the tarsus (1), flexors of the tarsus and extensors of the digits (2), extensors of the tarsus (3), and the extensors of the tarsus and flexors of the digits (4).

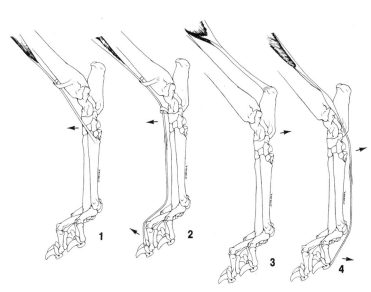

Fig.5.37. Action of crural muscles on the pes.

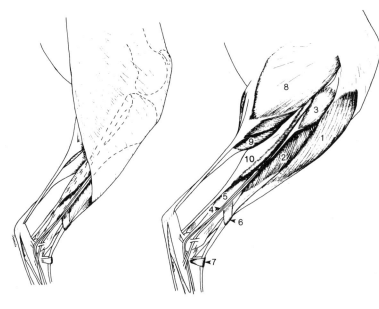

Fig.5.38. Muscles of the right crus, lateral view.

The flexors of the tarsus and extensors of the digits form the craniolateral muscles of the crus (Fig. 5.38). The **CRANIAL TIBIAL** (1), **LONG DIGITAL EXTENSOR** (2), **FIBULARIS** (peroneus) **LONGUS** (3), **LATERAL DIGITAL EXTENSOR** (4), and **FIBULARIS BREVIS** (5) form the craniolateral muscular mass. The tendons of insertion of the cranial tibial and long digital extensor muscles pass deep to a thickening of the deep fascia, the **CRURAL EXTENSOR RETINACULUM** (6), on the distal cranial surface of the crus.

A second fascial band on the dorsal surface of the tarsus, the **TARSAL EXTENSOR RETINACULUM** (7), binds down the long digital extensor tendon.

The large cranial tibial muscle, which is the most cranial of the craniolateral muscle group, arises from the lateral surface of the tibial tuberosity; the tendon of insertion passes deep to the crural extensor retinaculum, arches around the medial surface of the tarsus, and inserts on the proximal plantar surface of metatarsals I and II.

The long digital extensor muscle (2) is caudolateral and partially deep to the cranial tibial muscle. It crosses the genual articulation and all joints distal to the stifle, arising from the extensor fossa of the femoral bone and inserting by means of four tendons on the proximal dorsal surfaces of the distal phalanx of digits II, III, IV, and V. Both crural and tarsal extensor retinacula retain the tendon of insertion in place, proximal to where the tendon separates into its four cords.

The extensors of the tarsus and flexors of the digits form the caudal muscles of the crus; this caudal muscle mass is formed by the gastrocnemius (8), superficial digital flexor (9), deep digital flexor (10), caudal tibial, and popliteus (pop-lit' e-us) muscles.

(DIFFERENCES TO BE NOTED IN THE CAT: A muscle in the proximal lateral portion of the feline crus is the SOLEUS (sole'us). It arises from the fibular head and inserts as part of the common calcanean tendon on the calcanean tuberosity. The soleus and gastrocnemius muscles are collectively named the triceps surae (su' rye, sing. sura; calf).)

The short-bellied fibularis longus muscle (1, Fig. 5.39) is caudal and superficial to the long digital extensor muscle (2). The fibularis longus arises from the lateral collateral ligament (3), lateral tibial condyle, and head of the fibula; the distal tendon of the fibularis longus muscle crosses the lateral surface of the tarsocrural articulation and divides into two tendons at the level of tarsal bone IV. One tendon inserts on the proximal dorsolateral surface of metatarsal bone IV; the other passes to the plantar surface of the pes through a groove in tarsal bone IV and inserts on the proximal plantar surface of one or more metatarsal bones.

The slender lateral digital extensor muscle (4), which is deep and caudal to the fibularis longus muscle, arises from the fibula proximally and inserts either on the proximal dorsal surface of the proximal phalanx of digit V or in common with the lateral tendon of the long digital extens muscle.

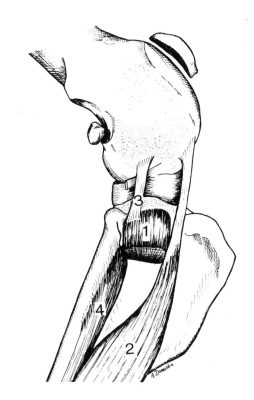

Fig.5.39. Deep muscles of the crus, lateral view of proximal portion.

The fibularis brevis muscle arises from the lateral surface of the fibula and tibia, near their midlength, and inserts on the proximal dorsolateral surface of metatarsal V (Fig. 5.40).

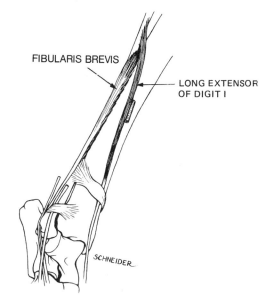

FIBULARIS BREVIS

LONG EXTENSOR OF DIGIT I

SCHNEIDER

Fig.5.40. Fibularis brevis and extensor muscle of digit 1, lateral view.

103

A small **LONG EXTENSOR MUSCLE OF DIGIT I** may be observed deep against the tibia; it arises from the fibula and passes distally through the crural extensor retinaculum, deep to the long digital extensor muscle.

The **MEDIAL** (1) and **LATERAL** (2) **HEADS** of the **GASTROCNEMIUS MUSCLE** (Fig. 5.41) arise from the medial and lateral supracondylar tuberosities of the femoral bone, respectively. The common tendon of insertion attaches to the tuber calcanei.

The **SUPERFICIAL DIGITAL FLEXOR MUSCLE** (3) arises from the lateral supracondylar tuberosity of the femoral bone, deep to the gastrocnemius. The superficial digital flexor muscle and lateral head of the gastrocnemius muscle are difficult to separate

proximally; distally, the tendon of insertion of the superficial digital flexor (4) crosses the medial surface of the gastrocnemius tendon (5) to become superficial near the tuber calcanei.

The superficial digital flexor tendons insert on the tuber calcanei and on the proximal plantar surface of the middle phalanx of digits II, III, IV, and V (arrows, Fig. 5.42).

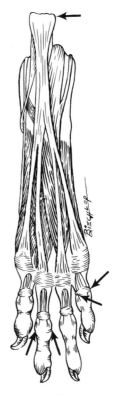

Fig.5.42. Plantar surface of the left pes.

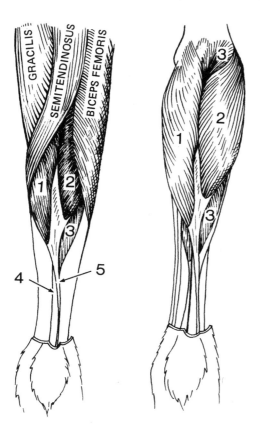

Fig.5.41. Caudal muscles of the right crus, caudal view.

The **POPLITEUS MUSCLE** (1, Fig. 5.43A) arises from the popliteal muscle fossa of the lateral femoral condyle. The belly of the popliteus is oriented distomedially across the caudal surface of the articular capsule to insert on the proximal caudal surface of the tibial diaphysis.

The deep digital flexor is composed of **LATERAL** (2) and **MEDIAL** (3) **DIGITAL FLEXOR MUSCLES.** The larger lateral head arises from the caudal surface of the fibula and tibia; the smaller medial head arises from the caudal border of the tibia between the popliteus and lateral head of the deep digital flexor muscles.

The lateral deep digital flexor tendon passes through the **TARSAL CANAL**, medial to the tuber calcanei; distal to the tarsal canal, the two digital flexor tendons unite on the plantar surface of the tarsus to form a common tendon (4). This tendon is separated distally into four units (Fig. 5.43B).

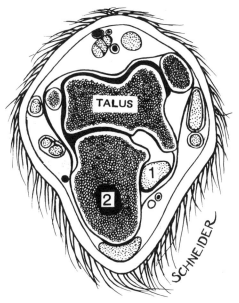

Fig.5.44. Tarsal canal, transverse section through the left pes.

The osseous tarsal canal (Fig. 5.44), through which the tendons of the deep digital flexor (1) pass, is a space medial to the calcaneus (2) on the plantar surface of the tarsus. Vessels, nerves, and tendons within the tarsal canal are held in place by the flexor retinaculum (superficially) and the fibrous membrane of the articular capsule (deeply).

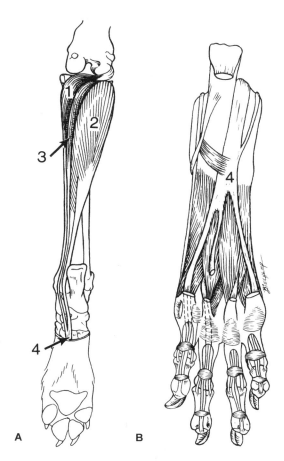

Fig.5.43. Popliteus and deep digital flexor muscles, caudal view of right pes (A).
Deep digital flexor tendons in the left pes, plantar surface (B).

The individual tendons of the deep digital flexor muscle (1, Fig. 5.45) pass through the superficial digital flexor tendons (2) at the level of the metatarsophalangeal articulation. Each deep digital flexor tendon inserts on the proximal plantar surface of each distal phalanx (of digit II, III, IV, or V). Strong deep fascial thickenings retain the tendons in position.

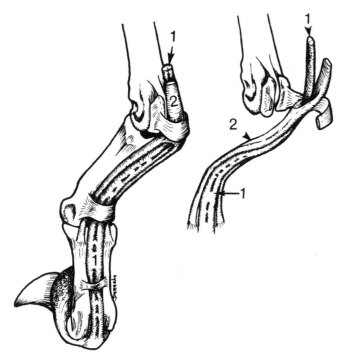

Fig.5.45. Relationship between superficial and deep digital flexor tendons in the digits.

The common tendon (Fig. 5.46) of the gastrocnemius (1), superficial digital flexor (2), biceps femoris (3), semitendinosus (4), and gracilis (5) muscles, which inserts on the tuber calcanei, is termed the **COMMON CALCANEAN TENDON** (6).

The **CAUDAL TIBIAL MUSCLE**, with a small body and a long, thin tendon, is positioned between the medial digital flexor and popliteus muscles. It arises from the fibula and inserts on the medial surface of the tarsus.

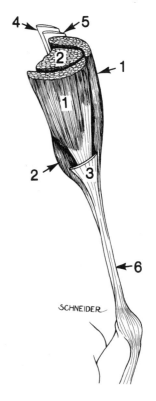

Fig.5.46. Common calcanean tendon, caudomedial view.

JOINTS OF THE PELVIC LIMB

The fibrocartilaginous junction formed midventrally between bones of the pelvis midventrally is an example of a symphysis (Fig. 5.47; see Table 4.1).

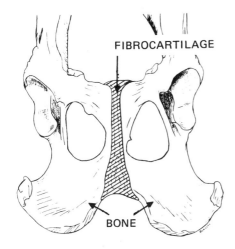

FIBROCARTILAGE

BONE

Fig.5.47. Pelvic symphysis, ventral view.

The **COXAL ARTICULATION** (hip joint) is a spheroidal type of synovial joint (Fig. 5.48).

An intracapsular ligament, the **LIGAMENT OF THE FEMORAL HEAD**, attaches the fossa of the femoral head to the acetabular fossa.

INTRACAPSULAR LIGAMENTS pass between two bones of a joint within an articular cavity, deep to the fibrous portion of the articular capsule. Such ligaments are not in the synovial fluid since they are surrounded by a synovial membrane sheath. Intracapsular ligaments assist in maintaining alignment of bones of a joint and provide a pathway across the articular cavity for vessels and nerves.

An extracapsular **TRANSVERSE ACETABULAR LIGAMENT** completes the **ACETABULAR LIP** (ventromedially) by spanning the acetabular notch. The articular capsule is relatively large, attaching from the peripheral margins of the acetabular lips to the neck of the femoral bone.

Radiographic examination of the coxal articulation may reveal a slipped proximal femoral epiphysis (common in smaller breeds), fractures of the femoral head, and/or dislocations.

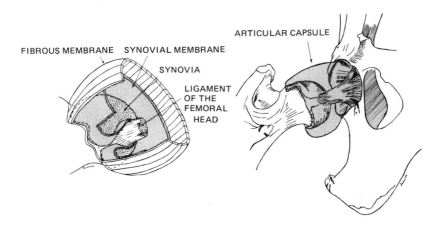

FIBROUS MEMBRANE   SYNOVIAL MEMBRANE

SYNOVIA

LIGAMENT OF THE FEMORAL HEAD

ARTICULAR CAPSULE

Fig.5.48. Coxal articulation.

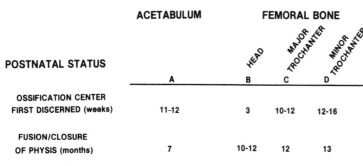

POSTNATAL STATUS	OSSEOUS ELEMENT			
	ACETABULUM	FEMORAL BONE		
		HEAD	MAJOR TROCHANTER	MINOR TROCHANTER
	A	B	C	D
OSSIFICATION CENTER FIRST DISCERNED (weeks)	11–12	3	10-12	12-16
FUSION/CLOSURE OF PHYSIS (months)	7		10-12	12	13

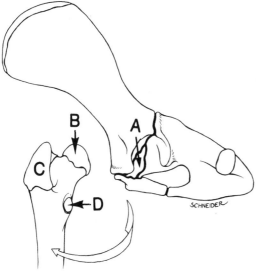

Fig.5.49. Ossification of bones in the proximal, femoral region.

The acetabulum is completely ossified in a 7-month-old dog (Fig. 5.49). The head of the femoral bone develops a center of ossification by 3 weeks and is fused to the diaphysis by 12 months. Both major and minor trochanters begin ossifying by 4 months and are fused to the diaphysis by 13 months postnatally.

The **STIFLE** (sti' fl) **JOINT**, or **GENUAL ARTICULATION** (Fig. 5.50) includes the **FEMOROPATELLAR** (1), **FEMOROTIBIAL** (2), and **PROXIMAL TIBIOFIBULAR** (3) **ARTICULATIONS**; since the articular surfaces of the three bones are present within a single interconnecting articular capsule, the **GENU** (je' nu; knee) is a composite articulation.

Movement of the genual articulation occurs primarily in one plane, characteristic of a ginglymus; however, rotation of 5–6 degrees laterally or medially does occur. Freedom for medial rotation increases to 19 degrees during flexion.

Four sesamoids are present in the genual region (Fig. 5.50): the **PATELLA** (4) in the tendon of insertion of the quadriceps femoris, the **LATERAL** (5) and **MEDIAL** (6) **FABELLAE** (fah-bel' lee; sing. fabella; little bean) in the tendons of origin of the heads of the gastrocnemius, and a **SESAMOID** (7) in the **TENDON OF THE POPLITEUS MUSCLE.**

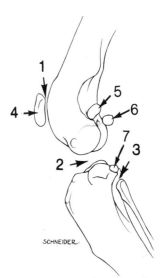

Fig.5.50. Left genual articulation, lateral view.

The osseous patella bears lateral and medial extensions, the **PARAPATELLAR FIBROCARTILAGES** (1, Fig. 5.51) that articulate with the lateral and medial trochlear lips of the femoral bone. **MEDIAL** and **LATERAL PATELLAR RETINACULA** (2) connect the parapatellar fibrocartilages to the medial and lateral fabellae, respectively.

During radiographic examination of the genual articulation, the appearance of normal structures must be differentiated from incidences of distal femoral epiphyseal separation, dislocation of the patella, proximal tibial epiphyseal separation (relatively common), and separation of the tibial tuberosity.

The distal epiphysis of the femoral bone has three centers of ossification (medial and lateral condyles and trochlea), which are present by 3 weeks of age (Fig. 5.52). By the age of 4 months the trochlea fuses with the condyles, and by 13 months the distal epiphysis is fused with the diaphysis. The proximal epiphysis of the tibia develops three centers of ossification by 11 weeks of age: the medial and lateral condyles and the tibial tuberosity. The condyles are fused to the tuberosity by 8 months of age and to the diaphysis by 13 months. The head of the fibula is fused to the diaphysis by 11 months of age.

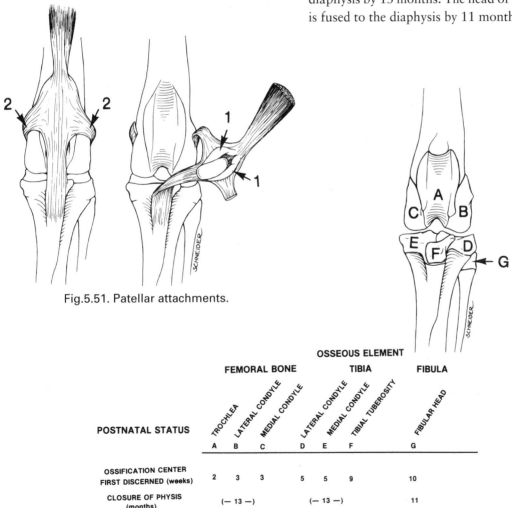

Fig.5.51. Patellar attachments.

POSTNATAL STATUS	FEMORAL BONE			TIBIA			FIBULA
	TROCHLEA	LATERAL CONDYLE	MEDIAL CONDYLE	LATERAL CONDYLE	MEDIAL CONDYLE	TIBIAL TUBEROSITY	FIBULAR HEAD
	A	B	C	D	E	F	G
OSSIFICATION CENTER FIRST DISCERNED (weeks)	2	3	3	5	5	9	10
CLOSURE OF PHYSIS (months)	(— 13 —)			(— 13 —)			11

Fig.5.52. Ossification of bones forming the genual articulation.

Two intracapsular ligaments attach the tibia to the femoral bone (Fig. 5.53). These cruciate ligaments, which cross each other, are named according to their distal attachment on the tibia.

The **CRANIAL CRUCIATE** (kroo' she-ate; cross shape) (1) stretches between the caudolateral surface of the intercondylar fossa of the femoral bone and the cranial intercondylar area of the tibia.

The **CAUDAL CRUCIATE** (2) stretches from the craniomedial surface of the femoral intercondylar fossa, past the medial surface of the cranial cruciate, to the caudolateral surface of the tibial medial condyle. The cruciate ligaments are ensheathed by synovial membrane.

The lateral and medial femoral condyles do not articulate directly with the lateral and medial tibial condyles; instead, a pair of fibrocartilaginous pads, termed **MENISCI** (sing. meniscus) (3, 4), separate the two bones. The peripheral margin of the **MEDIAL MENISCUS** (3) is attached to the articular capsule. A **MENISCOFEMORAL LIGAMENT** (5) attaches the caudal surface of the **LATERAL MENISCUS** (4) to the intercondylar fossa of the femoral bone.

Medial and lateral menisci are attached to each other cranially and to the cranial and caudal intercondylar areas of the tibia.

The articular capsule encloses a large articular cavity that separates the patella from the femoral bone, the femoral condyles from the tibial condyles, and the lateral tibial condyle from the fibular head. Cranial to the articular cavity, the two layers of the articular capsule,

fibrous and synovial, are separated by an **INFRAPATELLAR FAT BODY** (6). Thickenings in the fibrous membrane portion of the articular capsule (laterally and medially) form the lateral and medial collateral ligaments. The **LATERAL COLLATERAL LIGAMENT** (7) attaches to the lateral femoral epicondyle (proximally) and to the head of the fibula and lateral tibial condyle (distally).

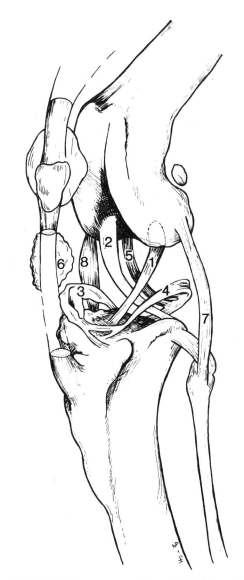

Fig.5.53. Ligaments and menisci of the left genual articulation, craniolateral "exploded" view.

110

The tendon of origin of the popliteus muscle is deep to the lateral collateral ligament. The **MEDIAL COLLATERAL LIGAMENT** (8) attaches to the medial femoral epicondyle (proxi-mally) and to the medial surface of the medial tibial condyle (distally). Injuries to the genual articulation frequently involve the cranial cruciate, medial collateral ligament, and medial meniscus. The femoral attachment of both cranial and caudal cruciate ligaments is caudal to the joint axis during flexion.

The cranial cruciate, the tibial attachment of which is cranial to the axis, is taut during extension of the genual articulation and also partially taut during flexion. The cranial cruciate ligament assists in preventing both hyperextension (148 degrees +) and hyperflexion of the stifle.

If the cranial cruciate is completely ruptured, cranial movement of the tibia relative to the femur (slight during extension, 2 mm) is marked during flexion (9.5 mm). Cranial displacement of the tibia on the femur is known clinically as "cranial drawer movement."

When the entire caudal cruciate is ruptured, a caudal movement of the tibia (slight during extension, 2 mm) is marked during flexion of the genual articulation (8 mm). Caudal displacement of the tibia is termed "caudal drawer movement."

Medial rotation of the tibia is prevented primarily by both cranial and caudal cruciates as they twist against each other. Lateral rotation of the tibia is prevented primarily by the collateral ligaments.

The **TARSAL ARTICULATION** (Fig. 5.54) includes the **TARSOCRURAL** (1), **TARSOMETATARSAL** (2), and various intertarsal articulations. The fibrous membrane of the articular capsule extends distally from the distal end of the tibia and fibula to the proximal end of the metatarsal bones; between its proximal and distal extent, the fibrous tissue is fused to the superficial surface of the tarsal bones. Synovial membranes, attaching to the peripheral margins of articular cartilage, span the distance from one osseous element of the tarsal articulation to another. The synovial sac of the tarsocrural joint is continuous with that of the proximal intertarsal articulations forming a single articular cavity. The synovial cavities of the distal intertarsal and tarsometatarsal articulations also interconnect.

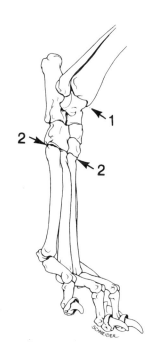

Fig.5.54. Right tarsal articulation, lateral view.

The distal epiphyses of the tibia and fibula are fused to their respective diaphyses in dogs 11 months of age (Fig. 5.55). Most of the tarsal bones develop ossification centers postnatally; a secondary ossification center develops in the tuber calcanei.

Ossification is complete in the calcaneus by 7 months of age. The diaphyses of the metatarsal and phalangeal bones are ossified at birth. The distal ends of the metatarsal bones (heads) and the proximal ends of the phalanges (bases) develop ossification centers by 6 weeks and ossify to the diaphyses by the time the dog is 9 months old.

Trauma of the tarsal bones frequently includes fracture of the talus and central tarsal bone and epiphyseal separation of the tuber calcanei. Fracture of the central tarsal bone often occurs in racing Greyhounds.

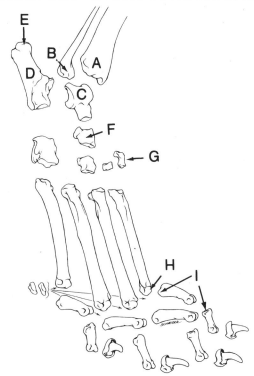

Fig.5.55. Ossification of bones forming the pes.

OSSEOUS ELEMENT – TARSUS

POSTNATAL STATUS	TIBIA DISTAL EPIPHYSIS	FIBULA DISTAL EPIPHYSIS	TALUS	CALCANEUS	TUBER CALCANEUS	CENTRAL TARSAL	TARSAL I-IV	METAATARSUS HEADS	PHALANGES BASES
	A	B	C	D	E	F	G	H	I
CLOSURE OF PHYSES (MONTHS)	3	6	1	1	8	5	3-7	4	6
	11	9	–	–	7	–	–	9	7

Chapter 6

HEAD

Objectives: Be able to identify structural features of bones, muscles, and joints in radiographs and dissected specimens, and be able to locate their positions in the intact animal.

Regions: Facial and Cranial

Surfaces, Margins, Prominences, Foramina, etc. of bones of the skull including those of the **Occipital, Parietal, Frontal, Temporal, Sphenoid, Ethmoid, Pterygoid, Vomer, Nasal, Maxillary, Incisive, Palatine, Lacrimal, and Zygomatic Bones, and Ventral Nasal Concha, Hyoid Apparatus, and Mandible**

Muscles of the Head including: Platysma, Orbicularis Oris, Orbicularis Oculi, Zygomaticus, Buccinator, Levator Nasolabialis, Masseter, Temporalis, Medial and Lateral Pterygoid, Digastricus, Mylohyoideus, Thyrohyoideus, Geniohyoideus, Genioglossus, Hyoglossus, Styloglossus, and the rostral, dorsal, and caudal Auricular Muscle groups

Temporomandibular and Intermandibular articulations, Auricular, Annular, and Scutiform Cartilages; Angle of Mouth; Palpebral Fissure

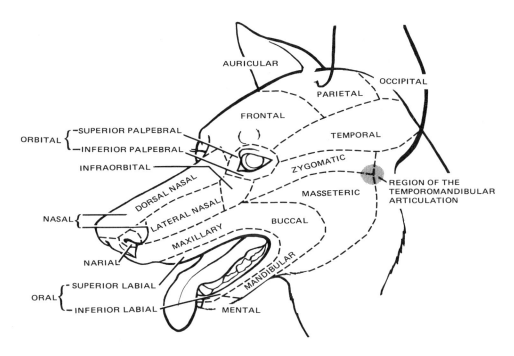

Fig.6.1. Regions of the face and cranium.

The **FACIAL REGION**, which overlies the bones that make up the face, is subdivided into 13 regions (Fig. 6.1): nasal, oral, mental, buccal, orbital, infraorbital, temporomandibular articulation, masseteric, maxillary, mandibular, zygomatic, intermandibular, and subhyoid.

The **NASAL REGION** overlies the nasal cavity and is subdivided into **NARIAL** and **DORSAL** and **LATERAL NASAL REGIONS**. The region of the **NARIS** is the surface area around the external opening into the nasal cavity. The **ORAL REGION** is subdivided into **SUPERIOR** and **INFERIOR LABIAL REGIONS**. The **MENTAL REGION** is the surface over the chin. The **BUCCAL REGION** refers to the cheek, which it overlies. The **ORBITAL REGION** is the area superficial to the bony socket that protects the eye; the **SUPERIOR** and **INFERIOR PALPEBRAL REGIONS** are subdivisions of the orbital region. Beneath and rostral to the orbit is the **INFRAORBITAL REGION**, named after the bony canal and foramen deep to the surface.

The joint between the lower jaw and the skull lies deep to the **REGION OF THE TEMPOROMANDIBULAR ARTICULATION**. The **MASSETERIC** (mass " e-ter' ik) **REGION** is superficial to the masseter muscle, a muscle of mastication. The **MAXILLARY** and **MANDIBULAR REGIONS** are superficial to facial bones with the same names. The **ZYGOMATIC REGION** overlies the zygomatic bone and zygomatic salivary gland. The ventral facial subregion, between right and left mandibles, is the **INTERMANDIBULAR REGION**. The **SUBHYOID REGION**, situated between intermandibular and laryngeal regions, is superficial to the hyoid apparatus and root of the tongue.

The **CRANIAL REGION**, superficial to the cranial bones that encase the brain, is subdivided into **OCCIPITAL, PARIETAL, TEMPORAL, AURICULAR,** and **FRONTAL REGIONS**. The **SUPRAORBITAL FOSSA** is a depression in the

115

temporal region above and behind the eye; this fossa is not as pronounced in dogs as it is in larger domestic mammals.

BONES OF THE HEAD

The **SKULL**, a bony case, houses the brain, inner ear, and the upper respiratory and digestive systems. It also partially encloses and protects the eye and larynx. The skull will be described prior to considering the soft structures of the head. Dentition is discussed with the remainder of the digestive system (pp. 207–09); foramina of the skull are described more fully in the chapters on the vessels and nerves of the head (see Chaps. 20, 26). The skull may be divided into cranial and facial bones, which provide support and protection for the brain and face, respectively.

The **CRANIUM** (Fig. 6.2) is composed of the following bones: occipital (1), parietal (2), frontal (3), temporal (4), pterygoid (ter' i-goid; winglike) (5), basisphenoid (6), presphenoid (7), ethmoid (8), and vomer.

The ossification of frontal and parietal bones may not yet be completed in a young puppy; thus this area may be soft and nonradiopaque.

Such osseous gaps between bones of the cranium are called **FONTANELLES** (fon " tah-nelz'). A fontanelle (1, Fig. 6.3) will also normally be observed in the adult Chihuahua where ossification of these bones is not complete.

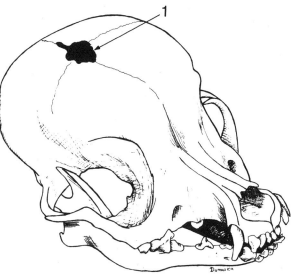

Fig.6.3. Fontanelle of a mature Chihuahua.

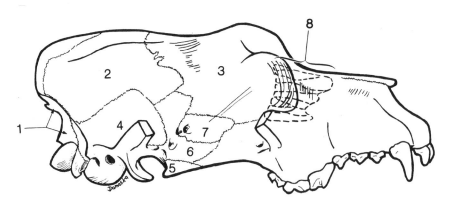

Fig.6.2. Right cranial bones.

The following external openings and prominences should be identified in the **OCCIPITAL BONE** (Fig. 6.4): the **FORAMEN MAGNUM** (1), the osseous border of which encircles the spinal cord; the paired **OCCIPITAL CONDYLES** (2), which articulate with the 1st cervical vertebra; the **NUCHAL** (nu' kal) **CREST** (3), which provides for attachment of certain neck muscles; the **EXTERNAL OCCIPITAL PROTUBERANCE** (4), which is the dorsocaudal prominence with which right and left nuchal crests merge; the **INTERPARIETAL PROCESS** (5), positioned dorsomedially, which arises as a separate bone and fuses prenatally with the occipital bone; and the bilateral **JUGULAR PROCESSES** (6), which provide for attachment of several muscles, one of which (the digastricus) functions to open the jaw.

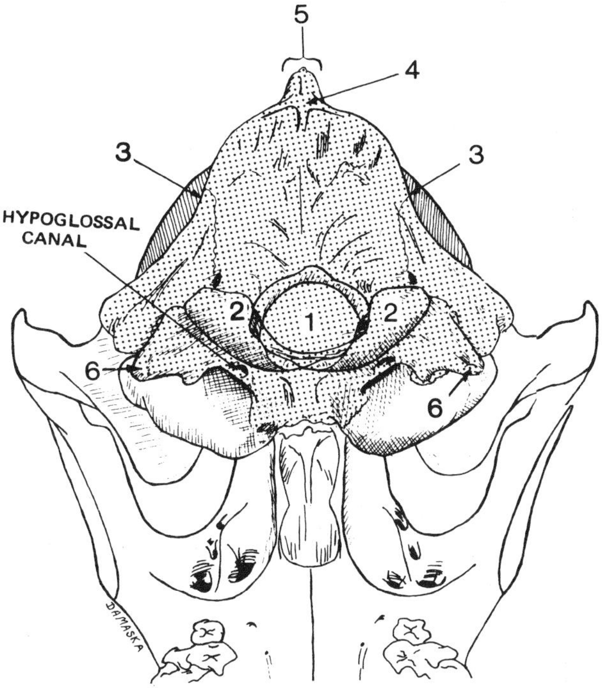

On the internal surface of the occipital bone, the **TENTORIUM PROCESS** (1, Fig. 6.5) projects rostroventrally into the cranial cavity from the dorsocaudal osseous wall.

Fig. 6.4. Occipital bone, caudoventral view.

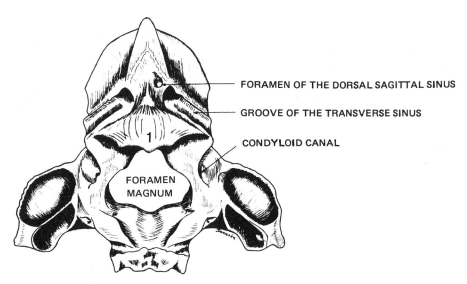

Fig. 6.5. Internal surface of occipital bone, rostral view.

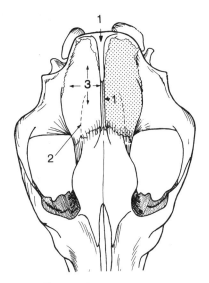

Fig.6.6. Parietal bones.

The **PARIETAL BONE** forms much of the dorsal and lateral walls of the cranium (Fig. 6.6). The **EXTERNAL SAGITTAL CREST** (1), as a dorsal median spine, is continuous in many dogs from the external occipital protuberance (caudally) to the frontal bones (rostrally).

Brachycephalic breeds, dogs with dome-shaped cranial vaults, and young dogs with weakly developed jaw muscles may have paired **TEMPORAL LINES** (2) in place of the external

sagittal crest. The **TEMPORAL SURFACE** (3) is a convex surface that serves as the area of origin for the temporalis muscle; the temporal and frontal bones (to be described later) also provide a portion of the temporal surface and temporal line. Intracranially, the parietal bone forms a

portion of the bony tentorium process, which projects rostroventrally between the cerebrum and cerebellum.

Much of the **FRONTAL BONE** (Fig. 6.7) is separated into a superficial (1) and a deep (2) bony layer by an air space termed the **FRONTAL SINUS** (3). The air-filled cavity of the frontal sinus, like all paranasal sinuses, opens into that of the nasal cavity.

The **ZYGOMATIC PROCESS OF THE FRONTAL BONE** (4) is a ventrolaterally projecting process from the external surface of the frontal bone.

The **TEMPORAL BONE** forms much of the caudolateral portion of the skull (Figs. 6.8, 6.9). The **ZYGOMATIC PROCESS OF THE TEMPORAL BONE** (1) forms a protective cover for more deeply situated nerves and vessels and provides an area of origin for the masseter muscle. The ventral proximal portion of the zygomatic process of the temporal bone has a concave **MANDIBULAR FOSSA** (2), a surface that articulates with the mandible. The large, rostroventrally directed **RETROARTICULAR PROCESS OF THE TEMPORAL BONE** (3) forms much of the articular surface.

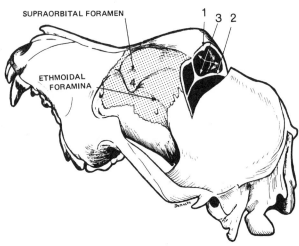

Fig.6.7. Frontal bones.

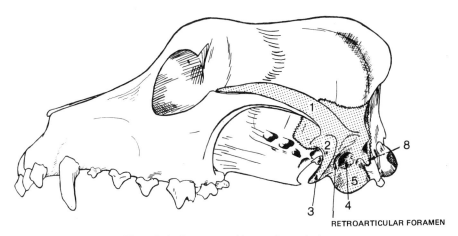

Fig.6.8. Left temporal bone, lateral view.

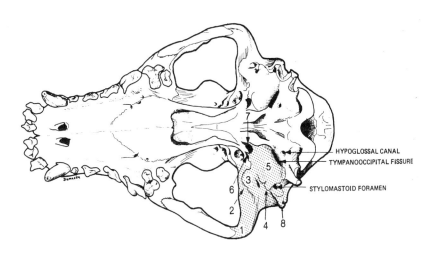

Fig.6.9. Right temporal bone, ventral view.

The **EXTERNAL ACOUSTIC MEATUS** (4) is the large opening immediately caudal to the retroarticular process; sound waves are transmitted through the external acoustic meatus to the middle ear.

The **TYMPANIC BULLA** (bul' ah, pl. bullae) (5), a rounded prominence situated between the retroarticular and jugular processes, contains the middle ear cavity.

The **MUSCULOTUBAL CANAL** (6, Fig. 6.9) is separated from the larger, more medial **CAROTID CANAL** (7) by a slender, bony

septum. The musculotubal canal contains the tendon of a tensor muscle and the **AUDITORY** (**Eustachian**) **TUBE**, which functions to allow air to pass between the pharynx and middle ear equalizing air pressure on each side of the ear drum.

The **MASTOID PROCESS** (8) is a blunt eminence dorsolateral to the tympanic bulla and rostrodorsal to the jugular process. It provides a point of attachment for the hyoid apparatus and the sternomastoideus, cleidomastoideus, and splenius muscles.

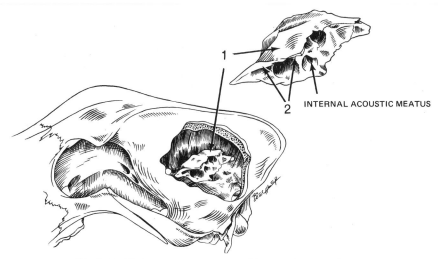

Fig.6.10. Right petrous temporal bone, deep surface.

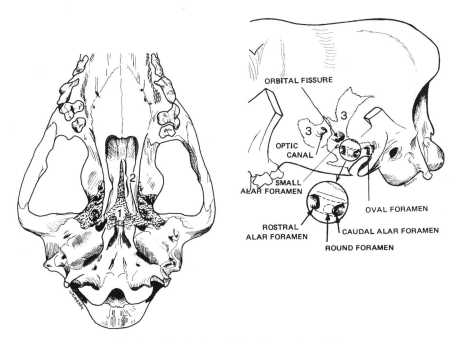

Fig. 6.11. Basisphenoid and presphenoid.

On the internal surface of the skull (Fig. 6.10) the **PETROUS** (pet' rus; rocklike) **PORTION OF THE TEMPORAL BONE** (1) projects into the cranial cavity, partially separating the cerebrum from the cerebellum. The **PETROSAL CREST** (2) is continuous with the tentorium process of the occipital and parietal bones.

The **BASISPHENOID** and **PRESPHENOID BONES** (Fig. 6.11) each consist of a body and two wings (alae). The body of the basisphenoid (1) and the body of the presphenoid (2) form much of the ventral floor of the cranium. The external surface of the wings of the sphenoid bones (3) contain a number of important foramina through which nerves and vessels pass.

120

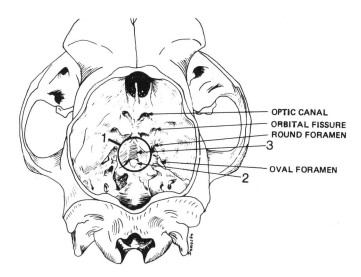

OPTIC CANAL
ORBITAL FISSURE
ROUND FORAMEN

OVAL FORAMEN

Fig.6.12. Deep surface of the sphenoid bone.

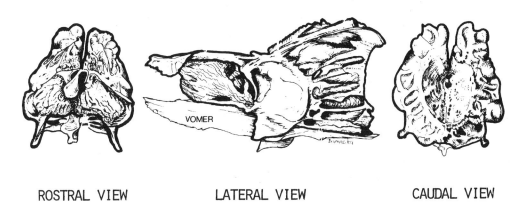

VOMER

ROSTRAL VIEW   LATERAL VIEW   CAUDAL VIEW

Fig.6.13. Ethmoid bone.

The **SELLA TURCICA** (sel' ah tur' sik-ah; Turkish saddle) (1, Fig. 6.12) is on the internal surface of the basisphenoid; it forms an osseous cradle for the hypophysis (pituitary). The **DORSUM SELLAE** (2) is a bony projection forming the caudal part of the cradle; the **HYPOPHYSEAL FOSSA** (3) is the depression that supports the hypophysis.

The **ETHMOID BONE** (Fig. 6.13) is a complex structure situated deep within the skull between the nasal and cranial cavities. It is discussed with the respiratory system.

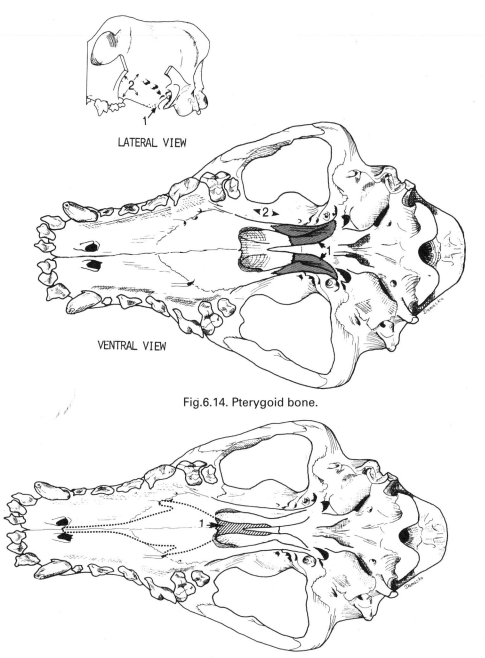

LATERAL VIEW

VENTRAL VIEW

Fig.6.14. Pterygoid bone.

Fig.6.15. Vomer, ventral view.

The **PTERYGOID BONE** (1, Fig. 6.14), which forms part of the lateral wall of the air passageway dorsal to the soft palate, also serves as a point of origin for the medial pterygoid muscle, a muscle of mastication. Portions of a number of important nerves and vessels are present laterally, adjacent to the palatine bone; this area containing muscle, nerves, and vessels is termed the **PTERYGOPALATINE FOSSA** (2).

The **VOMER** (1, Fig. 6.15) may be observed on the ventral surface of the skull, where it forms part of the dorsal wall of the nasopharyngeal meatus, and within the nasal cavity (dotted lines), where it forms a median U-shaped trough. A ventral extension from the vomer partially divides the air passage near the caudal portion of the hard palate.

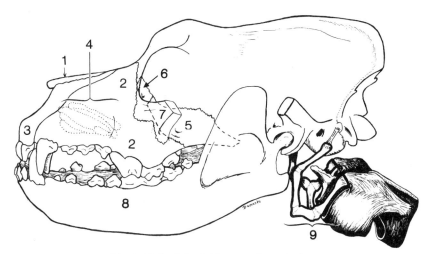

Fig.6.16. Left facial bones, lateral view.

Bones of the face (Fig. 6.16) are nasal (1), maxilla (2), incisive (3), ventral nasal concha (kong' kah, pl. conchae; shell) (4), palatine (5), lacrimal (6), zygomatic (7), mandibles (8), and the hyoid apparatus (9). The zygomatic bone and zygomatic process of the temporal bone form much of the **ZYGOMATIC ARCH.**Nasal, ventral nasal concha, lacrimal,and zygomatic bones will not be discussed further.

The **MAXILLA** (1, Figs. 6.17, 6.18) forms a major part of the hard palate and osseous lateral walls of the nasal cavity. The **LACRIMAL CANAL** is a tunnel through the maxillary bone extending from the **FOSSA OF THE LACRIMAL SAC** (in the lacrimal bone) to the nasal cavity; the nasolacrimal duct, which conveys lacrimal fluid or tears from the surface of the eye to the nose, is partially situated within the lacrimal canal (see p. 17).

The **INCISIVE BONE** (2, Figs. 6.17, 6.18) supports the six upper incisors and contributes to the formation of the **PALATINE FISSURE** (3, Fig. 6.17).

The **PALATINE BONE** (4, Fig. 6.17; 3, Fig. 6.18) forms part of the hard palate and pterygopalatine fossa.

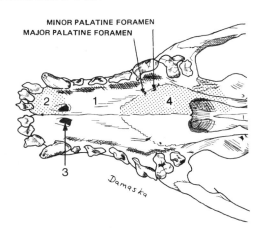

Fig.6.17. Incisive, maxillary and palatine bones, ventral view.

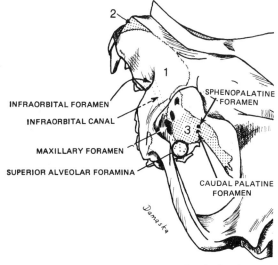

Fig.6.18. Incisive, maxillary, and palatine bones, caudolateral view.

123

Each **MANDIBLE** (Fig. 6.19) bears three processes on its proximal part: the coronoid process (1), the condylar process (2), and the angular process (3). The **CONDYLAR PROCESS** articulates with the mandibular fossa of the temporal bone at the **TEMPORO-MANDIBULAR ARTICULATION** (4).

The **CORONOID PROCESS** of the mandible, positioned between the zygomatic arch and the medial osseous wall of the orbit, provides a surface area for insertion by the powerful temporalis muscle.

The **ANGULAR PROCESS** forming the caudoventral portion of the mandible provides a point of insertion for another muscle of mastication, the masseter. The depression on the lateral surface of the mandible near the base of the coronoid process is the **MASSETERIC FOSSA** (5), which serves as an area of insertion for the masseteric muscle.

The **INTERMANDIBULAR ARTICULATION** (Fig. 6.20), between right and left mandibles, is formed by cartilaginous and fibrous connective tissue.

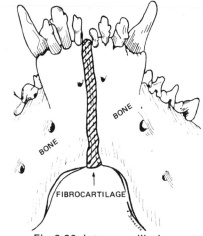

Fig.6.20. Intermandibular articulation.

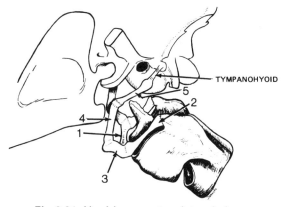

Fig.6.21. Hyoid apparatus, lateral view.

The **HYOID APPARATUS** (Fig. 6.21) is composed of a number of bones that articulate at one point with the mastoid process of the skull, at another point with the larynx, and third by means of connective tissue with the tongue.

The individual bones of the hyoid apparatus are a single **BASIHYOID** (1) and on each side a **THYROHYOID** (2), a **CERATOHYOID** (ser' ah-to-hioid) (3), an **EPIHYOID** (4), and a **STYLOHYOID** (5). The **TYMPANOHYOID** is usually cartilaginous, as may be a number of the other hyoid components in young animals.

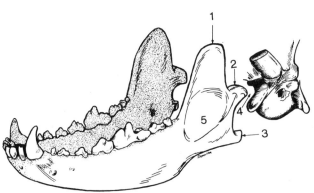

Fig.6.19. Mandibles, dorsolateral view.

MUSCLES OF THE HEAD

The muscles of facial expression function to move the lips, nasal alae, and the ears. Muscles of the face include the platysma; zygomaticus; orbicularis oris; buccinator; levator nasolabialis; orbicularis oculi; and rostral, dorsal, caudal, and ventral groups of auricular muscles.

The **PLATYSMA** (plah-tiz' mah) (1, Fig. 6.22) is a cutaneous muscle that passes from the middorsal **RAPHE** (ra' fe; seam) of the neck, across the parotid and masseteric regions, to the angle of the mouth, where it radiates into the **ORBICULARIS ORIS MUSCLE** (2). The platysma, which acts to pull the commissure of the lips cranially, is a superficial muscle covering the ventrolateral surface of the head.

The **ZYGOMATICUS MUSCLE** (1, Fig. 6.23) extends cranioventrally from the **SCUTIFORM** (sku ti-form; shield) **CARTILAGE** (2) of the ear to the caudal edge of the superior lip, where its fibers radiate into the orbicularis oris muscle (3). The scutiform cartilage is a small, flat cartilage interposed in the rostral auricular muscle group, rostromedial to and separate from the cartilage of the external ear. The orbicularis oris is a superficial muscle, the fibers of which are situated between the skin of the outer surface of the lips and the mucous membrane of the inner surface of the lips.

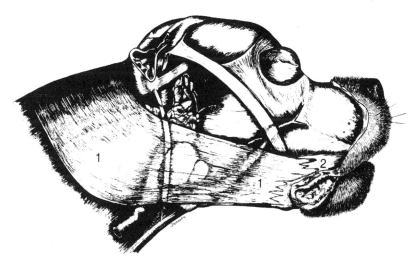

Fig.6.22. Superficial facial muscles, right lateral view.

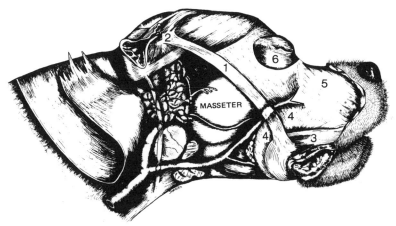

Fig.6.23. Facial muscles, right lateral view.

125

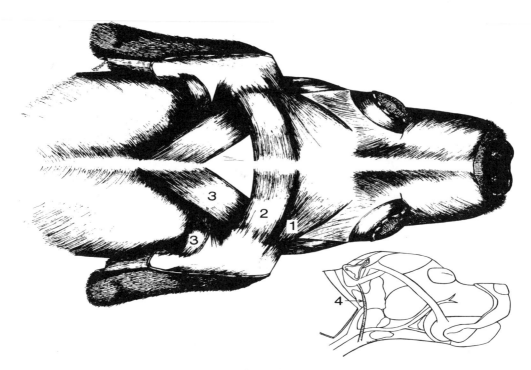

Fig.6.24. Auricular muscles.

As the orbicularis oris extends from the superior lip to the inferior lip around the **ANGLE OF THE MOUTH**, its purse-string action results in a closing of the lips.

Fibers of the orbicularis oris muscle intermingle with the larger and more deeply situated **BUCCINATOR MUSCLE** (4). The buccinator muscle lies deep to the zygomaticus muscle and between the rostral margin of the masseter muscle and the caudal margin of the orbicularis oris muscle. It functions to make the cheek taut.

The **LEVATOR NASOLABIALIS** (5) is a flat muscle that arises from the frontal region between the eyes and inserts on the superior lip and nasal ala; it elevates the superior lip and dilates the nostril.

The **ORBICULARIS OCULI** (6) is composed of a group of muscle fibers that encircle the eye, situated partially within the eyelids. Contraction of the orbicularis oculi closes the **PALPEBRAL FISSURE** (space between the free margins of the eyelids).

The muscles that move the external ear (Fig. 6.24) are divided into four groups: rostral, dorsal, caudal, and ventral auricular.

The **ROSTRAL AURICULAR MUSCLES** (1) arise from the forehead, rostromedial to the ear, and insert on the cartilaginous skeleton of the external ear.

The **DORSAL AURICULAR MUSCLES** (2) extend from the medial raphe of the caudal half of the head to insert on the cartilaginous skeleton of the external ear.

The **CAUDAL AURICULAR MUSCLES** (3) are a group of muscles that extend from the dorsum of the neck to the cartilaginous skeleton of the ear.

The small **PAROTIDOAURICULAR MUSCLE** (4) is the larger of two **VENTRAL AURICULAR MUSCLES**.

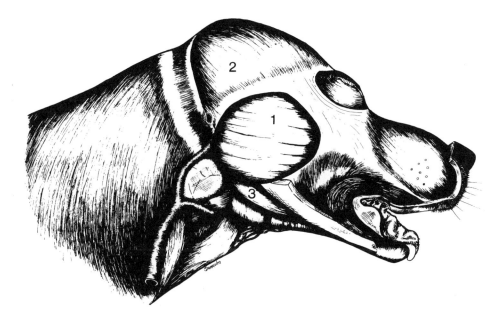

Fig.6.25. Muscles of mastication, right lateral view.

Muscles of mastication (Fig. 6.25) include the orbicularis oris, buccinator, masseter (mas-se' ter) (1), temporalis (2), medial pterygoid, lateral pterygoid, and digastricus (di-gas " trik' us; two bellies) (3). The orbiculars oris and buccinator muscles keep food within the oral cavity by means of their purse-string action.

The **MASSETER MUSCLE**—a large muscular mass located ventral to the zygomatic arch, rostral to the parotid salivary gland, and caudal to the facial vein—arises from the zygomatic arch and inserts in the masseteric fossa on the lateral surface of the mandible.

The **TEMPORALIS** is a thick muscle located between the sagittal crest of the skull (dorsally) and the zygomatic process of the frontal bone (rostrally). Deep to the rostral, dorsal, and caudal auricular muscles, the temporalis muscle arises from the temporal fossa of the skull and inserts on the medial surface of the coronoid process of the mandible. Both the temporalis and

the masseter muscles, the fibers of which intermingle at the zygomatic arch, act to close the mouth by elevating the lower jaw.

Deep to the zygomatic arch and the coronoid process of the mandible, the **MEDIAL PTERYGOID MUSCLE** (1, Fig. 6.26), covered with glistening deep fascia, is observed deep and medial to a number of vessels and nerves that course through the pterygopalatine fossa. The medial pterygoid muscle arises from the pterygopalatine fossa and inserts on the medial surface of the mandible, ventral to the area of insertion by the temporalis muscle.

The **LATERAL PTERYGOID MUSCLE** (2), which is smaller than the medial pterygoid, arises from the sphenoid bone and passes caudolaterally to insert on the medial surface of the mandibular condyle. Both the medial and lateral pterygoid muscles aid the masseter and temporalis muscles in closing the jaw.

127

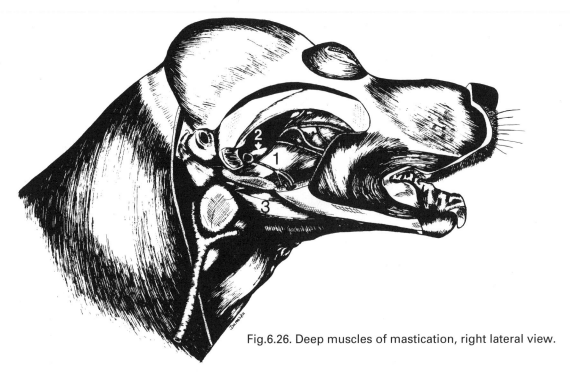

Fig.6.26. Deep muscles of mastication, right lateral view.

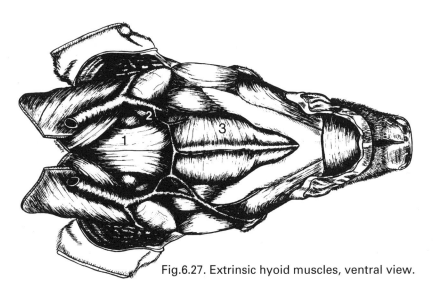

Fig.6.27. Extrinsic hyoid muscles, ventral view.

bones, pharynx, and esophagus. These structures are discussed in chapters covering the upper respiratory and digestive organs.

Extrinsic muscles of the hyoid apparatus (Fig. 6.27) include the sternohyoideus (1), thyrohyoideus (2), mylohyoideus (3), and geniohyoideus. The sternohyoideus and sternothyroideus muscles are also described with the muscles of the neck.

The **DIGASTRICUS MUSCLE** (3), which is located along the caudoventral surface of the mandible, arises from the jugular process of the occipital bone and inserts on the caudoventral portion of the body of the mandible. The digastricus functions to open the jaw.

Deglutition (swallowing) is a complex action involving the tongue, soft palate, larynx, hyoid

The **MYLOHYOIDEUS MUSCLE** is a thin sheet of transversely directed fibers situated superficially between the body of the right and left mandibles. The fibers of the mylohyoideus muscle arise from the medial surface of the body

128

of the mandible and insert on the contralateral muscle in the midline between the mandibles; the paired muscle thus forms a sling ventral to the tongue. A small vein (submental) courses rostrally from the venous hyoid arch along the raphe of the mylohyoideus muscle.

The **STERNOHYOIDEUS** (1, Fig. 6.28) and **THYROHYOIDEUS MUSCLES** exert a caudally directed force on the hyoid apparatus. The paired **GENIOHYOIDEUS** (3) is a straplike muscle, deep (dorsal) to the mylohyoideus (4),

that extends from the hyoid bone to the mandibular symphysis.

The extrinsic muscles of the tongue (Fig. 6.29) include the styloglossus (1), the hyoglossus (2), and the genioglossus (3). The fibers of the paired **GENIOGLOSSUS** (glossa: glos' ah; tongue) **MUSCLE** pass from the medial surface of the mandible (caudodorsally) into the body and root of the tongue, forming an inverted V-shaped mass dorsal to the geniohyoideus.

The **HYOGLOSSUS MUSCLE** passes from the hyoid bone into the body of the tongue, lateral to the caudodorsal extent of the genioglossus and dorsal to the mylohyoideus.

The **STYLOGLOSSUS** is a straplike muscle extending from the stylohyoid bone to the body of the tongue; it is located lateral to the distal end of the hyoglossus muscle and medial to the body of the mandible.

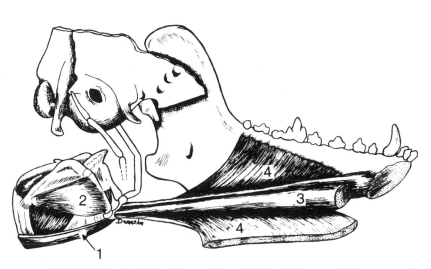

Fig.6.28. Extrinsic hyoid muscles with the right mandible removed, right lateral view.

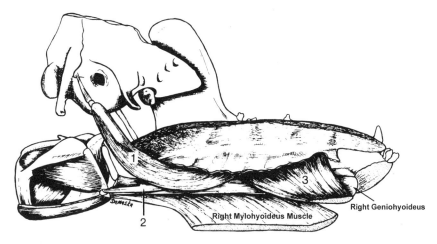

Fig.6.29. Extrinsic tongue muscles, with the right mandible removed, right lateral view.

Chapter 7
TRUNK

Objectives: Be able to identify structural features of bones, muscles, and joints in radiographs and dissected specimens, and be able to locate their positions in the intact animal.

Regions: Cervical, Pectoral, Abdominal, Dorsal, and Pelvic

Surfaces, Margins, Prominences, Foramina etc., of Vertebrae, Sternebrae, and Ribs

Sternocephalicus Muscles

Epaxial Muscles: Serratus Dorsalis, Splenius, Iliocostalis, Longissimus, Spinalis, Semispinalis, Multifidi, Rotator Muscles, Interspinalis, and Rectus Capitus Dorsalis Muscles

Hypaxial Muscles: Rectus Capitus Ventralis, Longus Capitis, Longus Colli, Psoas Minor, Quadratus Lumborum, Psoas Major, Iliopsoas, Sacrocaudalis Ventralis, Scalenus, External and Internal Intercostals, Levator Costarum, External and Internal Abdominal Obliques, Cremaster, Transversus Thoracis and Transversus Abdominis Muscles, Sternohyoideus, Sternothyroideus, Rectus Thoracis and Rectus Abdominis

Linea Alba, Inguinal Arch, Superficial Inguinal Ring, Umbilicus

Joints, Ligaments, and Disks: Atlantooccipital, Atlantoaxial, Intervertebral Symphyses, Costal Head and Costotransverse Articulations, Sacroiliac Articulation, and Sternocostal Articulation; Intervertebral Disks; Intercapital, Nuchal, Supraspinous, Dorsal Longitudinal, and Ventral Longitudinal Ligaments; Ligamenta Flava

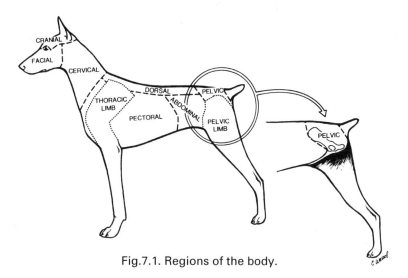

Fig.7.1. Regions of the body.

The trunk is a general term for that portion of the body not including the head or limbs. The surface of the trunk is divided into cervical, pectoral, abdominal, dorsal, and pelvic regions (Fig. 7.1).

The **CERVICAL REGION** is subdivided into parotid, dorsal cervical, lateral cervical, and ventral cervical regions (Fig. 7.2). The **PAROTID REGION** is the area ventral to the base of the ear that is superficial to the parotid salivary gland. The **DORSAL CERVICAL REGION** is dorsal to the cervical vertebrae. The **LATERAL**

CERVICAL REGIONS form the lateral surfaces of the neck.

The **VENTRAL CERVICAL REGION** is again subdivided into **LARYNGEAL** and **TRACHEAL REGIONS**. The external jugular vein separates the lateral and ventral cervical regions. The **JUGULAR FOSSAE** are depressions on each side of the base of the neck where right and left external jugular veins course deep to enter the thorax.

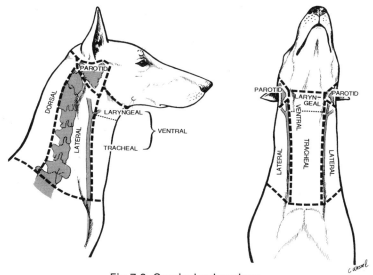

Fig.7.2. Cervical subregions.

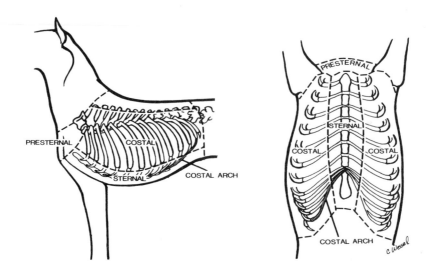

Fig.7.3. Pectoral subregions.

The **PECTORAL REGION** is composed of **PRESTERNAL, STERNAL,** and **COSTAL REGIONS** (Fig. 7.3). The sternal and costal regions are named according to location of the underlying sternum and ribs, respectively. The **CARDIAC REGION** is a subregion superficial to the heart. The **COSTAL ARCHES,** one on each side of the animal, are arches formed by cartilage of three of the most caudal four pairs of ribs.

The **ABDOMINAL REGION** is divided into nine regions by two transverse and two sagittal lines on the surface of the abdomen as a result of imaginary planes passed through the abdomen.

CRANIAL, MIDDLE, and **CAUDAL ABDOMINAL REGIONS** are formed by two transverse planes passing through the trunk; one transverse plane passes through the caudal border of the costal arch and the other passes through the cranial border of the hip bones (Fig. 7.4).

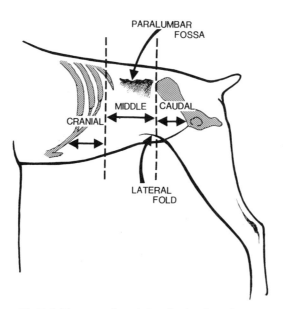

Fig.7.4. Three major abdominal subregions.

The cranial, middle, and caudal abdominal regions are each subdivided into three smaller regions by passing two sagittal planes through the trunk (Fig. 7.5); the sagittal planes, one on each side of the ventral median line, are located approximately half way between the median plane and the lateral surface of the animal.

The cranial abdominal region is thus divided into **RIGHT** and **LEFT HYPOCHONDRIAC** (under cartilage) **REGIONS** and a **XIPHOID** (zif' oid; swordlike) **REGION**.

The middle abdominal region is subdivided into **RIGHT** and **LEFT LATERAL ABDOMINAL REGIONS** and a midventral **UMBILICAL REGION**. In thin animals, a depression may be observed in the dorsal portion of the lateral regions termed the **PARALUMBAR FOSSA**. A fold of skin connects the thigh (cranially) with the abdomen; this **LATERAL FOLD** occurs in each lateral abdominal region.

The caudal abdominal region is subdivided by the sagittal planes into **RIGHT** and **LEFT INGUINAL REGIONS** and a midventral **PUBIC REGION**. The **PREPUTIAL REGION**, or area of the sheath of the penis, is a subregion of the male pubic region.

The **DORSAL REGION** is the area dorsal and superficial to the trunk vertebrae; it is subdivided into a **THORACIC VERTEBRAL REGION** and a **LUMBAR** (loin) **REGION** (Fig. 7.6).

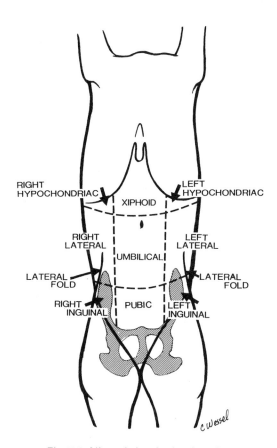

Fig.7.5. Nine abdominal subregions.

The portion of the thoracic vertebral region between the dorsal borders of the scapulae is the **INTERSCAPULAR REGION**; it is the most dorsal portion of the back.

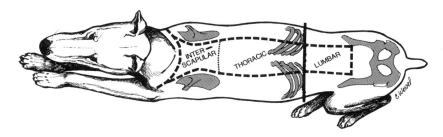

Fig.7.6. Dorsal subregions.

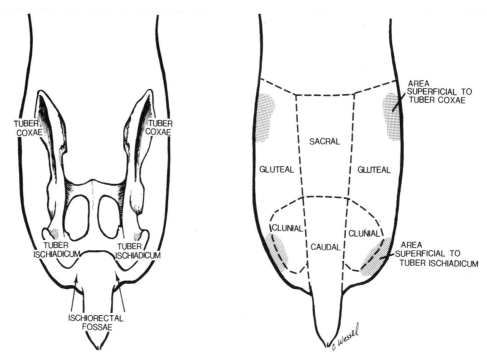

Fig.7.7. Pelvic subregions.

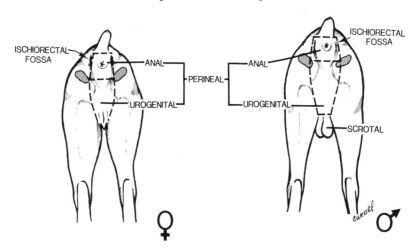

Fig.7.8. Perineal subregions.

The **PELVIC REGION** is subdivided into sacral, caudal, gluteal, clunial, tuber coxae, tuber ischiadicum, perineal, and scrotal or supramammary entities (Figs. 7.7, 7.8).

The **SACRAL, CAUDAL,** and **GLUTEAL REGIONS** overlie the sacral and caudal vertebrae and gluteal muscle groups, respectively. The **CLUNIAL** (kloo' ne-al;

buttocks) **REGION** is the area dorsal to the caudal extent of the pelvis. A depression in the clunial region, the **ISCHIORECTAL** (is' ke-o-rek' tal) **FOSSA,** may be observed in gaunt animals.

The regions of the **TUBER COXAE** and **TUBER ISCHIADICUM,** which are superficial to osseous enlargements of the bony pelvis, are located cranial and caudal to the hip joint, respectively.

The **PERINEAL** (per" i- ne' al) **REGION** extends ventrally from the base of the tail to the caudal attachment of the scrotum in the dog or to the ventral margin of the external genitalia in the bitch. The perineal region is subdivided into **ANAL** (dorsally) and **UROGENITAL** (ventrally) **REGIONS** by a transverse line connecting the ischiatic tuber of each side. ln the dog the **SCROTAL REGION** extends from the

urogenital region (dorsally) to the pubic region (cranially); the corresponding region in the bitch is the **SUPRAMAMMARY REGION.**

The head, trunk, and tail are positioned along the long axis of the body; the bones providing support and protection for these parts are collectively termed the **AXIAL SKELETON** (Fig. 7.9). Skeletal muscles associated with the axial skeleton are termed **AXIAL MUSCLES.**

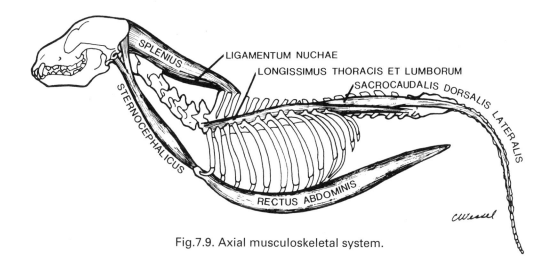

Fig.7.9. Axial musculoskeletal system.

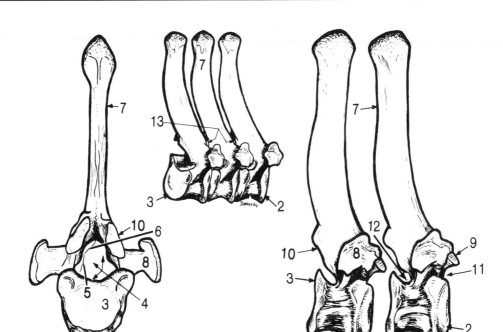

caudal view

lateral view

Fig.7.10. Vertebrae, structures in common.

BONES OF THE TRUNK

A **VERTEBRA** (pl. vertebrae) (Fig. 7.10)
typically is characterized by having a **BODY** (1);
a CRANIAL (2) and a CAUDAL (3)
EXTREMITY; a VERTEBRAL FORAMEN
(4), which forms one unit of the **VERTEBRAL
CANAL**; a VERTEBRAL ARCH, consisting of
ventral **PEDICLES** (5) and dorsal **LAMINAE**
(sing. lamina) (6); a **SPINOUS PROCESS** (7);
a pair of **TRANSVERSE PROCESSES** (8);
paired **CRANIAL** (9) and CAUDAL (10)
ARTICULAR PROCESSES; CRANIAL (11)
 and CAUDAL (12) **VERTEBRAL NOTCHES**
(each forms half of an **INTERVERTEBRAL
FORAMEN** when articulated with
adjacent vertebrae); and an
INTERARCUATE SPACE (13).

Cranial and caudal extremities begin to ossify 2
months postnatally and fuse with the body
between 7 and 10 months. Nutrient for

amina are usually present in the dorsal and
ventral surfaces of the vertebral bodies.

The presence of **7 CERVICAL VERTEBRAE**
(Fig. 7.11) is characteristic of most mammalian
species. The 1st (most cranial) cervical
vertebra is the **ATLAS** (1), which articulates
cranially with the occipital condyles and
caudally with the **AXIS** (2), or 2nd cervical
vertebra. The 7th cervical vertebra articulates
with the first (most cranial) thoracic vertebra
and with the head of the 1st pair of ribs.

TRANSVERSE FORAMINA (1, Fig. 7.12) are
present in the transverse processes of the
cranial six cervical vertebrae; blood vessels and
nerve fibers course along the vertebral column
through the transverse foramina.

The atlas (Fig. 7.13), lacking both a body and
spinous process, may be identified as a cervical
vertebra by the presence of transverse foramina

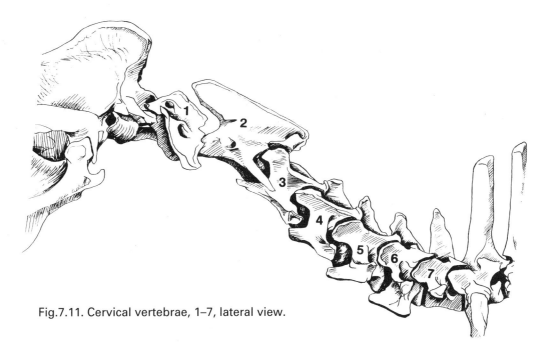

Fig.7.11. Cervical vertebrae, 1–7, lateral view.

(1). The transverse processes (2) are large lateral projections, which may be palpated in the live animal.

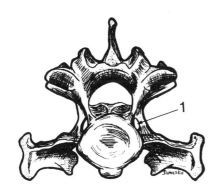

Fig.7.12. Transverse foramina of cervical vertebrae 1–6.

A second pair of foramina, the **LATERAL VERTEBRAL FORAMINA** (3), are present in the cranial portion of the dorsal vertebral arch; the first pair of spinal nerves pass out from the spinal cord through the lateral vertebral foramina (blood vessels pass through these foramina also). The typical vertebral body and extremities are not present in the atlas; instead, a **VENTRAL ARCH** (4) is present. The thickest portion of the atlas is its **LATERAL MASS** (5), which includes the transverse process, and the **CRANIAL** (6) and **CAUDAL** (7) **ARTICULAR FOVEAE**.

The cranial margin of the transverse process is notched, owing to the presence of blood vessels and a branch of the 1st spinal nerve; this notch is the **ALAR INCISURE** (8).

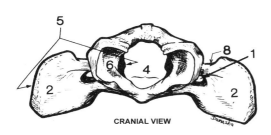

CRANIAL VIEW

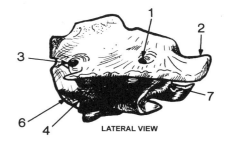

LATERAL VIEW

Fig.7.13. Atlas.

139

Small processes that project into the vertebral foramen provide attachment for a transverse ligament that divides the vertebral foramen into a dorsal and a ventral portion. The spinal cord occupies the dorsal portion; the ventral portion contains a tooth-shaped process of the 2nd cervical vertebra.

The axis (Fig. 7.14), the 2nd cervical vertebra, is also highly modified from the shape of a typical vertebra. The two most pronounced identifying features are the cranially extending **DENS** (1) and the well-developed elongated **SPINOUS PROCESS** (2). The spinous process

serves as a point of attachment for a number of neck muscles and for a strong ligament, the **LIGAMENTUM NUCHAE**. A transverse foramen (3) is located in the base of each slender transverse process (4).

Cervical vertebrae 3–5 are similar morphologically (Fig. 7.15). Each is characterized by the presence of transverse foramina (1), bifurcated transverse processes (2), and relatively small spinous processes (3).

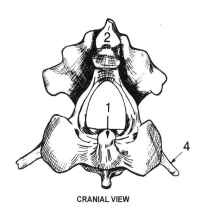

CRANIAL VIEW

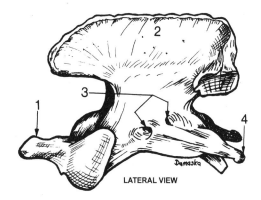

LATERAL VIEW

Fig.7.14. Axis.

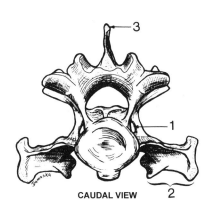

CAUDAL VIEW

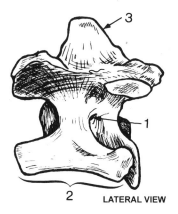

LATERAL VIEW

Fig.7.15. Cervical vertebrae 3–5.

The 6th cervical vertebra (Fig. 7.16) appears similar to cervical vertebrae 3–5 except for a pronounced extension of the bifurcated transverse processes (1).

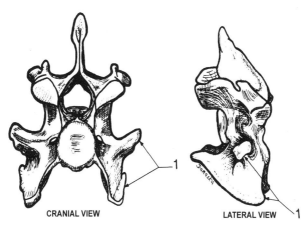

CRANIAL VIEW   LATERAL VIEW

Fig.7.16. Sixth cervical vertebra.

The 7th cervical vertebra (Fig. 7.17) has an elongated spinous process (1); bears **CAUDAL COSTAL FOVEAE** (2); and lacks transverse foramina. The caudal costal fovea provides part of the articular surface with the head of the 1st rib.

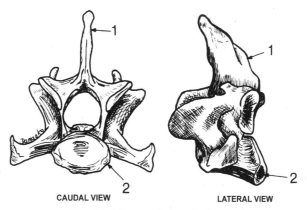

CAUDAL VIEW   LATERAL VIEW

Fig.7.17. Seventh cervical vertebra.

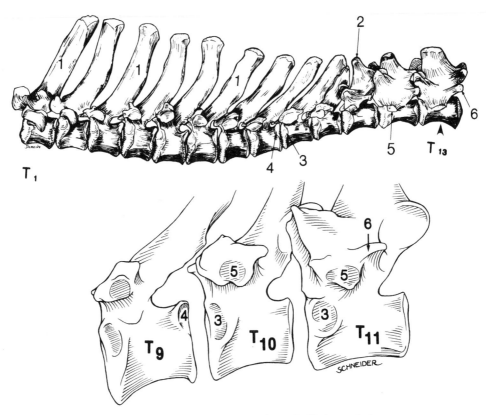

Fig.7.18. Thoracic vertebrae 1–13, lateral view.

Thirteen **THORACIC VERTEBRAE** (Fig. 7.18) are present in the dog. The first (cranial) 10 thoracic vertebrae have spinous processes (1) directed caudodorsally.

The thoracic vertebra with spinous process perpendicular to the long axis of the vertebral column, the **ANTICLINAL** (an" ti-klie' nal) **VERTEBRA** (2), is usually the 11th; spinous processes of the 12th and 13th thoracic vertebrae are directed craniodorsally.

Each side of the first 10 thoracic vertebrae bears two surfaces for articulating with the heads and one surface for articulating with the tubercles of ribs. The articular surfaces for the costal head are the **CRANIAL COSTAL FOVEA** (3) and the caudal costal fovea (4), present on the vertebral bodies.

The articular surface for each costal tubercle is the **COSTAL FOVEA OF THE TRANSVERSE PROCESS** (5), present on the lateral surface of each transverse process. The 11th, 12th, and 13th thoracic vertebrae usually have only two costal articular surfaces per side, the transverse (5) and cranial costal fovea (each rib, 11–13, articulates with only one vertebra).

Each of the 11th, 12th, and 13th thoracic vertebrae has an **ACCESSORY PROCESS** (6) on each side.

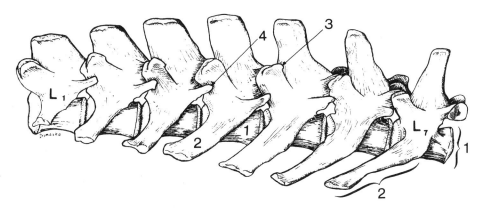

Fig.7.19. Lumbar vertebrae 1–7, lateral view.

The vertebral column of the dog contains seven **LUMBAR VERTEBRAE** (Fig. 7.19). A lumbar vertebra has a large body (1), long, cranioventrally directed transverse processes (2), and small **MAMILLARY PROCESSES** (3). Mamillary processes are also present on a number of thoracic vertebrae. Accessory processes (4) are also present on a number of lumbar vertebrae.

The **SACRAL BONE** (Fig. 7.20) is composed of three **SACRAL VERTEBRAE**, which fuse together within a few months postnatally.

The sacrum has **DORSAL** (1) and **PELVIC** (2) **SURFACES**, a **LATERAL PART** (3), a **BASE** (4), and an **APEX** (5). The dorsal surface bears a **MEDIAN SACRAL CREST** (6) of fused spinous processes and **DORSAL SACRAL FORAMINA** (7). The pelvic surface bears **VENTRAL SACRAL FORAMINA** (8) and a **PROMONTORY** (9). The promontory, present on the pelvic (ventral) surface of the sacral base, may create difficulties during parturition, particularly in dogs with dome-shaped crania.

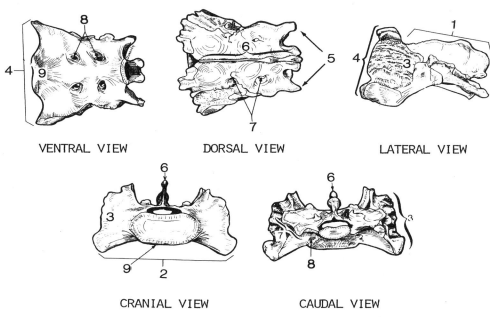

VENTRAL VIEW   DORSAL VIEW   LATERAL VIEW

CRANIAL VIEW   CAUDAL VIEW

Fig.7.20. Sacrum.

143

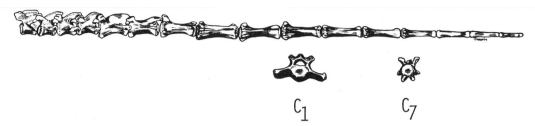

Fig.7.21. Caudal vertebrae.

CAUDAL VERTEBRAE (Fig. 7.21) vary in number and shape. A vertebral arch (and therefore a vertebral foramen and canal) is not present caudally past the 6th or 7th caudal vertebra.

Eight bones, or **STERNEBRAE**, and seven **INTERSTERNEBRAL CARTILAGE** segments form the **STERNUM** (Fig. 7.22). The sternebra situated farthest cranially is the **MANUBRIUM** (I); the following six sternebrae are termed the **BODY**, and the last sternebra is the **XIPHOID PROCESS** (2). **XIPHOID CARTILAGE** projects caudally from the xiphoid process.

There are 13 pairs of **RIBS** in the thorax (Fig. 7.23). The first (most cranial) 9 pairs of ribs are termed **STERNAL RIBS** (1) since they each attach directly to the sternum. The last 4 pairs of ribs are named **ASTERNAL RIBS** (2), although the ventral tips of the 10th, 11th, and 12th pairs

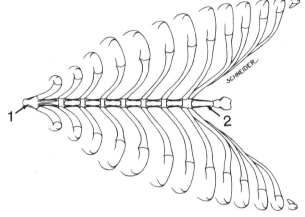

Fig.7.22. Sternum, ventral view.

of ribs attach to preceding ribs and thus to the sternum. Each rib is composed of **COSTAL BONE** (3) and **COSTAL CARTILAGE** (4). The costal cartilages of the 9th, 10th, 11th, and 12th ribs form the **COSTAL ARCH** (5). The ventral portion of the 13th rib is not attached to the preceding rib or sternum; thus it is often described as "floating."

The 1st costal cartilage articulates with the 1st sternal segment; the following eight costal cartilages articulate with cartilage between sternal segments, with the 8th and 9th costal cartilages sharing an intersternebral point of attachment.

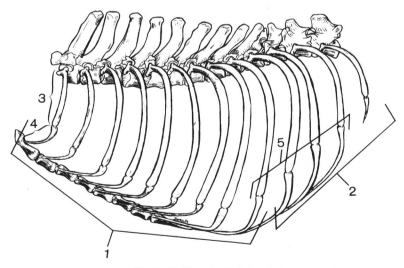

Fig.7.23. Ribs 1-13, lateral view.

144

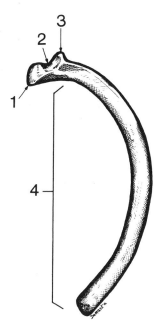

Fig.7.24. Costal bone.

MUSCLES OF THE TRUNK

Trunk muscles may be described as belonging in one of two major groups: epaxial or hypaxial muscles. **EPAXIAL MUSCLES** are those muscles dorsal to the long axis of the vertebral column; bilateral contraction of epaxial muscles results in extension of the vertebral column. **HYPAXIAL MUSCLES**, those muscles ventral to the long axis of the vertebral column, have a number of functions; however, most hypaxial muscles contribute to flexion of the vertebral column. Specialized muscles concerned with respiration, digestion, urination, and copulation are discussed later with the specific body systems concerned.

Each costal bone (Fig. 7.24) consists of a **HEAD** (1), **NECK** (2), **COSTAL TUBERCLE** (3), and **BODY** (4). The costal tubercles of all 13 pairs of ribs articulate with the transverse processes of thoracic vertebrae of corresponding number. The heads of the first 10 or 11 ribs articulate with surfaces on the caudal edge of the body of each preceding vertebra and on the cranial edge of the body of each correspondingly numbered vertebra.

The epaxial (extensor) group is composed of a number of complex muscles that are difficult to separate and identify. The epaxial muscles may be divided into the following divisions: splenius, erector spinae, transversospinalis, interspinalis, and intertransversarius muscles.

To observe the epaxial muscles in the cervical and thoracic regions, the **STERNO-CEPHALICUS MUSCLE** (1, Fig. 7.25), the pectoral limb, and the serratus dorsalis muscle need to removed. The sternocephalicus muscle has two parts, both of which arise from the

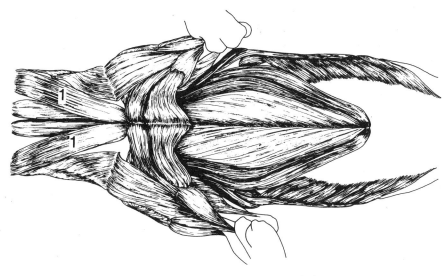

Fig.7.25. Sternocephalicus, ventral view.

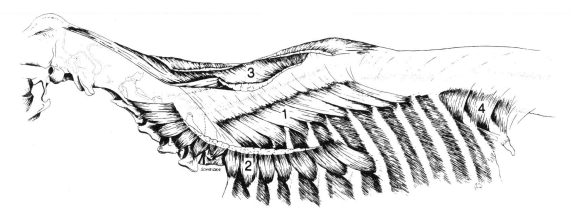

Fig.7.26. Muscles overlying the cranial portion of the epaxial muscle system.

manubrium of the sternum. A cranioventral part of the sternocephalicus muscle inserts on the mastoid process of the skull and a caudodorsal part inserts on the nuchal crest of the skull.

The **SERRATUS DORSALIS CRANIALIS MUSCLE** (1, Fig. 7.26), which is deep to the serratus ventralis (2) and rhomboideus (3) muscles, arises from the dorsal cervical raphe and the spinous processes of thoracic vertebrae; its fibers are directed caudoventrally to insert on ribs 2–10. The very small **SERRATUS DORSALIS CAUDALIS MUSCLE** (4) is oriented in a cranioventral direction from the thoracolumbar fascia to the last several ribs.

The **SPLENIUS CERVICIS** (1, Fig. 7.27) is a flat muscle that attaches caudally to the dorsal midline from the 1st cervical to the 3rd thoracic vertebrae and cranially to the nuchal crest. The three subdivisions that form the **ERECTOR SPINAE MUSCLE** are the iliocostalis, longissimus, and spinalis muscles, from ventrolateral to dorsomedial in position. The **ILIOCOSTALIS MUSCLE** is present as a series of short muscle fascicles occurring in the lumbar and thoracic regions as the **ILIOCOSTALIS LUMBORUM** (2) and **ILIOCOSTALIS**

THORACIS (3) **MUSCLES.** The iliocostalis lumborum muscle attaches caudally to the wing of the ilium and cranially to the last ribs. The iliocostalis thoracis muscle attaches ribs to ribs and to the transverse process of the last cervical vertebra.

The **LONGISSIMUS** (lon-jis' i-mus) **MUSCLE** (Fig. 7.27) is present as a series of short muscle fascicles, located dorsal to the iliocostalis system, that occur in the lumbar, thoracic, and cervical regions. The **LONGISSIMUS LUMBORUM MUSCLE** (4) extends from iliac crest and spinous processes of lumbar vertebrae (caudally) to the vertebral arch and accessory processes of lumbar vertebrae (cranially).

The **LONGISSIMUS THORACIS MUSCLE** (5) is a thoracic continuation of the longissimus that inserts on accessory and transverse vertebral processes and on ribs adjacent to the costal tubercles. The **LONGISSIMUS CERVICIS MUSCLE** (6), as a cervical continuation, inserts on the transverse processes of the last four cervical vertebrae.

The **LONGISSIMUS CAPITIS MUSCLE** (7) is that portion of longissimus, dorsomedial to the longissimus cervicis muscle and deep to the

146

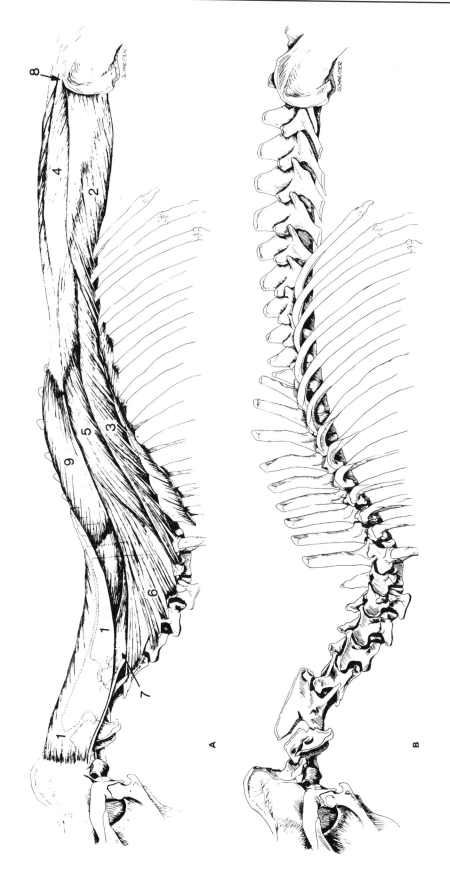

Fig. 7.27. Superficial epaxial muscles, with extrinsic limb muscles and serratus dorsalis removed (A); epaxial skeleton for visual comparison (B), lateral view.

splenius muscle, that extends from the transverse processes of the first three thoracic vertebrae and the caudal articular processes of the last five cervical vertebrae to the mastoid process of the temporal bone. A caudal continuation of the longissimus muscle into the tail is named, descriptively, the **SACROCAUDALIS DORSALIS LATERALIS MUSCLE (8)**.

The **SPINALIS MUSCLE** is composed of thoracic and cervical portions, with the thoracic portion fused to fibers of the semispinalis thoracis. The fused muscle, **SPINALIS AND SEMISPINALIS THORACIS** (9, Fig. 7.27), arises from the thoracolumbar fascia and the dorsomedial surface of the longissimus thoracis muscle. The spinalis and semispinalis thoracis muscle inserts on the spinous processes of the last two cervical and first six thoracic vertebrae.

The **SPINALIS CERVICIS MUSCLE** (1, Fig. 7.28) arises from the spinous process of the 1st thoracic vertebra and inserts cranially on spinous processes of the 2nd to 5th cervical vertebrae.

The **TRANSVERSOSPINALIS MUSCLE** division is a series of deep epaxial muscles and includes the semispinalis, multifidi, and rotator muscles.

The **SEMISPINALIS MUSCLES** consists of thoracic, cervical, and capital portions. The thoracic portion of the semispinalis muscle, fused with the spinalis, has been described (9, Fig. 7.27). Another segment of the semispinalis muscle, the **SEMISPINALIS CAPITIS**, composed of biventer cervicis and complexus, is superficial to the spinalis cervicis muscle (Fig. 7.28).

The **BIVENTER** (two bellies) **CERVICIS MUSCLE (2)** arises medial to the longissimus muscle from the transverse processes of the 2nd to 4th thoracic vertebrae and inserts on the skull near the external occipital protuberance. The **COMPLEXUS MUSCLE (3)**, ventrolateral to the biventer cervicis, arises from the caudal articular processes of the last 5 cervical and 1st thoracic vertebrae; the c omplexus muscle inserts on the nuchal crest of the skull.

The **MULTIFIDI** (mul-tif'i-die, sing. multifidus) **MUSCLES** (4, Fig. 7.28; 1, Fig. 7.29) are a series of short muscles that attach caudoventrally to mamillary, transverse, or articular processes, pass craniodorsally over two vertebrae, and usually attach to spinous processes of other vertebrae. Muscles belonging to the multifidi subdivision are present from the caudal vertebrae to the skull. The multifidus series is continued cranially in the region of the first two cervical vertebrae (Fig. 7.28) as the caudal and cranial capital oblique muscles.

The **CAUDAL CAPITAL OBLIQUE MUSCLE** (5) arises from the spinous process of the axis and inserts craniolaterally on the transverse process of the atlas.

The **CRANIAL CAPITAL OBLIQUE MUSCLE** (6) arises on the transverse process of the atlas and inserts craniodorsally on the nuchal crest of the skull. The multifidi continue caudally into the tail as the **SACROCAUDALIS DORSALIS MEDIALIS**.

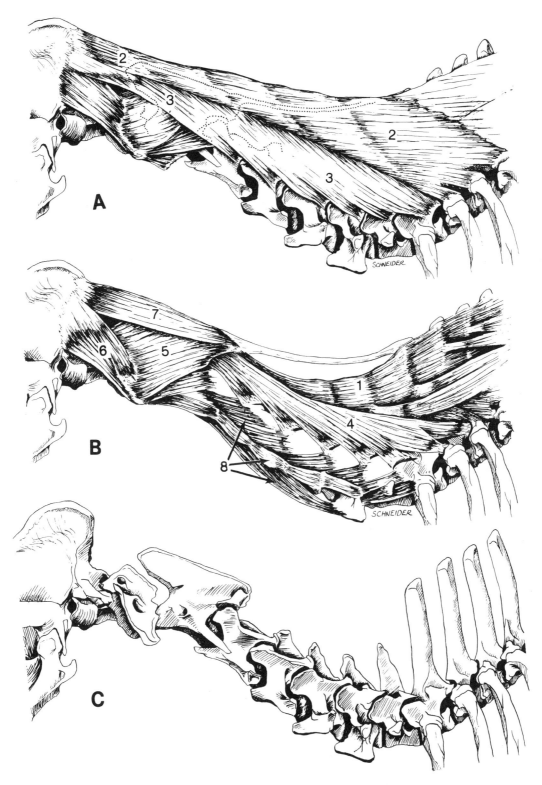

Fig.7.28. Deep epaxial muscles of the cervical region, lateral view: splenius, longissimus cervicis, and longissimus capitis muscles removed (A); semispinalis muscle also removed (B); all muscles removed (C).

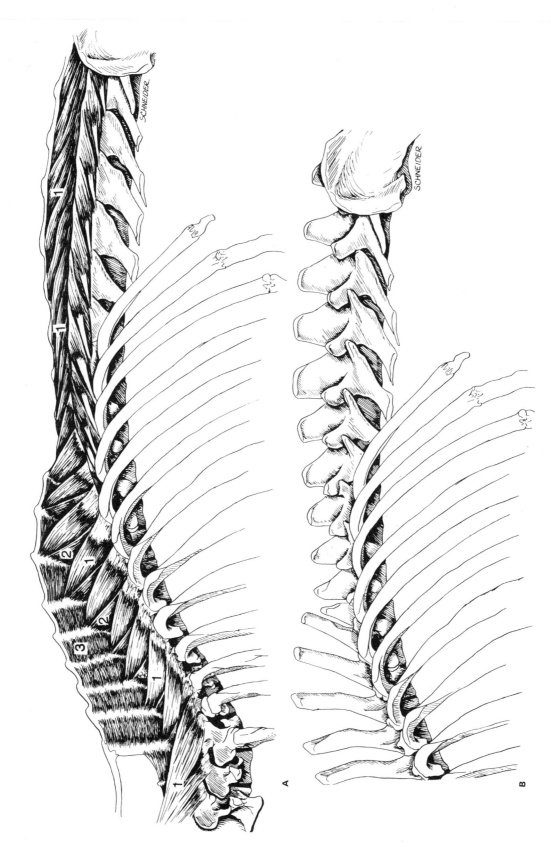

Fig.7.29. Deep epaxial muscles of the thoracic and abdominal regions, lateral view, with iliocostal and logissimus muscles removed (A); skeleton deep to the deep epaxial muscles of the thoracic and abdominal region.

In the cranial thoracic region, short muscle groups are present that act to pivot or rotate the thoracic vertebrae around their long axes. These **ROTATOR MUSCLES** (2, Fig. 7.29) occur as short and long fascicles. The short rotator muscles pass between the transverse process of one thoracic vertebra to the spinous process of the next preceding (cranial) vertebra; long rotator muscles pass by one vertebra from their origin to their point of insertion.

INTERSPINALIS muscles (3, Fig. 7.29) are segmental muscles that attach to the spinous processes of adjacent vertebrae. Muscles that may be considered modified interspinalis muscles are the **RECTUS CAPITIS MUSCLES**, which arise on the dorsal surface of the axis or atlas and insert on the skull near the nuchal crest.

The **RECTUS CAPITIS DORSALIS MAJOR MUSCLE** (7, Fig. 7.28; 1, 2, Fig. 7.30) arises on the spinous process of the axis and inserts on the occipital bone.

This major dorsal straight muscle of the head is comprised of two parts, a more superficial part (1, Fig. 7.30) which arises from the caudal portion of the spinous process and a deeper part (2, Fig. 7.30) which arises from the cranial portion of the spinous process.

The **RECTUS CAPITIS DORSALIS MINOR MUSCLE** (3) arises from the dorsal arch of the atlas and inserts on the occipital bone directly dorsal to the foramen magnum.

INTERTRANSVERSE MUSCLES, occurring from head to tail, are best developed in the cervical (8, Fig. 7.28) and caudal vertebral regions. These muscles arise from mamillary, articular, accessory, or transverse processes, pass over one or more vertebrae, and insert on transverse processes of other vertebrae.

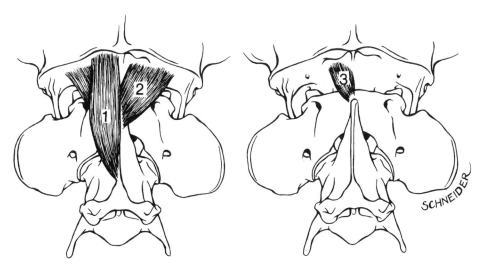

Fig.7.30. Rectus capitis dorsalis muscles, dorsal view.

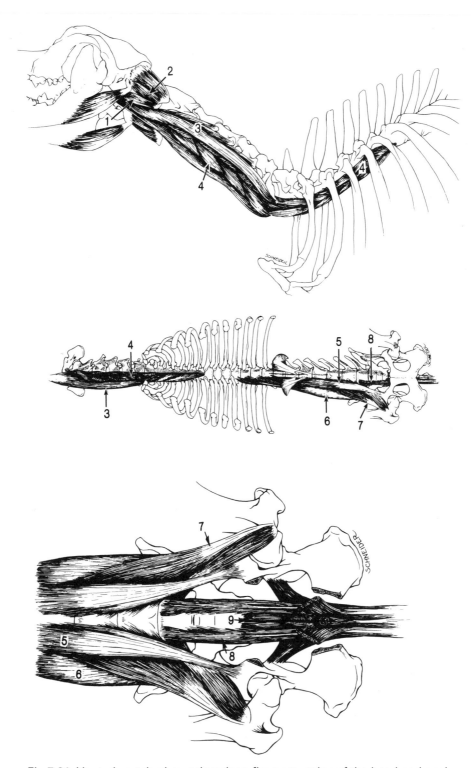

Fig.7.31. Ventral vertebral muscles: deep flexor muscles of the head and neck, ventrolateral view (A); deep flexor muscles of the trunk, ventral view (B); deep flexor muscles of the lumbar, sacral, and caudal vertebrae, ventral view (C).

For consideration of muscles ventral to the long axis of the vertebral column, these hypaxial muscles may be divided into three groups: deep flexors of the vertebral column, lateral thoracic and abdominal muscles, and ventral trunk muscles.

The deep vertebral (subvertebral) muscles (Fig. 7.31) include the rectus capitis ventralis, rectus capitis lateralis, longus capitis, longus colli, psoas minor, quadratus lumborum, psoas major, sacrocaudalis ventralis lateralis, and sacrocaudalis ventralis medialis.

The **RECTUS CAPITIS VENTRALIS MUSCLE** (1) attaches from the ventral arch of the atlas to the ventral surface of the occipital bone. Lateral to the rectus capitis ventralis, the **RECTUS CAPITIS LATERALIS MUSCLE** (2) attaches the transverse process of the atlas to the jugular process of the skull.

The **LONGUS CAPITIS MUSCLE** (3) arises from transverse processes of cervical vertebrae and inserts on the ventral surface of the occipital bone.

The **LONGUS COLLI MUSCLE** (4) in the thorax arises from the ventral surfaces of the first six thoracic vertebrae and inserts on the transverse processes of the last two cervical vertebrae; in the neck, the longus colli muscle arises from the transverse process of one vertebra and inserts on the ventral surface of the preceding (cranial) vertebral body. The longus colli muscle is situated medial to the longus capitis muscle.

The **PSOAS MINOR MUSCLE** (5, Fig. 7.31) arises from the ventral surfaces of the last thoracic and first four or five lumbar vertebrae and inserts as a cordlike tendon on the ilium adjacent to the iliopubic eminence.

The **QUADRATUS LUMBORUM MUSCLE** (6) arises dorsal to the psoas minor muscle from the ventral surfaces of the bodies of the last three thoracic vertebrae; it inserts on the transverse processes of the lumbar vertebrae and the medial surface of the wing of the ilium.

The **PSOAS MAJOR MUSCLE** (7) arises from the last six lumbar vertebrae and inserts, in common with the **ILIACUS MUSCLE** as the **ILIOPSOAS**, on the minor trochanter of the femoral bone (see p. 104).

The ventral tail muscles are the **SACROCAUDALIS VENTRALIS LATERALIS** (8, Fig. 7.31) and **MEDIALIS** (9). The major artery to the tail is situated in a depression between right and left sacrocaudalis ventralis medialis muscles.

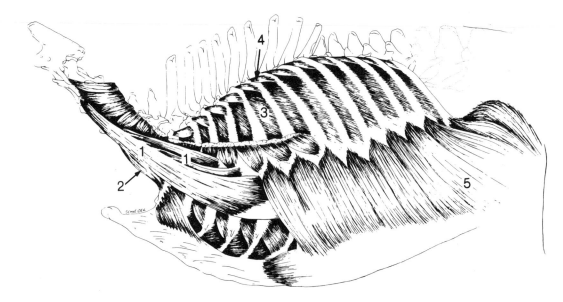

Fig.7.32. Superficial layer of hypaxial muscles, lateral view.

The lateral thoracic and abdominal muscles occur in three layers from superficial to deep. The superficial muscle layer of the lateral thorax (Fig. 7.32) includes the scalenus, external intercostals, levator costarum and external abdominal oblique. The superficial muscle of the abdomen is the external abdominal oblique.

The muscle fibers of all four muscles are oriented in a caudoventral direction. The scalenus has superficial and deep parts that form the **DORSAL** (1) and **MIDDLE** (2) **SCALENUS MUSCLES**; the fascicles of the scalenus muscle attach the 1st, 3rd, 4th, and 8th or 9th ribs to the last five cervical vertebrae.

The **EXTERNAL INTERCOSTAL MUSCLES** (3) arise from the caudal surface of a rib and insert on the cranial surface of the next rib (caudally). The short, fusiform-shaped **LEVATOR COSTARUM MUSCLES** (4) are deep to the longissimus thoracis muscle; 12 levator muscles attach the transverse processes of thoracic vertebrae to cranial borders of adjacent ribs.

The **EXTERNAL ABDOMINAL OBLIQUE MUSCLE** (5) arises from the superficial surfaces of ribs 4–13 and from the thoracolumbar fascia; it inserts by means of a wide aponeurosis on the linea alba and the prepubic tendon.

The **LINEA ALBA** (al' bah; white) (1, Fig. 7.33), or white line, is the combined aponeuroses of the abdominal muscles that extends along the ventral median line from the xiphoid process of the sternum to the pelvic symphysis.

The cranial pubic ligament (2) is a thickening of connective tissue that attaches the iliopubic eminence of one side to the pubic symphysis on the ventral median line and then to the iliopubic eminence of the other side.

A thickening in the dorsocaudal portion of the external abdominal oblique muscle's aponeurosis forms a part of the **INGUINAL ARCH** (3), which spans the distance from the tuber coxae to the iliopubic eminence. The **SUPERFICIAL**

154

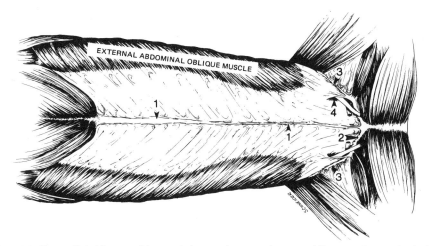

Fig.7.33. Superficial layer of hypaxial muscles, tendons and ligaments, ventral view.

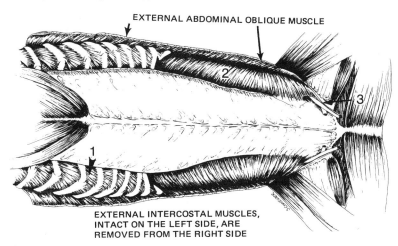

Fig.7.34. Middle layer of hypaxial muscles, ventral view.

INGUINAL RING (4) is a slitlike opening in the aponeurosis of the external abdominal oblique muscle. The peritoneal outpocketing, vessels, and reproductive structures that pass through the superficial inguinal ring are described on pages 254–255, 294–296, and 314.

The middle layer of lateral thoracic and abdominal muscles (Fig. 7.34) includes the **INTERNAL INTERCOSTAL** (1), **INTERNAL ABDOMINAL OBLIQUE** (2), and **CREMASTER** (to suspend) (3) muscles. The muscle fibers of both the internal intercostals and internal abdominal oblique muscles are oriented cranioventrally at right angles and deep to the superficial layer of muscles.

The internal intercostal muscles attach the cranial surface of individual ribs to the caudal surface of adjacent ribs. The internal abdominal oblique muscle arises from the thoracolumbar fascia, the tuber coxae, and the inguinal arch; it inserts on the 12th and 13th ribs and by an aponeurosis on the linea alba. The cremaster muscle, which is derived from the internal abdominal oblique, is described with the male reproductive system (see p. 253).

155

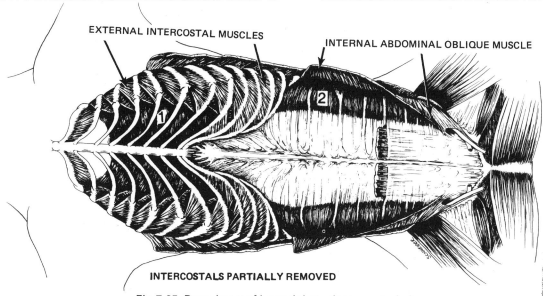

Fig.7.35. Deep layer of hypaxial muslces, ventral view.

The deep layer of lateral thoracic and abdominal muscles (Fig. 7.35) includes the transversus thoracis and transversus abdominis muscles. These two muscle groups are characterized by having muscle fibers oriented transversely to the long axis of the axial skeleton. Deep to the ribcage, the **TRANSVERSUS THORACIS MUSCLE** (1) arises from the sternum and inserts on the deep surfaces of the 2nd to 7th costal cartilages. The **TRANSVERSUS ABDOMINIS MUSCLE** (2) arises from the medial surfaces of the last five ribs, the transverse processes of the lumbar vertebrae, and the tuber coxae; it inserts by an aponeurosis on the linea alba.

The ventral trunk muscles include the rectus thoracis; the rectus abdominis; and the rectus cervicis complex, formed by the sternohyoideus, sternothyroideus, thyrohyoideus, and geniohyoideus muscles (see p. 129).

The **STERNOHYOIDEUS** is a straplike muscle that arises from the manubrium of the sternum and the 1st costal cartilage and inserts on the basihyoid.

The **STERNOTHYROIDEUS MUSCLE** arises with the sternohyoideus from the 1st costal cartilage and inserts on the lateral surface of the thyroid cartilage of the larynx. The sternothyroideus muscle is immediately deep to the sternohyoideus muscle. To approach the trachea along the ventral median line, an incision would be made between the sternohyoideus and the sternothyroideus of one side and the same muscles of the other side.

The **THYROHYOIDEUS** is a short muscle that attaches the thyroid cartilage to the thyrohyoid bone.

The **RECTUS THORACIS MUSCLE**, the fibers of which are oriented caudoventrally, attaches the costal cartilage of the 2nd to 4th ribs to the 1st rib.

The **RECTUS ABDOMINIS MUSCLE** is a long, straplike muscle that arises cranially by an aponeurosis from the sternum and 1st rib and inserts caudally on the cranial pubic ligament via the prepubic tendon. The paired recti abdomini muscles are separated at the ventral median line by the linea alba.

Depending upon location of an incision in the abdominal wall, different layers of tissue will be encountered. In the cranial part of the abdominal wall, the aponeuroses of the two oblique muscles of each side come together to form a sheath that surrounds each rectus abdominis muscle (Fig. 7.36).

Caudally, in the inguinal region, the rectus abdominis muscle is deep, next to the peritoneum, with the aponeuroses of the other three abdominal muscles superficial to it.

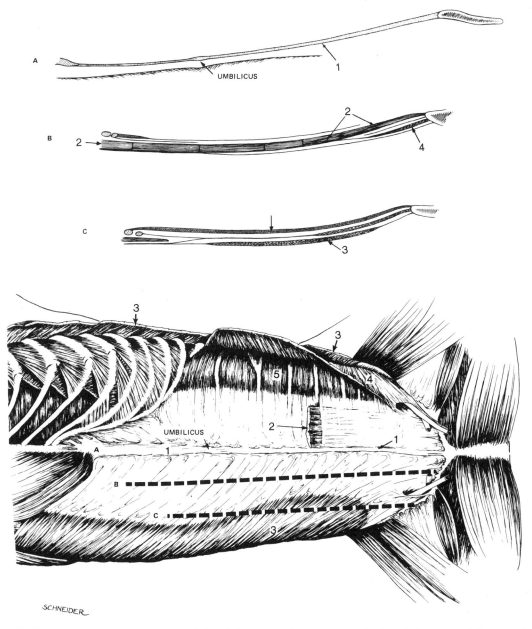

Fig.7.36. Change in position of rectus abdominis muscle in the abdominal wall, from cranial to caudal.

The linea alba (1), situated along the ventral median line between right and left rectus abdominis muscles (2), demarcates a line at which right and left sheaths are fused; at this point of fusion (A) an incision needs to pass through only one fused layer of deep fascia to reach the peritoneum. A sagittal incision a few centimeters to one side of the linea alba (B) would pass progressively through 3–5 layers depending upon whether the site of incision is cranial or caudal to the **UMBILICUS**. A more lateral sagittal incision (C) would involve both oblique muscles, or their separate aponeuroses, and the transversus abdominis muscle (5).

JOINTS OF THE TRUNK

Synovial joints in the vertebral column are present between articular processes (cranial and caudal) of adjacent vertebrae and between vertebrae and ribs.

The **ATLANTOOCCIPITAL ARTICULATION** (Fig. 7.37) is a site commonly used for puncturing membranes to remove (tap) cerebrospinal fluid. An articular capsule (1), enclosing a synovia-filled cavity, passes from the circumference of the articular surface of the occipital bone to the circumference of the cranial articular surface of the atlas. Thus the U-shaped articular capsule is lateral and ventral to the spinal cord. The thin **VENTRAL ATLANTOOCCIPITAL MEMBRANE** (a part of the fibrous articular capsule) passes from the ventral arch of the atlas to the ventral edge of the foramen magnum. The **DORSAL ATLANTOOCCIPITAL MEMBRANE** (2) attaches from the dorsal arch of the atlas to the dorsal edge of the foramen magnum.

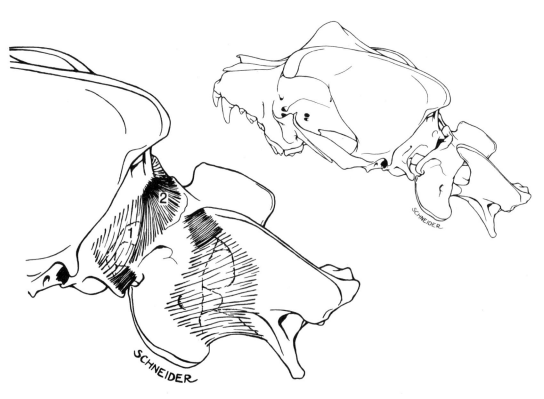

Fig.7.37. Atlantooccipital articulation, dorsolateral view.

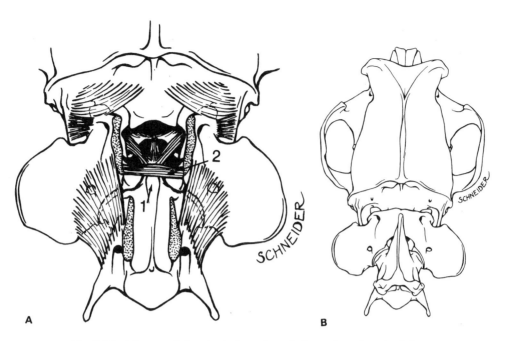

Fig.7.38. Atlantoaxial articulation, dorsal view: dorsal arch of the
atlas removed (A); muscles and articular capsule removed (B).

The articular cavity of the **ATLANTOAXIAL ARTICULATION** (Fig. 7.38) is continuous with the cavity of the atlantooccipital articulation. As in the atlantooccipital articulation, the articular cavity is lateral and ventral to the spinal cord, but not dorsal to it. The dens of the axis (1) is bound in the ventral part of the vertebral foramen of the atlas by the **TRANSVERSE ATLANTAL LIGAMENT (2).**

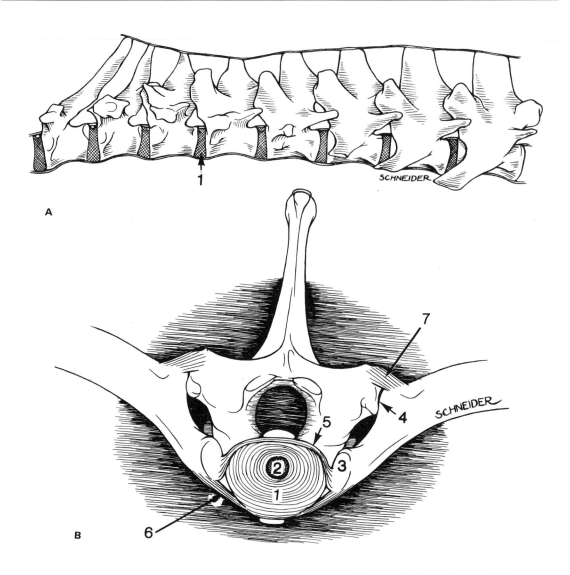

Fig.7.39. Intervertebral and costovertebral articulations. (A) lateral view; (B) cranial view.

The INTERVERTEBRAL SYMPHYSES (Fig. 7.39) are fibrocartilaginous joints between adjacent bodies of vertebrae. Each such symphysis contains a layer of fibers connecting the periphery of one vertebral body to the next; these crisscrossing fibers pass obliquely relative to the long axis of the vertebral column. A ring of fibrous tissue is thus formed around the space between adjacent vertebral bodies.

This ring, termed the **ANULUS FIBROSUS** (1), forms the outer portion of the **INTERVERTEBRAL DISC.**

Deep to the thick layers of the anulus fibrosus, a soft, gelatinous, glistening white material maintains separation of adjacent vertebral articular cartilage; termed the **NUCLEUS PULPOSUS** (2), it forms the center of the intervertebral disc.

Degenerative changes in the anulus fibrosus and/or a traumatic compression of the intervertebral disc may result in a herniation of the nucleus pulposus. If such a herniation occurs dorsally, a compression of the spinal cord and/or spinal nerves may result. Most intervertebral disc problems of the cervical region occur between C2 and C3; disc problems of the thoracolumbar region usually occur between Tl1 and L2. An intervertebral disc does not occur between Cl (atlas) and C2 (axis).

Ribs articulate with vertebrae at two synovial joints (Fig. 7.39): the **COSTAL HEAD ARTICULATION** (3), and the **COSTOTRANSVERSE ARTICULATION** (4). The head of each rib (110) articulates with costal articular surfaces on the bodies of two adjacent vertebrae and with an intervening intervertebral disc. The heads of each pair of ribs (2–10) are held tightly against their articular surfaces on the various vertebrae by an **INTERCAPITAL LIGAMENT** (5). Each intercapital ligament is a connective tissue band that is situated transversely across the dorsal surface of an intervertebral disc and attaches to the heads of right and left ribs.

The synovial membrane of the articular capsule on one side is continuous across the vertebral column, between the intercapital ligament and the intervertebral disc, with that of the articular capsule of the other side.

The **RADIATE LIGAMENT OF THE COSTAL HEAD** (6) attaches each rib head to the lateral surfaces of the bodies of two adjacent vertebrae (except for the last two or three pairs of ribs) and to the anulus fibrosus between them.

The costotransverse articulations are synovial joints between articular surfaces of costal tubercles and vertebral transverse processes. Peripheral to the synovial membrane, each costal tubercle is bound to a transverse process by a **COSTOTRANSVERSE LIGAMENT** (7).

A number of other articulations occur within the trunk: the **SACROILIAC ARTICULATION** (which craniodorsally is fibrocartilage and caudoventrally contains a synovial joint), the **STERNOCOSTAL ARTICULATIONS** (which are synovial joints), the **STERNAL SYNCHONDROSES** (joints between sternebrae without synovia), and the **COSTOCHONDRAL ARTICULATIONS** (joints between costal bone and costal cartilage without synovia).

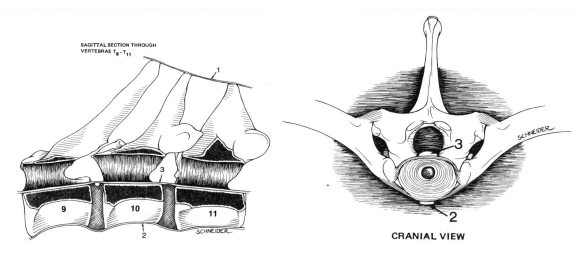

Fig.7.40. Intervertebral ligaments.

Each vertebra is united to adjacent vertebrae by various ligaments (Fig.7.40). A dorsal longitudinal band, the **SUPRASPINOUS LIGAMENT** (1) attaches to each spinous process between the 1st thoracic and 3rd caudal vertebrae.

The **NUCHAL LIGAMENT** is a cranial extension of the supraspinous ligament; it attaches to the spinous process of the 1st thoracic vertebra (caudally) and to the spinous process of the axis (cranially).

Two other longitudinal bands of connective tissue in the vertebral column are the ventral and dorsal longitudinal ligaments. The **VENTRAL LONGITUDINAL LIGAMENT** (2) is a slender band on the ventral surfaces of the vertebral bodies and intervertebral discs from the axis to the sacrum.

The **DORSAL LONGITUDINAL LIGAMENT** (3) is present on the dorsal surfaces of vertebral bodies and intervertebral discs from the axis to the caudal termination of the vertebral canal.

The intercapital ligaments of the ribs pass between the dorsal longitudinal ligament and the intervertebral discs.

The **LIGAMENTA FLAVA** (flav'ah; yellow) spans the distance between individual vertebrae, attaching vertebral arch to vertebral arch. This yellow ligament should not be confused with the more deeply situated dura mater, the outermost layer of the meninges.

Other connective tissue bands that may be encountered are **INTERSPINOUS** and **INTERTRANSVERSE LIGAMENTS**.

(DIFFERENCE TO BE NOTED IN THE CAT: A nuchal ligament is not present.)

162

Chapter 8
BIOMECHANICS

Objectives: To recognize that "soundness in conformation" and efficiency of movement are related and depend on laws of physics.

Stress: Compression vs. Shear

Gaits: Walk, Trot, Pace, and Gallop

Factors effecting afficiency of movement: Lateral Displacement and Single Tracking, Vertical Undulation of the Vertebral Column, Angulation of Limbs, and Position of Footpads relative to Long Axis of limb.

STRESS

The musculoskeletal system is designed for support and movement; its component parts are bone, cartilage, muscle, ligament, tendon, and fascia. Immobility results in a decrease in size of a muscle and loss of calcium from bones. This decrease in size of a structure is termed ATROPHY.

HYPERTROPHY is the opposite of atrophy and describes an enlargement resulting from exercise. Exercise places stress on bone through muscular activity. Muscles that attach on two opposite surfaces of a bone create stress in only one plane. This unidirectional stress, which stimulates the development of osseous tissue in one plane, contributes to the production of flat bone (Fig. 8.1).

The pull of muscles on their points of attachment on bone results in development of osseous projections that enlarge as the animal ages (Fig. 8.2).There is much variation in size and shape of osseous enlargements in various species since the same muscle in different species may perform different levels of activity and provide different degrees of tension on bone.

The weight of every part of the standing or moving dog is supported by the limbs. Most weight loads applied to long bones place stresses

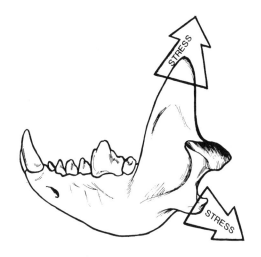

MANDIBLE

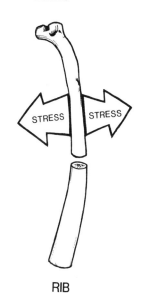

RIB

Fig.8.1. Contribution of stress to the production of flat bone.

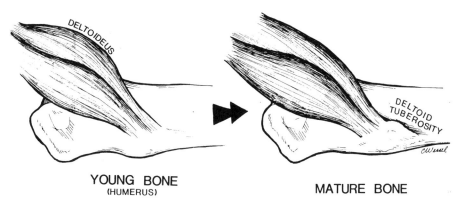

YOUNG BONE
(HUMERUS)

MATURE BONE

Fig.8.2. Contribution of stress to osseous projections.

on them that are parallel (COMPRESSION) and perpendicular (SHEAR) to their long axes. These stresses are greatly increased during running, when the pelvic limbs push against the ground or when the thoracic limbs catch and cushion the fall of the forward moving body after each pelvic thrust.

A series of bones placed end to end would be capable of carrying more weight than if they were placed at angles to each other because bone can withstand a greater compressive force than shear force. Bone that is slightly and temporarily deformed by stress develops STRESS LINES parallel to the weight load.

Stress is progressively less toward the central axis of a cylinder. The compact bone in the diaphyses of long bones is also strengthened by having a minimum of cavities, grooves, and notches that would weaken its structure. Thus, by being hollow and cylindrical, long bones have a greater strength (per unit weight) for resisting compression than solid or rectangular bones.

Due to the attachment of muscles to the epiphyses and metaphyses, the ends of long bones are subjected to bending forces; to resist bending, the ends of long bones are often oval in cross section, with thicker walls toward and away from the points of muscle attachment.

Forces transmitted by one bone to another across a partially flexed joint are carried through trabeculae in the epiphyses and metaphyses of each bone; the trabeculae are oriented linearly along the lines of stress.

An injury to bone or disuse of a muscle will result in an alteration of force and hence in a change in the direction and quantity of trabeculae.

Synovial joints (see pp. 71–81) permit long bones to move while under relatively little shearing stress.

The synovia, which lubricates the articular cavity, reduces friction and wear by molecular shearing that occurs within the fluid itself. The reciprocal surfaces of the articulating epiphyses are so morphologically incongruous that the film of lubricant between them is shaped like a wedge. Stress during movement forces the wedge of synovia between newly developing contiguous surfaces.

MOVEMENT

A Whippet is able to travel 55 km/hr (35 miles/hr); the coyote and red fox run at 69 and 72 km/hr (43.9 and 45.8 miles/hr), respectively.

Mammals with rapid cursorial locomotion are characterized by having elongated distal limb segments and points of muscular insertion close to the joints. This lengthening of the limb in relation to body size results in a longer stride; stride is a full cycle of limb movement or the total distance covered after all limbs have moved. Speed in movement is equal to length of stride times the rate of stride.

Muscles of various mammals do not vary greatly in speed of contraction. The rate of stride is dependent upon proximity of the points of muscle insertion to limb joints (Fig. 8.3). When a tendon is inserted close to the joint, a larger stride is achieved in a shorter time, since a shorter distance of contraction is required to produce the same movement than an insertion farther from the joint would necessitate. Insertion by a tendon farther from the joint provides greater strength.

The dog initiates movement with a thoracic limb; as movement occurs, the metacarpal and metatarsal pads make contact with the ground before the digital pads do. The shock of the limbs striking the ground is cushioned by overextension of the carpal joints and flexion of the tarsal joints.

The tendons of superficial and deep digital flexors, flexors carpi ulnaris and radialis, and the common calcanean tendon take on the stress of impact, cushioning and dampening the shock. The ulnar and genual articulations have limited movement or cushioning function. The digital lexor muscles of both manus and pes increasingly contract, resulting in greater flexion such that the body weight is transferred to the digital pads.

Muscles of a limb that are active during that portion of movement when the limb is supporting weight usually have a pennate fiber pattern and are thus powerful and contract a short distance. Limb muscles that are active during the period of the stride when the limb is swinging and not in ground contact usually have parallel fibers, are relatively weak, and shorten a greater distance.

A GAIT is a regularly repeated sequence of leg movements; the walk, trot, pace, and gallop are each characterized by a unique sequence of movements.

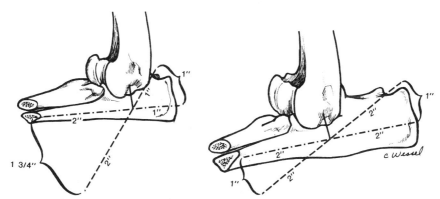

Fig.8.3. Strength/speed versus relative proximity of muscle insertion to the center of a joint.

167

The **WALK** (Fig. 8.4) is a gait in which each foot is in contact with the ground more than 50% of the time. Each foot moves independently (out of synchrony), and two or three feet provide support at all times.

The sequence of limb movements in one stride occurs as follows: right manus, left pes, left manus, right pes (or left manus, right pes, right manus, left pes).

The angle formed by the ground with a line passing through the acetabulum and supporting pad of a walking Greyhound is approximately 66 degrees both at the beginning and at the end of the support phase.

The **TROT** (Fig. 8.5) is a gait in which a thoracic limb and the opposite pelvic limb move nearly in unison (one diagonal followed by the other).

The trot may produce a rise and fall of the shoulders, which evidences a jolting gait; much of the shock will be absorbed by the thoracic limb if the scapula and long axis of the trunk are positioned at an angle of approximately 45 degrees to each other.

Some dogs, such as the German Shepherd, are able to trot rapidly enough to utilize their momentum for forward motion while all four feet are off the ground (**SUSPENSION**); the "flying trot" is characterized by suspension in two phases: one following movement of one diagonal and the other following movement of the other diagonal.

Animals are often moved at a trot while being diagnosed for lameness as abnormal movement becomes more apparent during this gait. The degree of flexion and extension is decreased and the swing and support phases of limb movement are shortened in an injured

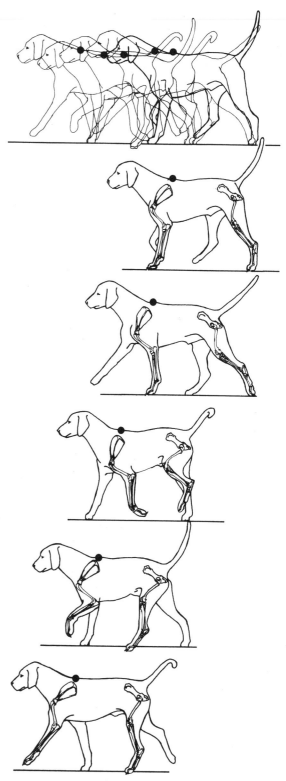

Fig.8.4. Walk.

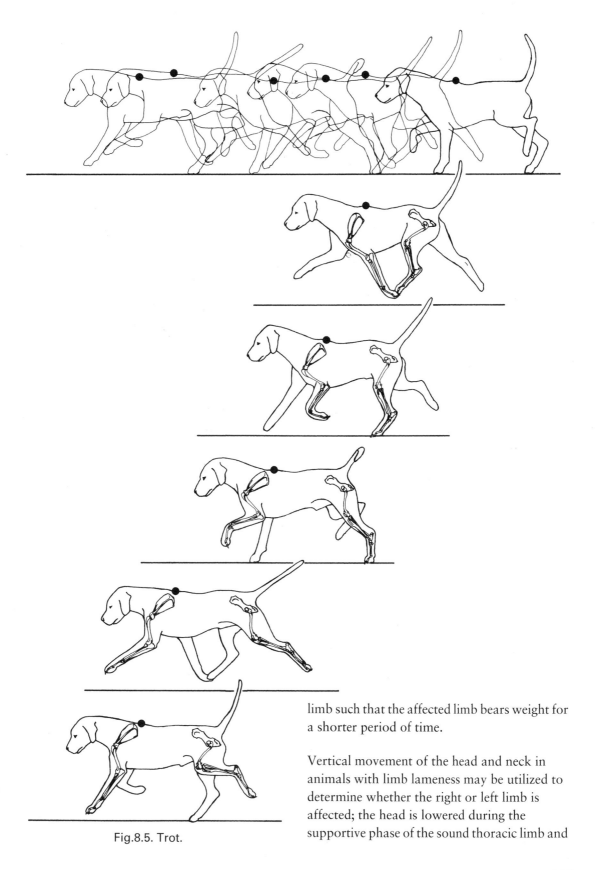

Fig.8.5. Trot.

limb such that the affected limb bears weight for a shorter period of time.

Vertical movement of the head and neck in animals with limb lameness may be utilized to determine whether the right or left limb is affected; the head is lowered during the supportive phase of the sound thoracic limb and raised during the supportive phase of the lame limb.

An animal with a lameness in a pelvic limb will carry its pelvis tilted such that less weight is applied to the injured limb.

The **PACE**, or amble, is a gait in which first one lateral (thoracic and pelvic) and then the other lateral move in unison. This gait is faster than the trot and is often utilized by a tired or unsound dog.

In the **GALLOP** (Fig. 8.6), the two pelvic limbs make contact with the ground out of synchrony and then the two thoracic limbs do likewise. There are various forms of galloping (sustained, normal, and leaping).

The sustained gallop (**CANTER**) is a sequence of three supports per stride: one pes, the opposite pes with its diagonal, and the opposite manus. The portion of the stride with the single support by the manus provides a catapultlike action; the body is propelled forward like that of a polevaulter by the extended thoracic limb. A scapula-thoracic angle of 45 degrees will permit optimum propulsion by this single support. The normal gallop is characterized by four distinct supports sequenced as follows: left pes, right pes, left manus, right manus.

The leaping gallop is characteristic of gazehounds (Greyhound, Whippet, Saluki, Borzoi, and Afghan) and Doberman Pinschers. The body loses all contact with the ground two times per stride. The first period of suspension is obtained by one thoracic limb; the second suspension is obtained two supports later by the diagonal pelvic limb. The sequence of supports in the leaping gallop is: right pes, left pes, left manus, and right manus.

BODY STRUCTURES– RUNNING

A dog's body may be specialized for many purposes such as digging, entering small underground tunnels, fighting, retrieving, or running down prey. The remainder of this chapter will be concerned only with certain factors related to the efficiency and effectiveness of the body structure for running.

Large dogs with body proportions similar to those of small dogs are not built as efficiently for locomotion as the smaller dogs (as the body length increases X times, body weight increases X^3 while muscular force increases only by X^2).

Efficiency in cursorial movement may be increased by (1) decreasing the vertical movement of the trunk, (2) decreasing the lateral movement of the body during forward motion, (3) reducing muscles that abduct, adduct, or rotate the limbs, (4) lengthening the distal limb segments relative to proximal segments, and (5) decreasing the vertical distance the distal ends of the limbs move from the ground. The presence of only a rudimentary clavicle in an animal enables greater movement of the scapula relative to the thorax than in animals with well-developed clavicles. A deep, narrow chest further contributes to freedom of the scapula to pivot cranially and caudally. Such a movement of the scapula increases the effective stride and thus the animal's speed.

For efficient movement, a dog's pelvic and thoracic limbs should be in a straight line (when viewed from the cranial or caudal surface) from the humeral or coxal articulation to the ground. Since each joint distal to the humeral and coxal joints acts as a hinge joint, a deviation of bone laterally or medially would require more muscular effort for support

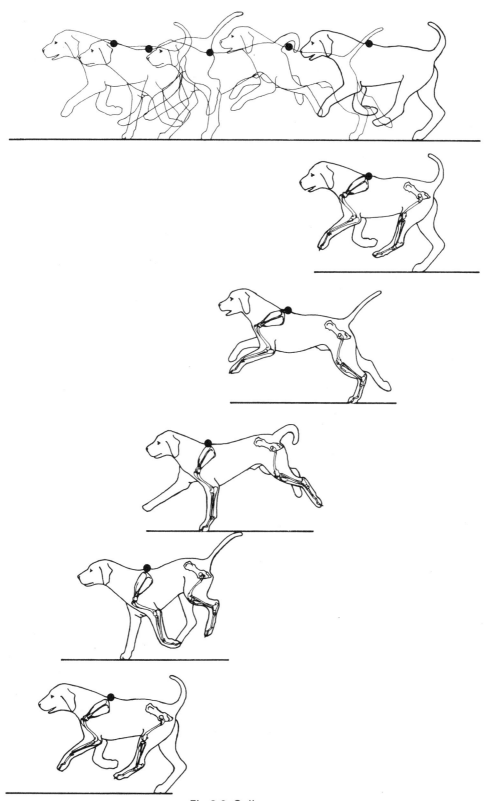

Fig.8.6. Gallop.

and hence would be more fatiguing. Both thoracic and pelvic limbs should move cranially and caudally in a straight line during locomotion.

A thrusting force by a limb against the ground results in a movement of the body both forward and toward the opposite side (i.e., the right foot pushes the body cranially and left laterally). Fighting this **LATERAL DISPLACEMENT** with opposing muscles results in fatigue. Most running dogs bring their feet in toward the median plane (**SINGLE TRACKING**), which reduces lateral displacement (i.e., the distance between right and left manus and right and left pes is less on a running dog than on a standing dog). The limbs, while forming a straight line (as observed cranially or caudally), incline medially. Many thick-chested, short-legged dogs (such as the Basset Hound) partially achieve this method of reducing lateral displacement by having a curved radius and ulna. By having widely separated feet, other dogs (such as the Bulldog) achieve stability at the expense of cursorial efficiency.

Vertical undulations of the vertebral column permit longer strides. Flexion of the vertebral column is accompanied by movement of the pelvic limbs, cranially. Extension of the vertebral column is associated with movement of the thoracic limbs cranially, with each step of a rapidly galloping dog, the thorax and pelvis both rotate in the same direction as the limbs they support are moving.

Although the limbs of a running dog are straight when viewed cranially or caudally, the limbs during their supportive portion of the stride should not be straight when viewed laterally. For efficiency in running, the scapula should be set at a 45 degree angle to the long axis of the trunk; the scapula may normally pivot approximately 15 degrees during rapid locomotion. The humerus, which is optimally positioned at

approximately a 90-degree angle to the scapula during the standing phase, may extend during locomotion to approximately a 150-degree angle with the long axis of the scapula. A vertical line drawn through the center of the scapula should intersect the metacarpal pad of a supporting limb. If the pad is cranial to the line the carpus would tend to sink, placing more strain on the carpal and digital flexors. If the pad is caudal to this vertical line, the dog will tend to travel on its toes, with continual danger of knuckling over or stumbling. The flexor angle of the cubital articulation would ideally approximate 130 degrees during the supportive phase of the stride. The flexor angle of the carpal articulation should be somewhat more than 180 degrees in order for this joint to take up the shock of ground contact (by sinking caudoventrally).

The pelvic limb of the dog functions to power the body forward. The pelvic limb is set to provide maximum thrust against the ground when the metatarsal pad is in a vertical line with the coxal articulation. The force that can be generated by the pelvic limb is determined by the ratio of the limb length with pad under coxal articulation and that of the fully extended limb. An angle of 150 degrees between the long axis of the lumbar vertebrae and that of the pelvis is nearly optimum. The flexor angle of the proximal femoral articulation should approximate 75–90 degrees. The longer the crus, relative to limb length, the more powerful the limb is likely to be. The pea should be at 90 degrees to the surface of the ground for optimum power (the dorsal surface of the German Shepherd pes is at a greater then 90-degree angle). A long metatarsus will provide greater power at the loss of endurance.

UNIT IV

Respiratory System

In the two chapters that follow, you will learn to understand the complex nasal structures, the larynx, the air conduction system, and the lungs, mediastinum, and pleural spaces.

Contents:

Chapter 9

RESPIRATORY SYSTEM—ROSTRAL PORTION

Objectives: Be able to identify the complex structures of the internal nose and larynx.

External Nose: Nasal Plane, Nasal Sulci, and Nasal Alae

Internal Nose: Nasal Cavity, Nasal Vestibule, Nasal Septum; Dorsal, Ventral, and Ethmoid Conchae; Alar Fold of Ventral Concha; Nasolacrimal Ostium and Duct; Dorsal, Middle, Ventral, and Common Nasal Meatuses; Maxillary Recess and Hiatus of Maxillary Recess; Aperture of the Frontal Sinus; Vomeronasal Organ; Incisive Duct; Choana

Nasopharynx and Nasopharyngeal Meatus; Soft Palate, Intrapharyngeal Ostium, Palatopharyngeal Arches, Pharyngeal ostia of Auditory Tubes, Pharyngeal Tonsils, and Medial Retropharyngeal Lymph Node

Laryngopharynx, Esophagus, and Larynx

Larynx: Piriform Recesses; Epiglottis; Aryepiglottic Fold; Arytenoid Cartilage, Vocal, Cuneiform and Corniculate Processes; Thyroid and Cricoid Cartilages; Caudal Thyroid Notch; Cricothyroid Ligament; Cricothyroideus, Cricoarytenoideus Dorsalis, Thyroarytenoideus, and Vocalis Muscles; Vocal Ligament and Vocal Fold; Laryngeal Vestibule, Lateral Laryngeal Ventricle, Glottis and Rima Glottidis

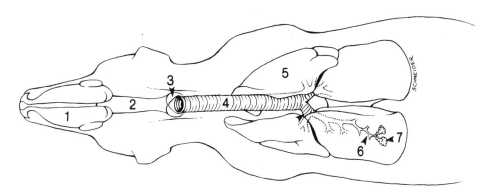

Fig.9.1. Schematic of the respiratory organs, dorsal view.

The respiratory system consists of organs that conduct gases (oxygen and carbon dioxide) between the blood and the external environment. The exchange of gases between the blood and the air around the organism is termed external respiration.

At rest, an average dog breathes in, and out, a volume of approximately 175 ml of air, 10–30 times per minute; this external respiration is a diffusion process, i.e., air molecules move from an area of higher concentration in the ambient air to an area of lower concentration in the lung tissue and then from an area of higher concentration in the lung to an area of lower concentration in the ambient air.

By increasing the volume of the thoracic cavity—which results in a changing lung volume—the concentration of air molecules is decreased within the lungs, resulting in inspiration, or a movement of air from a region of high pressure (atmosphere) to a region of low pressure (lung).

By decreasing the volume of the thoracic cavity—thereby decreasing the lung volume—the density of air molecules is increased, resulting in an outward diffusion of air molecules (expiration).

The respiratory organ system (Fig. 9.1) consists of the conducting airways—nasal cavity (1), nasopharynx (na " zo-far' inks) (2), laryngopharynx and larynx (lar' inks) (3), trachea (4), bronchi (5), and bronchioles (6)—and the gas exchange area, or alveoli (sing. alveolus; small hollow sac) (7).

The **NASAL CAVITY** (1, Fig. 9.2) is a paired space with constricted openings both rostrally and caudally. The paired vestibules form the rostral portion of the nasal cavity. Each **NASAL VESTIBULE** (antechamber) (2) is bounded and supported by cartilage; the surface of the nasal vestibule is a transitional zone

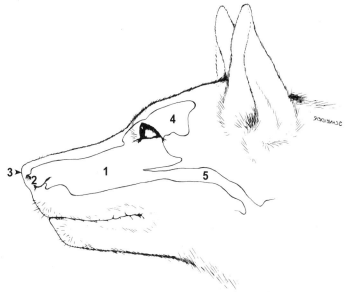

Fig.9.2. Schematic of the nasal cavity, lateral view.

between the pigmented skin of the **NASALPLANE** (3) and the mucous membrane of the nasal cavity proper.

Inspired air flows rapidly and at low pressure through the constricted orifice of the nasal vestibule; watery secretions from a number of nasal glands are discharged into the constricted orifice and are atomized into the air current. Small openings interconnect the caudodorsal portion of the nasal cavity with the frontal sinuses (4).

Caudoventrally, the nasal cavity is continuous with the **NASOPHARYNGEAL MEATUS** (5).

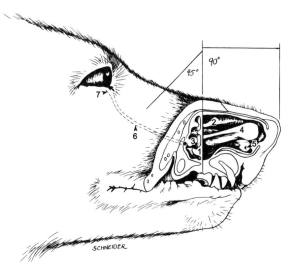

Fig.9.3. Nasal cavity, with a portion of the nasal septum and right wall removed.

The nasal cavity (Fig. 9.3) is divided by a median **NASAL SEPTUM** (1) into two fossae. Each **NASAL FOSSA** is subdivided by membrane-surfaced osseous projections into smaller air channels. Two of these osseous projections, named conchae, are present in the rostral portion of the nasal cavity. The **DORSAL CONCHA**, or nasoturbinate (2), is a ventral osseous projection from the nasal bone; the long dorsal concha is also a rostral projection of one of the ethmoid conchae. The greatly convoluted or scrolled **VENTRAL CONCHA**, or max-

illoturbinate (3), projects dorsomedially from the maxillary bone into the nasal fossa. The rostral noncoiled~ enlargement of the ventral concha is the **ALAR FOLD** (4).

An opening, the **NASOLACRIMAL OSTIUM** (5), is present in the ventromedial surface of the alar fold; the **NASOLA-CRIMAL DUCT** (6) drains orbital secretions from the **LACRIMAL SAC** (7) through the osseous lacrimal canal into the nasal vestibule.

A second ostium of the nasolacrimal duct may also be present.

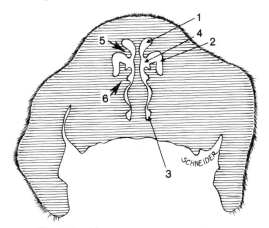

Fig. 9.4. Air passages or meatuses in the nasal cavity.

The rostral portion of each nasal fossa is subdivided by the conchae (Fig. 9.4) into dorsal (1), middle (2), ventral (3), and common (4) nasal meatuses. The **DORSAL NASAL MEATUS** (1) is the portion of the nasal fossa dorsomedial to the dorsal concha (5). The **MIDDLE NASAL MEATUS** (2) is the lateral airway situated between the dorsal concha and the ventral concha (6). The **VENTRAL NASAL MEATUS** (3) is the ventral air channel situated ventromedial to the ventral concha. The **COMMON NASAL MEATUS** (4) is the airway formed by the junction of dorsal, middle, and ventral meatuses.

The middle, ventral and common nasal meatuses

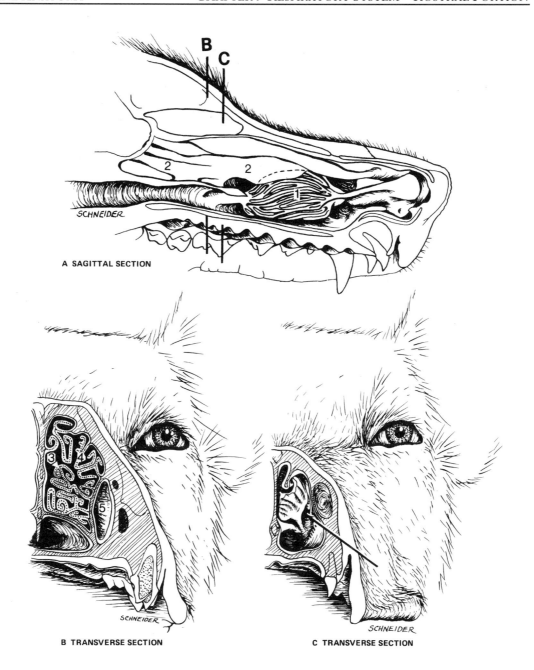

Fig.9.5. Conchae of the left nasal fossa: sagittal section (A) indicating levels of transverse sections B and C.

or the midportion of the nasal cavity are nearly occluded by the greatly branched ventral concha (1, Fig. 9.5); the membrane-covered branches (**LAMELLAE,** sing. lamella) of the ventral concha form many smaller airways, providing an increased surface area for more efficient filtering and warming of inhaled air.

The **ETHMOID CONCHAE** (2) are a series of turbinates or osseous scrolls that project rostrally from the **CRIBRIFORM LAMINA** of the ethmoid bone; they also attach laterally or dorsally to other lamina of the ethmoid bone. Ethmoid conchae are described as **ENDOTURBINATES** (3) or **ECTOTURBINATES** (4) based upon how far they extend medially toward the nasal septum (i.e., whether they are observable from the median plane with the septum removed). An endoturbinate is usually larger, projects farther medially, and is more easily observed within the nasal cavity from the median plane than an ectoturbinate.

Several of the larger endoturbinates project rostrally and are easily confused with the ventral concha. A few ectoturbinates project caudodorsally into the frontal sinus. Many air channels (ethmoid meatuses) occur between the ethmoid conchae; the apertures of three compartments of the frontal sinus open into the ethmoid meatuses.

Much of the caudomedial epithelial surface of the ethmoid conchae contains olfactory receptor cells.

The **MAXILLARY RECESS** (5, Fig. 9.5) is a large cavity situated between the orbital lamina of the ethmoid bone (medially) and the maxillary, lacrimal, and palatine bones (laterally). The thick membrane that surfaces the

maxillary recess is quite glandular.

The maxillary recess opens rostromedially into the nasal cavity between the rostral margin of the ethmoidal orbital lamina and conchae and the caudodorsal margin of the ventral conchae; the opening is termed the **HIATUS** (hi-a' tus; cleft) **OF THE MAXILLARY RECESS** (arrow, Fig. 9.5; 1, Fig. 9.6).

Much of the frontal bone is separated into a superficial and a deep bony layer by three air spaces (see p. 114) termed the frontal sinuses. As is true of all paranasal sinuses, the air-filled cavity of the frontal sinus opens into the nasal cavity; and is termed the **APERTURE OF THE FRONTAL SINUS.**

(*DIFFERENCES TO BE NOTED IN THE CAT: A single frontal sinus occurs in each frontal bone.*)

The portion of the nasal cavity that conducts as a single tube all the air inhaled through both nasal fossae (Fig. 9.6) extends caudally from the ventral nasal meatus (2) to the nasal part of the

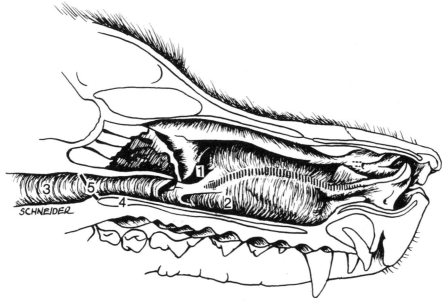

Fig.9.6. Left nasal fossa, with ventral concha and portions of the ethmoturbinates removed, sagittal section.

pharynx (3). The lumen of this portion situated dorsal to the caudal portion of the hard palate (4), is nearly the same size as the constricted lumen of the nasal vestibule.

The **CHOANA** (ko'a-nah, pl. choanae; funnel) (5) is the single opening formed by osseous structures separating the nasal cavity (rostrally) from the nasal part of the pharynx (caudally). The choana, formed by the palatine, vomer, and presphenoid bones, is dorsal to the caudal extent of the hard palate.

The rostral portion of the nasal septum (Fig. 9.7) contains cartilage (1). The osseous **PERPENDICULAR LAMINA** (2) of the ethmoid bone forms the skeleton of the caudal portion of the nasal septum.

The **VOMERONASAL** (vo" mer-o-na' sal) **ORGAN** (3) is a small, hollow, blind-ending structure that occurs bilaterally in the ventral portion of the nasal septum. This hollow tube, which is surfaced partially by olfactory epithelium, may be observed in a transverse section through the rostral portion of the nose. The vomeronasal organ opens rostrally into the **INCISIVE DUCT** (4); a vascular pumping mechanism may move fluid into and out of the vomeronasal organ. The incisive duct connects the ventral nasal meatus, via the palatine fissure, to the rostral portion of the oral cavity.

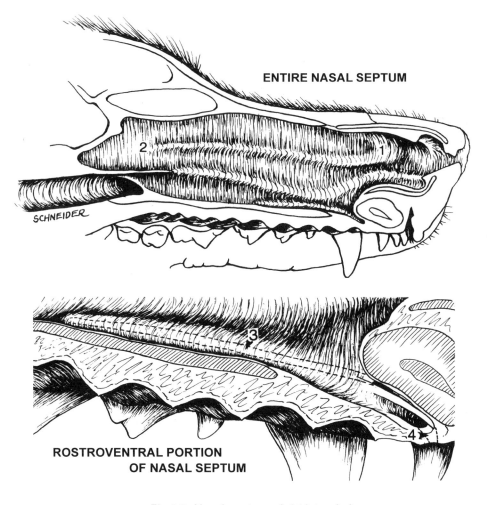

Fig.9.7. Nasal septum, right lateral view.

The **SOFT PALATE** (1, Fig. 9.8) is a caudal extension from the hard palate that separates the **PHARYNX** (far'inks; throat) into adorsal airway and a ventral food passageway.

The **NASOPHARYNX** (2) is that portion of the pharynx dorsal to the soft palate. It connects with the nasal cavity through the choana (3) and with the laryngeal portion of the pharynx through the **INTRAPHARYNGEAL OSTIUM**, which is a transverses opening formed by the free caudal margin of the soft palate (4), rostrally, and the **PALATO-PHARYNGEAL ARCHES** (5), laterally.

The soft palate, elevated against the dorsal wall of the nasopharynx during swallowing, prevents food from entering the nasal cavity.

The **PHARYNGEAL OSTIA** (6) of right and left **AUDITORY TUBES** are in the dorsolateral wall of the nasopharynx; the auditory tubes extend to the middle ear cavities and function in the equalization of air pressures on the vibrant partition (**TYMPANIC MEMBRANE**) between middle and external ears.

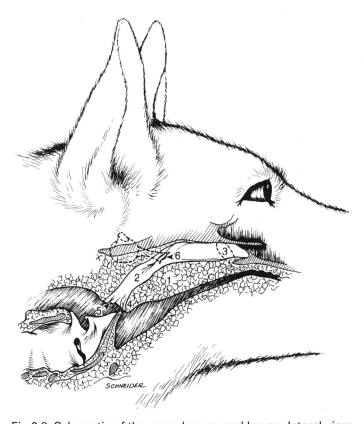

Fig.9.8. Schematic of the nasopharynx and larynx, lateral view.

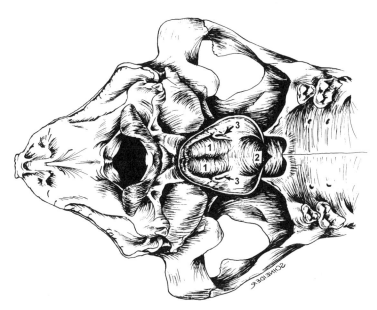

Fig.9.9. Rostrodorsal portion of the nasopharynx, all other soft tissue removed.

PHARYNGEAL TONSILS (1, Fig. 9.9) are inconspicuous paired lymphatic tissues situated on the dorsal surface of the nasopharynx (2) between and adjacent to the auditory tube openings (3). Pharyngeal tonsils have efferent lymph vessels that drain into the **MEDIAL RETROPHARYNGEAL** (behind the pharynx) **LYMPH NODES** (see p. 181). Tonsils do not have afferent lymph vessels since they are directly exposed to foreign substances present in the pharynx.

The **LARYNGOPHARYNX** (1, Fig. 9.10) is that portion of the pharynx dorsal to much of the larynx and between the **NASOPHARYNX** (2) and the cranial end of the **ESOPHAGUS** (3). The dorsal tip, or apex, of the **EPIGLOTTIS** (4) projects into the intrapharyngeal ostium (5) during quiet respiratory movements; during panting or labored breathing the soft palate is elevated, allowing air to pass in and out of the mouth, thus circumventing the greater air resistance of the nasal cavity.

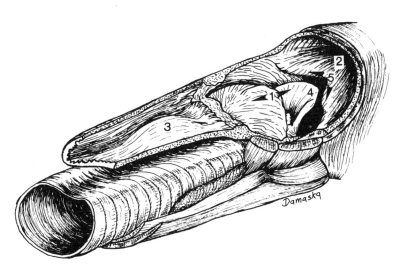

Fig.9.10. Pharynx, larynx, trachea, and esophagus with a portion of the pharynx and esophagus removed, dorsolateral view.

183

Brachycephalic dogs have soft palates that extend caudally past the epiglottis; air movement between nasopharynx and larynx is hampered by this relative extension of the soft palate.

The grooves in the ventral wall of the laryngopharynx (Fig. 9.11), one to each side of the epiglottis (I), are termed **PIRIFORM RECESSES** (2). These recesses are important in the conduction of food through the laryngopharynx such that food does not enter the larynx.

A fold of tissue, the **ARYEPIGLOTTIC FOLD** (3), connects the lateral margin of the epiglottis with the **CUNEIFORM** (ku-ne' i-form; wedge shape) **PROCESS** (4) of the arytenoid cartilage and assists in preventing food from entering the larynx.

The cartilaginous skeleton of the dog larynx (Fig. 9.12) consists primarily of one paired

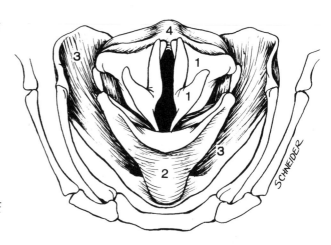

Fig.9.12. Laryngeal cartilages and the hyoid apparatus, rostral view.

cartilage: the arytenoid (ar " e-te' noid) cartilage (1), and three unpaired cartilages: the epiglottis (2), thyroid (shield shape) cartilage (3), and cricoid (kri' koid; ring shape) cartilage (4).

The epiglottis (1, Fig. 9.13) is the farthest rostrally of the laryngeal cartilages; it is described as having an **APEX** (1), a **BASE** (2), right and left **LATERAL MARGINS** (3), and **LARYNGEAL** (4) and **LINGUAL** (ling' gwal; tongue) (5, Fig. 9.14) **SURFACES**.

The **THYROID CARTILAGE** (6) is a U–shaped structure that forms the most lateral and ventral portion of the cartilaginous laryngeal skeleton. The right and left **THYROID LAMINAE** form the lateral walls of the U, with the open portion of the U directed dorsally. Rostral and caudal projections on the dorsal portion of the laminae are termed the **ROSTRAL** (7) and **CAUDAL** (8) **CORNU** (kor 'nu, pl. cornua; horn). The rostral cornu articulates with the thyrohyoid bone (9). The cranial laryngeal nerve enters the larynx ventral to the rostral cornu.

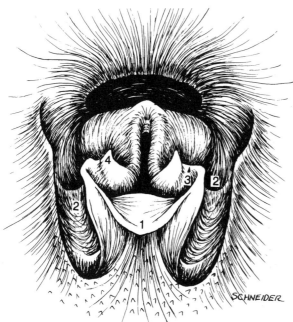

Fig.9.11. Laryngopharynx, rostral view.

184

The **LARYNGEAL PROMINENCE** (10) is palpable on the ventral surface of the thyroid cartilage.

The ventral portion of the thyroid cartilage is notched caudally; this median notch is named the **CAUDAL THYROID NOTCH** (11).

The **CRICOID** (ring form) **CARTILAGE** (12), the most caudal cartilage of the larynx, forms a complete ring around the airway. The cricoid cartilage is wide dorsally and narrow ventrally; the ventral portion is connected to the caudal

thyroid notch by the **CRICOTHYROID LIGAMENT** (an important structure in the horse for surgical entry into the larynx). Much of the dorsal and lateral portions of the cricoid cartilage is positioned medial to the lamina of the thyroid cartilage (6). A small thyroid articular surface (13) is present on each lateral surface of the cricoid for articulation with the thyroid cartilage. Another small arytenoid articular surface (14) is present rostrally on each dorsolateral surface for articulation with the bilaterally paired arytenoid cartilage.

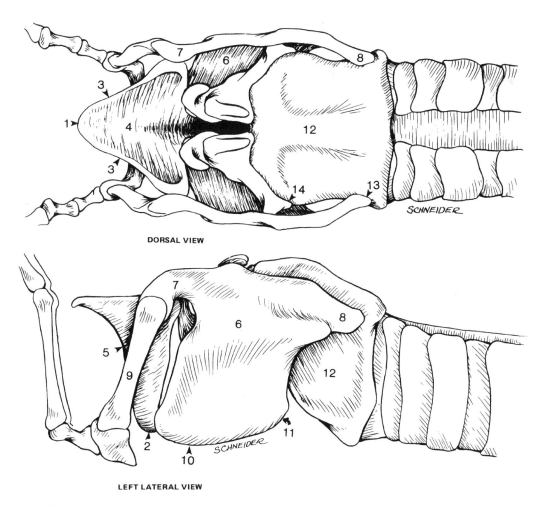

DORSAL VIEW

LEFT LATERAL VIEW

Fig.9.13. Hyoid apparatus laryngeal cartilages and a cranial portion of the trachea.

The **ARYTENOID** (laddle form) **CARTILAGE** (Fig. 9.14) is a paired cartilage situated medial to the lamina of the thyroid cartilage and between the epiglottic (rostrally) and the cricoid cartilage (caudally). Movement of the arytenoid cartilage relative to the other laryngeal cartilages results in the production of noise of various amplitudes (loudness) and frequency (pitch).

Four cartilaginous processes of each arytenoid cartilage, which are of great importance in the functioning of the larynx, are the cuneiform, corniculate, vocal, and muscular processes.

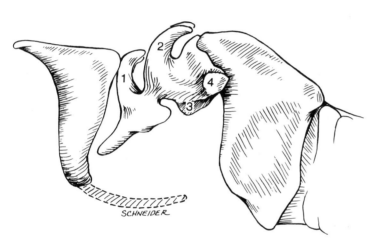

Fig.9.14. Epiglottis and left arytenoid and cricoid cartilages, left lateral view.

The **CUNEIFORM** (wedge form) **PROCESS** (1) is the most rostrodorsal projection of the arytenoid cartilage. The **CORNICULATE PROCESS** (2) is the conspicuous dorsal, hornlike process of the arytenoid. The vocal process (3) is a caudoventral projection of the arytenoid that provides an area of attachment for the vocal fold.

The **MUSCULAR PROCESS** (4) is on the lateral surface of the most caudal portion of the arytenoid cartilage, near the surface that articulates with the cricoid cartilage (3); it is a caudoventral projection of the arytenoid that provides an area of attachment for the vocal fold.

(DIFFERENCES TO BE NOTED IN THE CAT: The arytenoid cartilage of the cat lacks corniculate and cuneiform processes.)

The intrinsic muscles of the larynx attach to the laryngeal cartilages; contraction of an intrinsic muscle produces movement of one cartilage relative to another, resulting in closure or opening of the space between the vocal folds. Seven intrinsic laryngeal muscles are present in the dog, six of which arise or insert on the muscular process (4) of the arytenoid cartilage and hence have arytenoideus as part of their name.

The **CRICOTHYROIDEUS MUSCLE** (1, Fig. 9.15), which does not attach to the arytenoid cartilage, may be observed on the caudoventral surface of the larynx, deep to the sternohyoideus muscle (2). It arises from the ventrolateral surface of the cricoid cartilage (3) and inserts on the caudomedial surface of the thyroid lamina (4). Contraction of this muscle, through innervation by the cranial laryngeal nerve, pivots the ventral portion of the thyroid and cricoid cartilages toward each other, indirectly producing a stretching of the vocal folds.

186

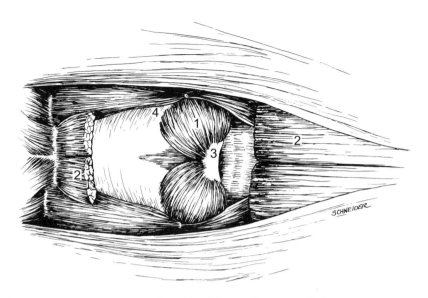

Fig.9.15. Laryngeal and hyoid muscles, ventral view.

Only two of the six muscles that attach to the arytenoid cartilages will be examined here; all six muscles are innervated by the caudal laryngeal nerve, a branch of the recurrent laryngeal.

The **CRICOARYTENOIDEUS DORSALIS MUSCLE** (1, Fig. 9.16) is located on the dorsal surface of the larynx, ventral to some caudal pharyngeal muscles (2) and the cranial portion of the esophagus. Arising on the dorsal surface

of the cricoid cartilage (3) and inserting on the muscular process of the lateral surface of the arytenoid cartilage, it is the only intrinsic laryngeal muscle responsible for enlarging (opening) the space between the vocal folds of each side. The dorsal cricoarytenoid muscle functions by drawing the arytenoid cartilage of each side dorsolaterally. Atrophy of this muscle, which results from damage to a recurrent laryngeal nerve (see p. 434), results in an inability to abduct the vocal folds of the airway.

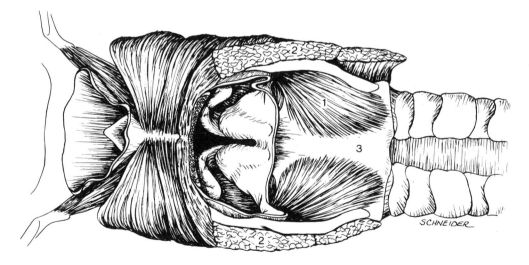

Fig.9.16. Laryngopharynx, larynx, and cranial portion of the trachea, with the caudodorsal portion of the pharynx and esophagus removed, dorsal view.

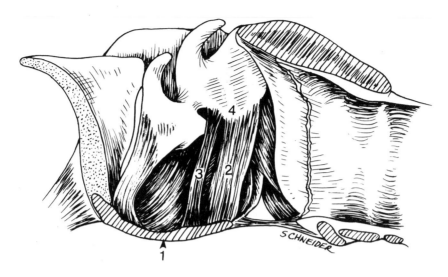

Fig.9.17. Right half of the larynx and cranial portion of the trachea, with the laryngeal mucosa removed, medial view.

Another intrinsic muscle is the **THYROARYTENOIDEUS MUSCLE,** which extends between the median plane of the thyroid cartilage (1, Fig. 9.17), ventrally, and the muscular process of the arytenoid cartilage, dorsally.

The **VOCALIS MUSCLE** (2) is a portion of the thyroarytenoideus that arises from the thyroid cartilage caudal and medial to the remainder of the thyroarytenoideus. The vocalis muscle is adjacent and caudolateral to the **VOCAL LIGAMENT** (3), which extends between the vocal process of the arytenoid (4), dorsally, and the thyroid cartilage, ventrally.

The **VOCAL FOLD** is the membrane that covers the inner surface of the vocal ligament. Vibrations of the vocal fold (bilaterally), resulting from air rushing past these membranes, produce noise, which is then modulated by the remainder of the larynx, pharynx, nose, and mouth into barking, whimpering, and growling sounds of various tones.

The **VESTIBULAR FOLD,** or false vocal fold (1, Fig. 9.18), extends from the base of the cuneiform process (2), dorsally, to the cranioventral portion of the thyroid cartilage (3), ventrally.

The **ADITUS LARYNGIS** (4), the opening into the larynx, is formed by the apical margin of the epiglottis, the aryepiglottic fold, and the membrane between the corniculate processes (5). The cavity of the larynx between the aditus laryngis (rostrodorsally) and the vestibular fold (caudally) is the **LARYNGEAL VESTIBULE** (6).

The **LARYNGEAL VENTRICLE** (7) of each side is a lateral cavity, situated medial to the lamina of the thyroid cartilage, that opens into the larynx between the vestibular and vocal folds (8).

(DIFFERENCES TO BE NOTED IN THE CAT: The vestibular fold is thin and membranous. The feline larynx does not possess a laryngeal ventricle.)

The **GLOTTIS** is the vocal apparatus and consists of the vocal folds and the opening between the folds; the opening is named the **RIMA GLOTTIDIS.** The size of the rima

188

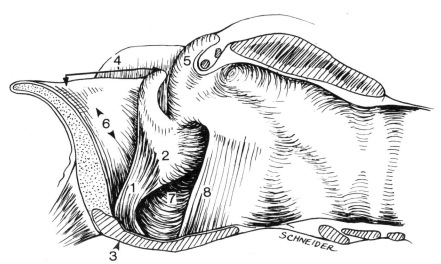

Fig.9.18. Right half of the larynx and cranial portion of the trachea.

glottidis varies with the respiratory cycle, widening during inspiration and narrowing during expiration. By adducting the vocal folds and closing off the rima glottidis during simultaneous contractions of the abdominal muscles, great pressures can be built up within the thoracic, abdominal, and pelvic cavities. These pressures are sufficient to cough up an irritant from the trachea into the mouth, sneeze an irritant out of the nose, force fecal material out the rectum, or aid in propelling a new puppy out into the world of the dog lover.

(DIFFERENCES TO BE NOTED IN THE CAT: The purring of a cat is a complex physiological mechanism present during both inspiratory and expiratory phases of respiration. Some 20–30 contractions per second by intrinsic laryngeal adductor muscles occur during purring. The rima glottidis is thus intermittently closed, periodically increasing then decreasing transglottal pressure. During inspiration in a purring animal, contractions by the thoracic diaphragm are interrupted 20–30 times. Laryngeal and diaphragmatic action potentials alternate. Air flow past the vocal folds produces the purring sound. Cats usually purr in the presence of humans although the sound may not be audible.)

Chapter 10

RESPIRATORY SYSTEM—CAUDAL PORTION

Objectives: Be able to identify structures of the conducting airways, gas exchange area, and pleura.

Trachea; Tracheal Cartilage and Annular Ligaments; Trachealis Muscle

Thoracic Diaphragm and Central Tendon of Diaphragm; Crura of the Diaphragm; Esophageal Hiatus, Aortic Hiatus, and Vena Caval Foramen

Thoracic Cavity; Cranial and Caudal Thoracic Apertures; Mediastinum and Mediastinal Pleura; Diphragmatic and Costal Pleura; Pleural Cavity

Tracheal Carina, Principal Bronchi, Lobar Bronchi

Right Cranial, Right Middle, Right Caudal, and Accessory Lung Lobes

Left Cranial and Left Caudal Lung Lobes

Pulmonary Cardiac Notch; Costal, Medial, Diaphragmatic, and Interlobar Surfaces of the Lung; Ventral and Basal Margins

Costodiaphragmatic and Mediastinal Recesses, Pleural Cupula, Pulmonary Ligament, and Plica Venae Cavae

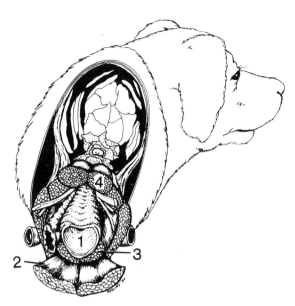

Fig.10.1. Transverse section through the neck.

The **TRACHEA** (1, Fig. 10.1) is situated dorsal to the sternohyoideus (2) and sternothyroideus (3) muscles and ventral to the longus colli muscles (4). It extends caudally from the cricoid cartilage (at the level of the axis) to the tracheal bifurcation into right and left principal bronchi (at the level of the 4th and 5th thoracic vertebrae). The level of the tracheal bifurcation varies somewhat with the phase of respiration.

In the cranial cervical region, the trachea (1, Fig. 10.2) is ventral to the esophagus (2); in the midcervical region it is situated to the right of

the esophagus; and near the base of the heart, it is again situated ventral to the esophagus.

The trachea (Fig. 10.3) consists of an outer wall of **TRACHEAL CARTILAGE (1), ANNULAR LIGAMENTS (2), TRACHEALIS MUSCLE (3)**, and an inner mucous membrane. The U-shaped bands of tracheal cartilage are completed dorsally by the transversely oriented trachealis muscle (3), which is composed of smooth muscle fibers that connect the dorsal free portion of each cartilage band to that of the other side. Contraction of the trachealis muscle results in a constriction of the tracheal lumen (a parasympathetic effect). Annular ligaments encircle the trachea between consecutive tracheal cartilages, attaching adjacent cartilages to each other.

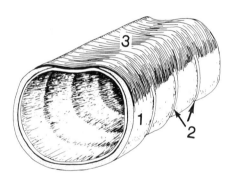

Fig.10.3. Tracheal segment, left craniolateral view.

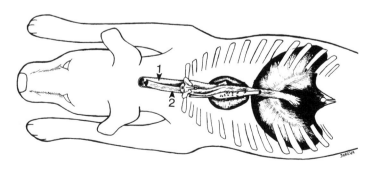

Fig.10.2. Relative positions of trachea and esophagus, dorsal view.

The **THORACIC CAVITY** is that potential space within the walls of the thorax, cranial to the diaphragm ("potential", because it is compactly filled by visceral structures). The internal layers of the thoracic walls are formed bilaterally by the ribs and intercostal muscles, dorsally by the thoracic vertebrae and intervertebral discs (plus the longus colli muscle in the cranial portion of the dorsal thoracic wall), and ventrally by the sternum and transversus thoracis muscles. The "inlet" and "outlet" of the thoracic cavity are termed the cranial and caudal thoracic apertures, respectively.

The **CRANIAL THORACIC APERTURE** (Fig. 10.4) is the oval "space" enclosed by the first pair of ribs and their costal cartilages (laterally), the 1st thoracic vertebra and longus colli muscles (dorsally), and the manubrium of the sternum (ventrally).

Structures that course through the cranial thoracic aperture include the trachea (1), esophagus (2), right and left vagosympathetic trunks (3), right and left common carotid arteries (4), right and left recurrent laryngeal nerves, right and left phrenic nerves, right and left ventral rami of thoracic spinal nerves 1 and 2, and a number of blood vessels.

The **CAUDAL THORACIC APERTURE** (Fig. 10.5) is the area within the line formed by the diaphragmatic attachment to the 3rd and 4th lumbar vertebrae (1), costal arch (2), and sternum (3).

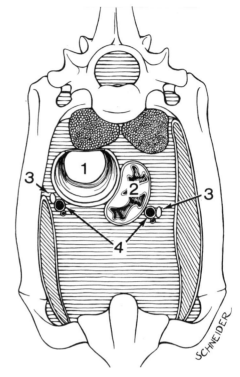

Fig.10.4. Cranial thoracic aperture, cranial view.

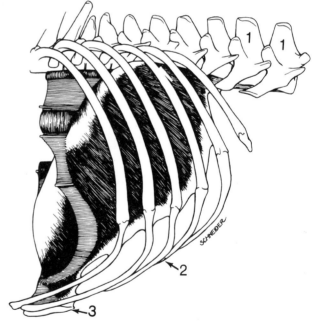

Fig.10.5. Caudal thoracic aperture, left lateral view.

194

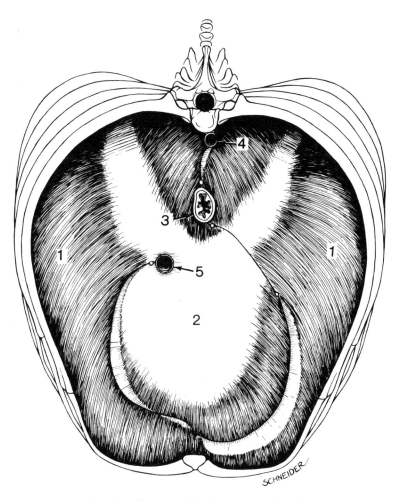

Fig.10.6. Thoracic diaphragm, cranial view.

The **THORACIC DIAPHRAGM** (Fig. 10.6) which divides the thoracic cavity from the abdominal cavity, is composed of a peripheral muscular portion (1) and a **CENTRAL TENDON** (2). A dorsal or lumbar part of the muscular portion attaches caudally to the lumbar vertebrae as the **RIGHT** and **LEFT CRURA OF THE DIAPHRAGM.**

Three openings in the diaphragm through which structures pass between the thoracic and abdominal cavities are the **ESOPHAGEAL HIATUS** (3), the **AORTIC HIATUS** (4), and the **VENA CAVAL FORAMEN** (5).

The cranial surface of the dome-shaped diaphragm projects cranially at the end of expiration approximately to the sixth intercostal space.

The apex of the dome is within the ventral portion of the thoracic cavity.

The diaphragm as the principal muscle of inspiration functions by lengthening the thoracic cavity; however, a paralyzed diaphragm does not critically debilitate an animal.

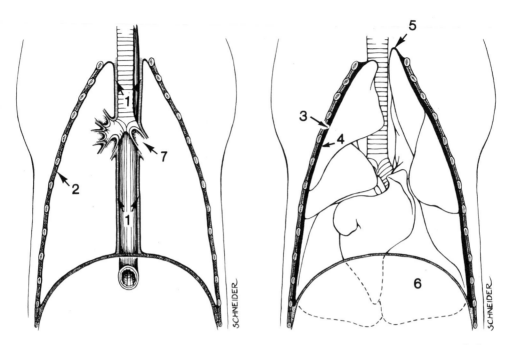

Fig.10.7. Schematics of the pleural cavities pleura, mediastinum, and lungs, ventral view.

The thoracic cavity is divided into right and left portions by a vertical connective tissue septum, the **MEDIASTINUM** (me" de-asti'num) (1, Fig. 10.7), which extends from the cranial thoracic aperture to the diaphragm at the caudal thoracic aperture.

The internal surface of the wall of each portion of the thoracic cavity is lined by a thin, glistening moist membrane, the **PARIETAL** (wall) **PLEURA** (2), named according to its location as the **DIAPHRAGMATIC, COSTAL,** or **MEDIASTINAL PLEURA.** The pleura is attached to the deep layer of the deep fascia (endothoracic fascia) by subserous fascia (see p. 31). Lobes of the right and left lungs project from the mediastinum out into the right and left portions, respectively, of the thoracic cavity. Each pulmonary lobe is surfaced with a visceral (sing. viscus, pl. viscera) layer (3) of pleura (**PULMONARY PLEURA**), which is also tightly bound to pulmonary tissue by means of

subserous fascia. The pulmonary and parietal pleura are held together by forces of capillary attraction and subatmospheric pressure. The normally nonexistent capillary "space" between pulmonary and parietal pleural layers is the **PLEURAL CAVITY** (4). When air is permitted to enter a pleural cavity (right or left), the bond is broken between the pleural linings of the thoracic wall and the pulmonary tissue; the lung and thoracic wall separate since each has a tension pulling it in opposite directions.

Each lung (right and left) has an apex, a base, and a hilus. The **PULMONARY APEX** (5) is the cranial portion that extends toward the cranial thoracic aperture;the left lung extends farther cranially in the dog than the right. The **PULMONARY BASE** (6) is the concave caudal portion of the lung that makes contact with the diaphragmatic parietal pleura. The **HILUS** (7) is the area of the lung through which vessels, nerves, and lobar bronchi enter the lung.

196

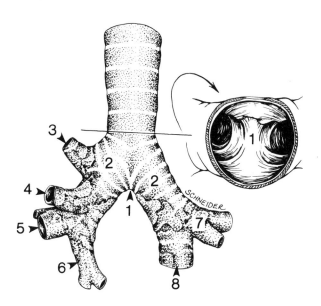

Fig.10.8. Tracheal birfurcation, principal and lobar bronchi

A ridge of cartilage forms part of the medial wall of the two principal bronchi at their origin (Fig. 10.8). The ridge, or **TRACHEAL CARINA** (kah-ri' nah; keel) (1), representing the last tracheal cartilage, is often utilized during intubation of the bronchi.

The right and left **PRINCIPAL BRONCHI** (sing. bronchus) (2) are short and have a structure similar to that of the trachea. Each divides into lobar bronchi, which enter the pulmonary tissue. The lobes of the lung are named in various species according to the presence of lobar bronchi, not according to the fissures present on the surface of the lungs.

The right lung of the dog has a **RIGHT CRANIAL LOBAR BRONCHUS** (3), a **RIGHT MIDDLE LOBAR BRONCHUS** (4), a **RIGHT CAUDAL LOBAR BRONCHUS** (5), and an **ACCESSORY LOBAR BRONCHUS** (6).

The left lung is supplied by a **LEFT CRANIAL LOBAR BRONCHUS** (7) and a **LEFT CAUDAL LOBAR BRONCHUS** (8). Each of the lobar bronchi subdivide into segmental bronchi within the lobes of the lungs.

The lungs are divided by fissures into lobes, each of which is named according to the lobar bronchus that supplies it with air (Fig. 10.9). The right lung is larger than the left. Four lobes are present on the right: **RIGHT CRANIAL** (1), **RIGHT MIDDLE** (2), **RIGHT CAUDAL** (3), and **ACCESSORY** (4).

Two fissures are present on the costal surface of the right lung, one between the cranial and middle lobes (**CRANIAL INTERLOBAR FISSURE**) and one between the middle and caudal lobes (**CAUDAL INTERLOBAR FISSURE**). One interlobar fissure, the caudal interlobar fissure, is present in the costal surface of the left lung dividing it into **CRANIAL** (5) and **CAUDAL** (6) **LOBES**. The cranial lobe is subdivided by an intralobar fissure into **CRANIAL** (5a) and **CAUDAL** (5b) **PARTS**.

The **PULMONARY CARDIAC NOTCH** (1, Fig. 10.10) in the ventral border of the lungs is more pronounced on the right side in the dog, where it is a wedge-shaped "space" situated between the cranial (2) and middle (3) lobes of the lung, deep to the fourth intercostal space. The heart is vulnerable to cardiac puncture via the cardiac notch with relatively little traumatizing of lung tissue. On the left side, a small cardiac notch is situated between cranial and caudal parts of the cranial lobe.

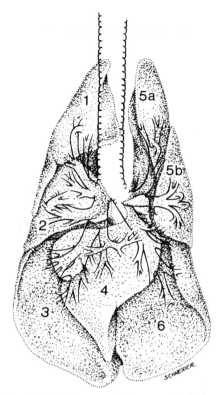

Fig.10.9. Pulmonary lobes, ventral view.

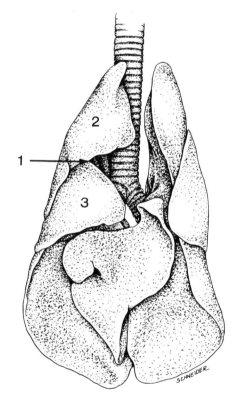

Fig.10.10. Pulmonary lobes, ventral view

Surfaces of the lung are the **COSTAL SURFACE** (1), **MEDIAL SURFACE** (2), **DIAPHRAGMATIC SURFACE** (3), and **INTERLOBAR SURFACES** (4), each of which is self-explanatory (Fig. 10.11). The diaphragmatic surface is the surface over the base of the lung.

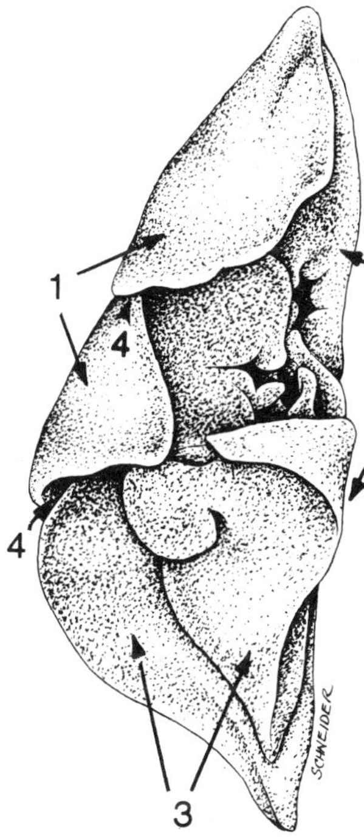

costal pleura (2) from the thoracic wall onto the diaphragm as diaphragmatic pleura (3). The costodiaphragmatic recess contains the basal margin of the lung. During inspiratory and expiratory movements the basal border of the lung slides caudally and cranially in contact with the parietal pleura of the costal and diaphragmatic surfaces. A surgical approach cranial to the line of reflection of the costodiaphragmatic recess would enter the pleural cavity; an incision caudal to the line of reflection would enter the peritoneal cavity of the abdomen.

The **MEDIASTINAL RECESS** (4) is the portion of the right pleural cavity, between the caudal mediastinum (5) and the plica venae cavae (6), that contains the accessory lobe of the right lung.

Fig.10.11. Right lung, ventral view.   Fig.10.12. Right lung.

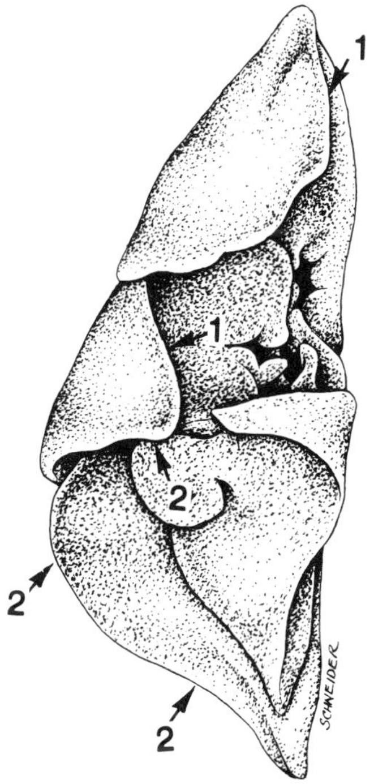

With the lungs fully expanded, the margins of lung tissue formed by the ventral junction of costal and medial surfaces, the **VENTRAL MARGIN** (1, Fig. 10.12), and the peripheral portion of the diaphragmatic surface, the **BASAL MARGIN** (2), form acute angles. The acutely angled ventral and basal margins are positioned in recesses formed by the parietal pleura.

The **COSTODIAPHRAGMATIC RECESS** (1, Fig. 10.13) is formed by the caudal reflection of

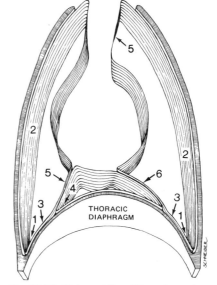

Fig.10.13. Schematic of the pleural reflections, dorsal view.

The **PLEURAL CUPULA** (ku'pu-lah; small cup) (1, Fig. 10.14) is a cup-shaped extension of the pleural cavity of each side that extends cranially through the cranial thoracic aperture. The left pleural cupula extends farther cranially than the right. The apex (2) of each lung (cranial lobe) is situated in contact with the pleural cupula.

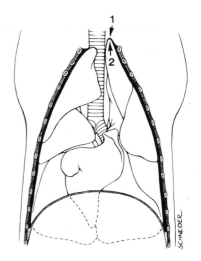

Fig.10.14. Schematic of the thoracic cavity, trachea, and lungs, ventral

The **PULMONARY LIGAMENT** (1, Fig. 10.15) of each lung is a caudodorsal reflection of the visceral or pulmonary pleura from the caudal lobe (2) to the dorsal portion of the mediastinum. It is a caudally tapering continuation of the pleura that attaches the hilus of the lungs to the mediastinum.

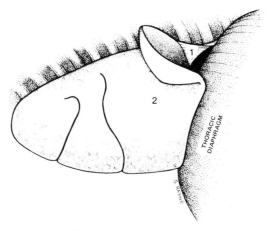

Fig.10.15. Left pulmonary ligament, lateral view

The **PLICA** (pli' kah; fold) **VENAE CAVAE** (1, Fig. 10.16) is a reflection of mediastinal pleura to the right and dorsally from the mediastinum (2); the dorsal extent of the plica vena cava forms a sheath around the caudal vena cava (3). The accessory lobe of the right lung is positioned in the space between the plica and the mediastinum; since the caudal mediastinum is deflected to the left, the accessory lobe appears to be on the left side.

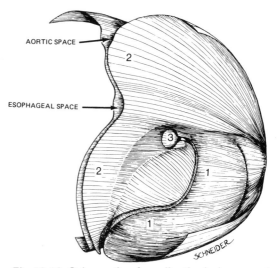

Fig.10.16. Schematic of mediastinal pleura and plica vena cava, right caudolateral view.

200

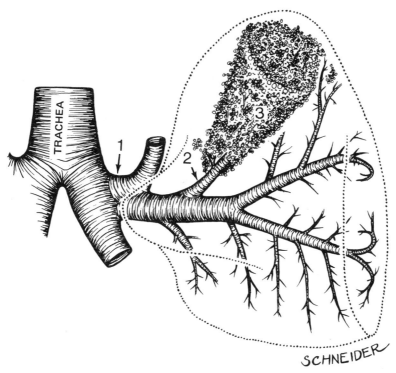

Fig.10.17. Caudal portion of the left cranial pulmonary lobe, ventral view.

Each lobar bronchus (1, Fig. 10.17) divides into many **SEGMENTAL BRONCHI** (2) within the lung tissue. Each segmental bronchus and the tissue it supplies with air is a **BRONCHOPULMONARY SEGMENT** (3), a cone-shaped structure with its apex directed toward the lobar bronchus.

Since the dog has relatively little pulmonary connective tissue, adjacent bronchopulmonary segments are not well separated and may evidence collateral ventilation. Within the bronchopulmonary segment, numerous consecutive branches occur, yielding smaller and smaller bronchi, each with less cartilaginous supportive content.

Airways smaller than 1 mm in diameter are named **BRONCHIOLES** (sing. bronchiole). Unlike the larger bronchi, bronchioles do not contain cartilage in their walls; they are completely encircled by smooth muscle.

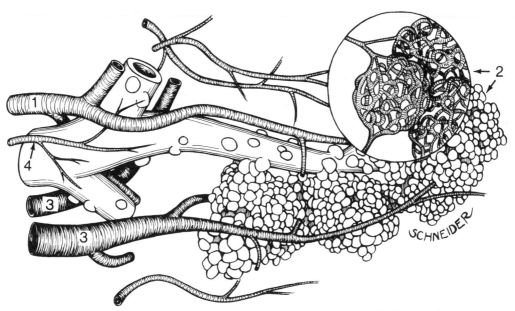

Fig.10.18. Schematic of the terminal airways and alveoli with their vasculature.

Pulmonary arteries (1, Fig. 10.18) carry blood toward the **GASEOUS EXCHANGE AREA**, or **PULMONARY ALVEOLI** (2), where it is oxygenated. Pulmonary veins (3) return the oxygenated blood to the left atrium for delivery to the body via the left ventricle.

The conducting airways are supplied by blood primarily through the bronchial branches (4) of the bronchoesophageal artery (see p. 284). Some shunting of blood occurs between the two arterial systems.

The lung is a vascular filter for large blood-borne particles; particles ranging between 10 and 75 μm are delayed if not retained by the lung capillaries. Physiological emboli such as conglutinated blood cells, fat, bone marrow particles, placental tissue, and tumor cells are often trapped in the lung.

Unit V

Digestive System

In the two chapters that follow, you will study the organization and identity of portions of the digestive tube and associated structures.

Contents:

Chapter 11
DIGESTIVE SYSTEM— ROSTRAL PORTION

Objectives: Be able to identify the structures of the oral cavity, teeth, salivary glands, and pharynx.

Oral Cavity: Oral Vestibule and Oral Cavity Proper

Teeth: Dental Arches, Incisors, Canines, Premolars and Molars; Dental Crown, Dental Neck, and Dental Roots; Dental Root Canal and Dental Cavity

Tongue: Apex, Body, and Root; Lingual Frenulum, Sublingual Caruncle, and Lingual Papillae

Salivary Glands: Parotid, Manibular, Sublingual, and Zygomatic Salivary Glands

Pharynx: Oropharynx, Laryngopharynx, and Nasopharynx; Palatoglossal Arches, Isthmus Faucium, Tonsilar Fossa and Palatine Tonsil

Pharyngeal Muscles: Hyopharyngeus, Thyropharyngeus, and Cricopharyngeus

The digestive system is composed of the digestive tract (mouth, pharynx, and alimentary canal) and associated glands (salivary glands, liver, and pancreas). The alimentary canal consists of the esophagus, stomach, and slender (small) and thick (large) intestines.

The mouth is composed of the oral cavity and surrounding walls: lips, teeth, hard palate, and rostral portion of the tongue.

The **ORAL CAVITY** (Fig. 11.1) consists of the **ORAL VESTIBULE** (1) and the **ORAL CAVITY PROPER** (2). The oral vestibule is the space external to the teeth and gums and internal to the lips and cheeks. The zygomatic and parotid salivary ducts open into the caudodorsal part of the vestibule. The walls of the oral cavity proper are the hard palate, dental arcades, tongue, and adjacent mucosa.

The teeth of the dog are present in two **DENTAL ARCHES, SUPERIOR** and **INFERIOR** (Fig. 11.2). Based upon structure,

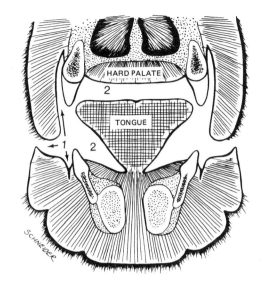

Fig.11.1. Schematic of the oral cavity, transverse section.

three types of teeth are present in the dog: **INCISORS** (1), **CANINES** (2), and **CHEEK TEETH**.

Cheek teeth consist of **PREMOLARS** (3) and **MOLARS** (4), which are difficult to differentiate morphologically.

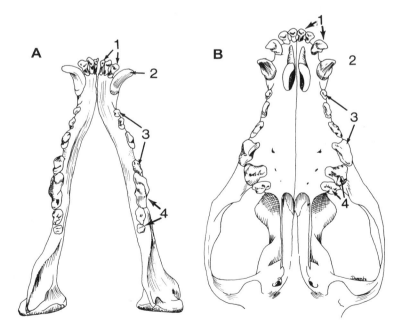

Fig.11.2. Dental arches, inferior and superior.

207

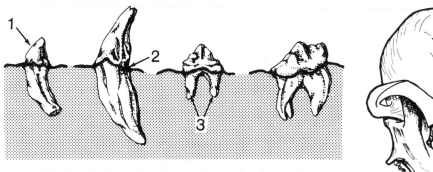

Fig.11.3. Schematic of teeth, illustrating free and embedded portions.

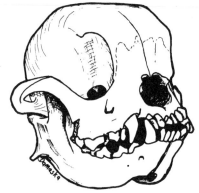

Fig.11.4. Brachycephalic skull.

Each tooth (Fig. 11.3) consists of the **DENTAL CROWN** (1), or free distal portion; the **DENTAL NECK** (2), a slightly constricted portion at the gum line; and the **DENTAL ROOT** or ROOTS (3), the embedded portion. From 5 to 50 apical foramina are present in the apex of each dental root; these foramina open into the **DENTAL ROOT CANAL**, which in turn connects with the **DENTAL CAVITY**. The large dental cavity and wide root canal of the young tooth are partially and gradually filled by **DENTINE**, thus narrowing the lumen.

The shape, position, and number of teeth vary in brachycephalic dogs with shortened faces (Fig. 11.4).

The dog, a **DIPHYODONT** (dif' i-o-dont; grow teeth twice) animal, has two sets of teeth: deciduous and permanent. The pup has no teeth during the first 3 weeks of life; in one half of each dental arch, three incisor, one canine, and three premolar teeth emerge through the gums between the ages of 3 and 6 weeks. The deciduous set of teeth does not contain molars. Thus the dental formula of the pup is 2(Di 3/3; Dc 1/1; Dp 3/3) = 28.

The deciduous teeth are replaced between the ages of 2 to 7 months by the permanent teeth: three incisors, one canine, and three premolars for each half of each dental arch (Table 11.1).

Permanent teeth develop along the **LINGUAL SURFACE** of the roots of deciduous teeth. The blood supply of the deciduous tooth is reduced by pressure of the adjacent growing permanent tooth; after a time the deciduous tooth becomes loosened and is lost.

The **BRACHYODONT** (brak' e-o-dont"; short tooth), or low-crowned, teeth are fully developed at the time of eruption through the gums; only the roots continue to grow, thrusting the crowns into their final position.

Permanent teeth for which no deciduous forerunners exist include the first premolar of each arcade, two molars of each half of the superior arcade, and three molars of each half of the inferior arcade. The dental formula of the permanent dentition is 2(I 3/3; C 1/1; P 4/4; M 2/3) = 42. The dog has its complete set of teeth by 8 months of age.

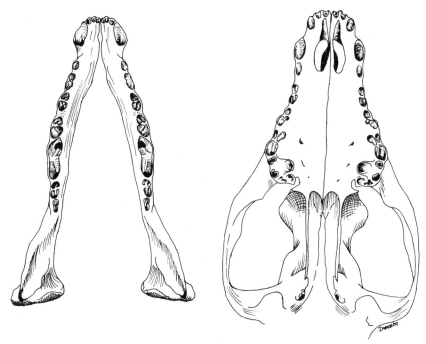

Fig.11.5. Dental alveoli, inferior and superior.

The permanent incisors, canines, first (most rostral) premolars of each arcade, and the most caudal inferior molar (M 3) all have one root each (Fig. 11.5). The root of the canine tooth is compressed laterally and is too large to be easily extracted from the alveolus.

The 2nd and 3rd premolars of both arcades plus the 4th inferior premolar and 1st and 2nd inferior molar teeth have two roots each. The superior 4th premolar is the **SECTORIAL (CARNASSIAL) TOOTH,** which shears against the inferior 1st molar (the sectorial tooth of the mandible).

The superior 4th premolar and each of the maxillary molars (M1 and M2) have three roots.

The relationship of the medial root of maxillary P4 should be noted in reference to the maxillary recess: an abscess in the two lateral roots may open through the maxilla and drain onto the surface of the face; an abscess of the medial root may drain into the maxillary recess.

(FELINE DENTAL FORMULAE. Kitten: 2 Di 3/3; Dc 1/1; Dp 3/2 = 26; adult: 2 I 3/3; C 1/1; P 3/2; M 1/1 = 30. The premolars are numbered 2–4 in the maxilla and 3 and 4 in the mandible. Only the superior fourth premolar has three roots.)

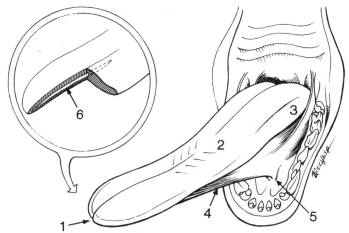

Fig.11.6. Tongue, right rostrolateral view.

The **TONGUE** forms much of the ventral surface of the oral cavity proper and the oropharynx (Fig. 11.6). The tongue is described as having an APEX (1), a BODY (2), and a ROOT (3).

The **LINGUAL FRENULUM** (4) is a median fold of mucosa connecting the free portion of the tongue (ventrally) to the floor of the oral cavity.

The **SUBLINGUAL CARUNCLE** (5), one on each side of the ventral portion of the lingual frenulum, may be observed projecting rostrally; the mandibular and monostomatic sublingual salivary ducts open into the oral cavity through the sublingual caruncles.

The **LYSSA** (lis' ah) (6) is a slender, wormlike structure oriented along the median plane in the apical portion of the tongue.

 LINGUAL PAPILLAE of five shapes are on the dorsal surface of the canine tongue (Fig. 11.7). These structures are filiform (thread shape), conical (cone

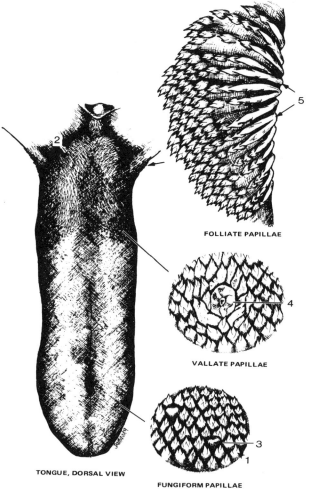

FOLLIATE PAPILLAE

VALLATE PAPILLAE

FUNGIFORM PAPILLAE

TONGUE, DORSAL VIEW

Fig.11.7. Lingual papillae.

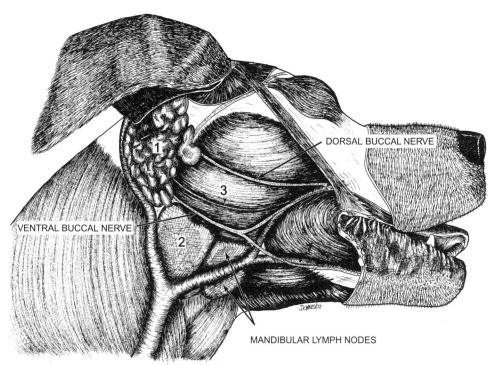

Fig.11.8. Dog head with skin and platysma muscle removed, lateral view.

shape), fungiform (mushroom shape), vallate (cup shape), and foliate (leaf shape). The **FILIFORM PAPILLAE**, (1) are on the rostrodorsal two-thirds of the tongue; they do not have taste receptors.

The **CONICAL PAPILLAE** (2), shaped similarly to the smaller filiform papillae, are over the caudal portion of the tongue; they also do not contain taste receptors.

The **FUNGIFORM PAPILLAE** (3) are primarily on the rostral two-thirds of the tongue; taste buds are present on the dorsal surface of the papillae.

VALLATE PAPILLAE (4) are four to six large, easily observable papillae arranged in a V shape on the dorsal surface of the tongue; the valate papillae demarcate the junction of the rostral two-thirds and caudal one-third of the tongue. Taste buds are also present in vallate papillae.

The **FOLIATE PAPILLAE** (5) are situated on the dorsolateral margins of the tongue, rostral to the palatoglossal arch; they also contain taste receptors. Tonsilar tissue is also present within the dorsal mucosa of the root of the tongue; however, this lymphatic tissue is not observable grossly.

(DIFFERENCES TO BE NOTED IN THE CAT: The filiform papillae have elongate, caudally directed spines composed of KERATIN. Foliate papillae lack taste buds.)

The extrinsic muscles of the tongue, which have already been studied (see p. 137), include the genioglossus, hyoglossus and styloglossus. The salivary glands include the parotid, mandibular sublingual, zygomatic, and buccal glands. The **PAROTID** (1, Fig. 11.8) and **MANDIBULAR** (2) **SALIVARY GLANDS** are most easily observed.

The **PAROTID DUCT** (3) crosses the surface of the masseter muscle and opens through the lip into the oral vestibule near the caudal surface of P4.

211

The **ZYGOMATIC SALIVARY GLAND** (1, Fig. 11.9), present in the orbit ventral to the eye and medial to the zygomatic arch, opens into the oral vestibule opposite the last molar tooth by means of four or five ducts; one major duct opening may be observed caudal to that of the parotid salivary duct. **VENTRAL BUCCAL SALIVARY GLANDS** (2), inconspicuous in most dogs, are present in the caudal and ventral portions of the cheek, adjacent to buccinator muscle fibers.

The mandibular salivary gland (1, Fig. 11.10) and the major portion of the sublingual salivary gland (2) are contained in a common connective tissue capsule; the ducts of both glands course rostrally between the mandible (laterally) and the tongue muscles (medially), to reach the sublingual caruncles (3). The major portion of the sublingual gland is part of the **MONOSTOMATIC** (one mouth) **SUBLINGUAL SALIVARY GLAND** (2). A series of salivary gland

lobules (4) are positioned along the **MAJOR SUBLINGUAL DUCT** and open into the oral cavity proper either through the major duct (monostomatic) or via numerous minor sublingual ducts. These lobules, which have separate ducts opening into the oral cavity, are collectively named the **POLYSTOMATIC SUBLINGUAL SALIVARY GLANDS.**

(DIFFERENCES TO BE NOTED IN THE CAT: The parotid duct opens opposite the second upper cheek tooth into the oral vestibule. The cat has a MOLAR SALIVARY GLAND in the submucosal fascia of the inferior lip, near the oral commissure.)

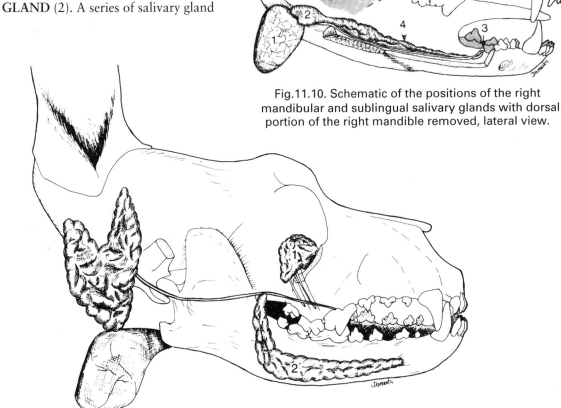

Fig.11.10. Schematic of the positions of the right mandibular and sublingual salivary glands with dorsal portion of the right mandible removed, lateral view.

Fig.11.9. Schematic of the positions of salivary glands, right side of the skull.

The **PHARYNX** (Fig. 11.11) is subdivided into oropharynx (1), nasopharynx (2), and laryngopharynx (3) (see p. 183).

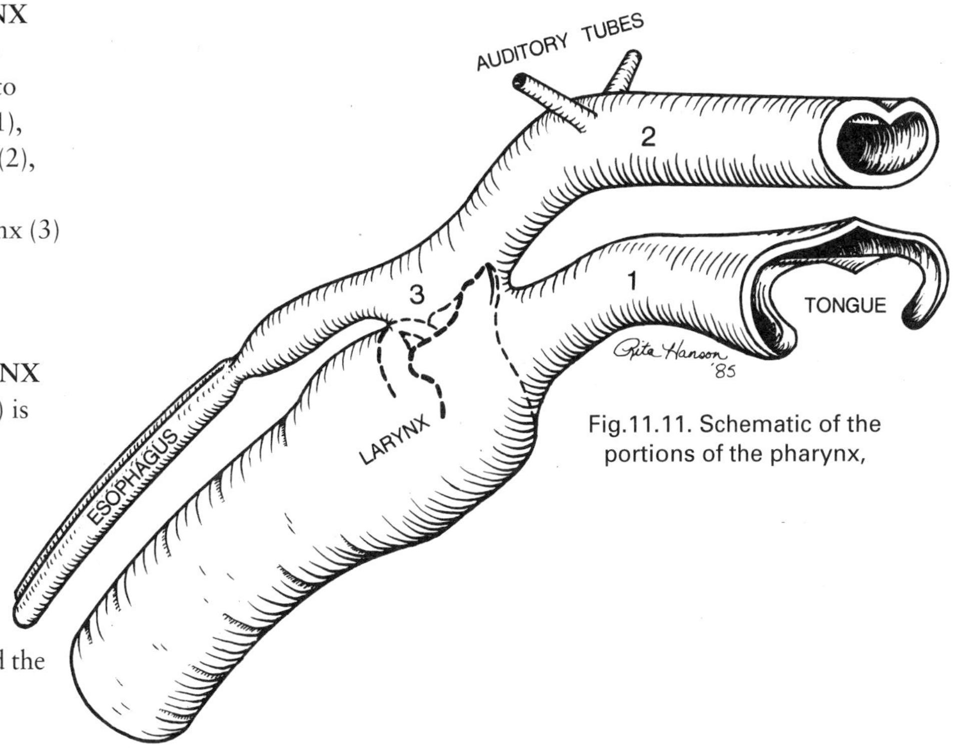

The **OROPHARYNX** (1, Fig. 11.12) is that portion of the pharynx between the oral cavity proper (2) and the **LARYNGOP HARYNX** (3). The **PALATOGLOSSAL ARCHES** (4), or membranous folds, extending between the base of the tongue and the rostral portion of the soft palate (more easily observed by pulling on the tongue), demarcate the caudal boundary of the oral cavity proper.

Fig.11.11. Schematic of the portions of the pharynx,

The **ISTHMUS** (is' mus) **FAUCIUM** (5), or opening into the pharynx, is the transversely oriented space between the palatoglossal arches. The caudal portion of the oropharynx merges with the laryngopharynx at the level of the epiglottis and caudal border of the soft palate.

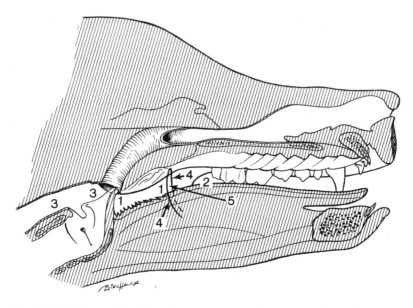

Fig.11.12. Schematic of the pharynx, larynx, trachea, and esophagus as observed in a sagittal section, medial view.

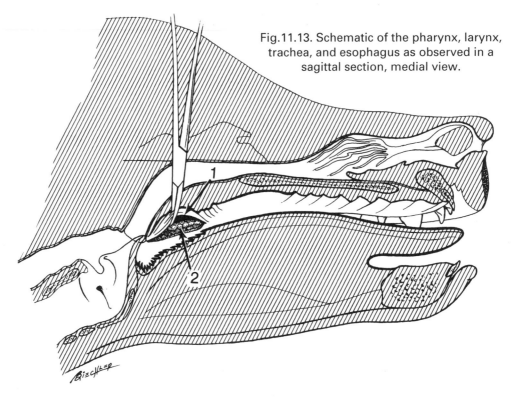

Fig.11.13. Schematic of the pharynx, larynx, trachea, and esophagus as observed in a sagittal section, medial view.

A **TONSILAR FOSSA** (1, Fig. 11.13) containing the **PALATINE TONSIL** (2) is present in the lateral wall of the oropharynx; the palatine tonsil drains by way of efferent vessels into the more caudally situated medial retropharyngeal lymph node (see p. 355).

Various palatine muscles (which act upon the soft palate) and pharyngeal muscles (which act upon the pharynx) are present in the dog; of these, only three pharyngeal constrictors are described here (Fig. 11.14).

The **HYOPHARYNGEUS** (1), **THYROPHARYNGEUS** (2), and **CRICOPHARYNGEUS** (3) are paired muscles that arise from the thyrohyoid, thyroid lamina, and cricoid cartilage, respectively.
The three muscles insert in series, from rostral to caudal, on the dorsal median raphe of the pharynx.

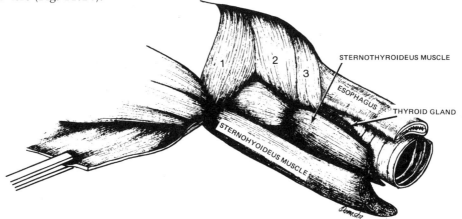

STERNOTHYROIDEUS MUSCLE

ESOPHAGUS

THYROID GLAND

STERNOHYOIDEUS MUSCLE

Fig.11.14. Left pharyngeal constrictor muscles, ventrolateral view.

The caudal portion of the laryngopharynx (1, Fig. 11.15) is situated dorsal to the cricoid cartilage of the larynx. An annular fold of the mucous membrane, the **PHARYNGOESOPHAGEAL LIMEN** (li' men; boundary) (2), indicates the rostral extent of the esophagus.

Deglutition (swallowing) is a complex act of moving food from the oral cavity to the stomach. Once food enters the oropharynx an involuntary act of swallowing is initiated.

The intrapharyngeal ostium is closed by elevation of the soft palate; the root of the tongue is raised against the soft palate; the larynx is drawn rostrodorsally, resulting in the epiglottis being passively hinged caudally; and the esophagus is dilated and drawn rostrally to receive the food.

Semiliquid or liquid food passes around each side of the epiglottis and aryepiglottic membranes through the piriform recesses to reach the esophagus. Solid food may be thrown over the dorsal surface of the epiglottis; closure of the vocal folds (reduction of the rima glottidis) is an additional safeguard for the respiratory system.

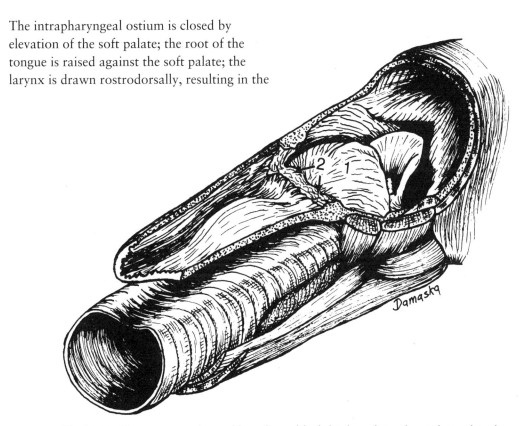

Fig.11.15. Pharyngoesophageal junction with right dorsolateral esophageal and pharyngeal walls removed.

Chapter 12

DIGESTIVE SYSTEM— CAUDAL PORTION

Objectives: Be able to identify and understand the normal positions of the esophagus, stomach, duodenum, ileojejunum, and ascending, transverse and descending colon. Also, be able to identify the major glands, ducts, and supportive membranes associated with the digestive tube.

Esophagus: Cervical, Thoracic and Abdominal Portions; Esophageal Hiatus

Peritoneum: Greater and Lesser Omenta; Mesogastrium, Mesoduodenum, Mesojejunoileum, Mesocolon; Omental Bursa and Omental Foramen

Stomach: Greater and Lesser Curvatures; Parietal and Visceral Surfaces; Cardiac and Pyloric Sphincters and Ostia; Cardia, Fundus, Body, and Pylorus; Angular Incisure, Pyloric Antrum, and Pyloric Canal

Duodenum: Cranial and Caudal Duodenal Flexures; Descending and Ascending Portions; Right Lobe of the Pancreas; Pancreatic and Common Bile Ducts; Duodenocolic Fold

Liver: Right Medial, Right Lateral, Quadrate, Left Medial and Left Lateral Lobes; Gall Bladder, Cystic Duct, and Hepatic Ducts; Falciform, Round, Coronary, and Triangular Hepatic Ligaments; Hepatogastric and Hepatoduodenal Ligaments

Pancreas: Right Lobe, Body, and Left Lobe

Slender Intestine: Duodenum and Jejunoileum; Root of the Mesentery; Ileal Spincter and Ostium

Thick Intestine: Cecum, Cecal Sphincter, and Cecocolic Ostium; Lymph Nodules; Ascending Colon, Right Colic Flexure, Transverse Colon, Left Colic Flexure, Descending Colon

Rectum, Anal Canal; Internal and External Anal Sphincters; Anal Sacs; Pelvic Diaphragm, Ischiorectal Fossa, Rectococcygeus Muscle

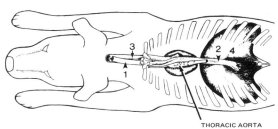

Fig.12.1 Esophagus, dorsal view.

The esophagus (Fig. 12.1) is divided into cervical (1), thoracic (2), and abdominal portions. The cervical portion arises from the laryngopharynx at the pharyngoesophageal limen. The cricopharyngeus muscle forms a physiological sphincter (not well enough developed to be regarded as an anatomical sphincter).

The cervical portion of the esophagus is at first (cranially) dorsal to the trachea (3) and then is situated to the left of the trachea (at the midcervical region). The esophagus is very close to the median plane in the midthoracic region, where it is situated within the mediastinum (between the right and left pleural cavities) and dorsal to the tracheal bifurcation.

After passing through the thoracic diaphragm via the esophageal hiatus (4), a very short segment of esophagus is situated within the abdominal cavity.

The serous membrane that surfaces the wall of the abdominal cavity and the viscera (Fig. 12.2) is termed **PARIETAL** (1) and **VISCERAL** (2) **PERITONEUM** (per" i-to-ne' um, pl. peritonea; stretching around), respectively.

The peritoneum provides a moist, slippery surface that facilitates digestive movements and prevents adhesions of viscera to the abdominal wall. Infections of the peritoneal cavity are minimized by the serous membrane (production of a fluid and cellular exudate in response to an infection) and lymphatic tissue (vessels, lymphatic foci, and nodes).

Embryologically the parietal peritoneum is connected to visceral peritoneum ventrally by **PRIMITIVE VENTRAL MESENTERY** (3) and dorsally by **PRIMITIVE DORSAL MESENTERY** (4). Most of the ventral mesentery is absent in the mature animal; a portion is present between the stomach and liver, between the liver and the ventral median line of the abdominal cavity, and between the urinary bladder and the ventral median line of the abdominal wall. The dorsal mesentery is intact in the mature animal and is named according to the structure it supports, e.g., mesoduodenum, mesojejunum, mesoileum, mesocolon, and mesorectum.

The mesojejunum and mesoileum are collectively known as the **MESENTERY**.

The **PERITONEAL CAVITY** is the space between parietal and visceral peritonea. This cavity normally is only

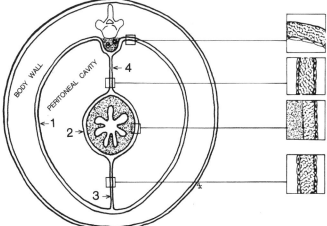

Fig.12.2. Schematic of the peritoneum and mesentery.

a potential space of microscopic thickness; the amount of space shown in Figure 12.2 and the dissected cadaver is very misleading.

The parietal peritoneum is attached superficially by subserous fascia to the deepest layer of deep fascia, the transversalis fascia (see p. 31). Fat is stored in the subserous fascia.

The transversalis fascia is continuous with the deep fascia of the thoracic cavity (endothoracic fascia) through the three openings in the thoracic diaphragm (esophageal hiatus, aortic hiatus, and vena caval foramen) and through the "spaces" dorsolateral to the diaphragmatic crura (lumbocostal arch).

Displacement of an abdominal structure through the esophageal hiatus is termed a **HIATAL HERNIA.**

The **DORSAL MESOGASTRIUM,** or portion of the mesentery between the dorsal body wall and the stomach, is commonly known as the **GREATER OMENTUM** (o-men' tum, pl. omenta; fat skin) (Fig. 12.3). It arises from the dorsal body wall as a double layer of serous membranes tightly adhered to each other by connective tissue (i.e., the dorsal parietal peritoneum reflects ventrally from the right and left sides of the abdominal cavity to form the transparent double serous–layered membrane).

A DEEP PART (1) of the greater omentum descends caudally to near the urinary bladder, then reflects or loops cranioventrally as the **SUPERFICIAL PART** (2); the "space" situated between the deep and superficial parts of the folded sheetlike greater omentum is the **OMENTAL BURSA** (3). Thus the greater omentum extends caudally as a folded sheet between the intestines and the ventral abdominal wall and between the intestines (craniodorsally) and the urinary bladder (caudoventrally).

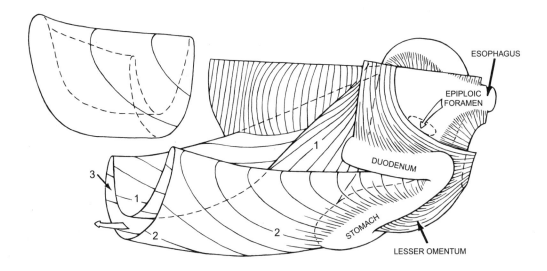

Fig.12.3. Greater omentum and omental bursa, right lateral view.

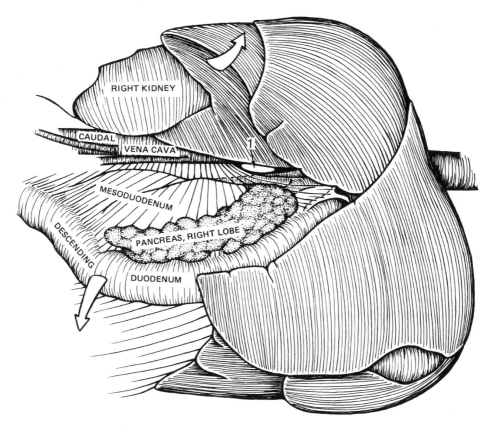

Fig.12.4. Liver, duodenum, pancreas, and epiploic foramen, right lateral view.

The superficial portion of the greater omentum attaches cranially to the greater curvature of the stomach.

The spleen and the left lobe of the pancreas are within and supported by the greater omentum. The spleen is in contact with the left abdominal wall.

The omental bursa is an extensive "space" that opens into the greater peritoneal sac through the **OMENTAL (EPIPLOIC)** (ep" i-plo' ik) **FORAMEN** (1, Fig. 12.4); the omental foramen is a small, cleft like opening situated between the caudal vena cava (dorsally) and the complex of common bile duct, hepatic portal vein, and gastroduodenal artery (ventrally).

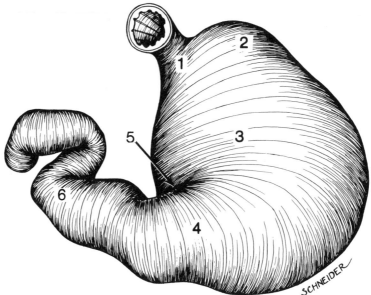

Fig.12.5. Stomach, cranial view.

The **STOMACH** (Fig. 12.5), the largest dilatation of the alimentary canal, extends from the esophagus to the small intestine. The four parts of the stomach are the cardiac portion, fundus, body, pyloric portion, and pylorus. The **CARDIAC** (car'de-ak; relating to heart) **PORTION** (1), which arises from the esophagus, is the part that contains the pacemaker cells; these cells establish the inherent contractions of the stomach, the rhythm of which is modified by the autonomic and endocrine systems.

The **GASTRIC FUNDUS** (2), a dome-shaped diverticulum adjacent and dorsal to the cardiac portion, is positioned dorsally on the left side of the abdominal region in serous contact with the diaphragm. The gastric fundus is apparent in radiographs since it is usually filled with air.

The **BODY** (3) of the stomach is that portion between the fundus and pyloric portion.

The **PYLORIC PORTION** (4) of the stomach is usually partly separated from the body by the

ANGULAR INCISURE (5). The **PYLORUS** (pi-lo' rus; gate) (6) is the caudal portion of the stomach from which the small intestine originates.

The stomach has a **GREATER CURVATURE** (1, Fig. 12.6), which makes contact with the diaphragm dorsally, left laterally, and ventrally. The **LESSER CURVATURE** (2) and the greater curvature of the stomach form nearly concentric arcs. The surface of the stomach directed dorsocranially toward the liver is the **PARIETAL**

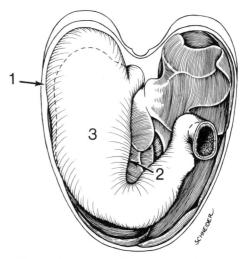

Fig.12.6. Stomach in situ, caudal view.

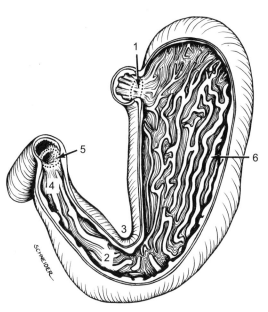

Fig.12.7. Stomach, with a portion of the
parietal surface removed, cranial view.

SURFACE. The **VISCERAL SURFACE** (3) is directed caudoventrally toward the intestines. When empty, the stomach is situated within the rib cage (cranial to the osseous caudal thoracic aperture); however, when full, the stomach distends and occupies the abdominal cavity as far caudally as the transverse level of the umbilicus.

Both the cardiac portion and pylorus of the stomach are structurally modified to regulate the passage of ingested matter. In the cardiac portion a circular layer of smooth muscle forms the **CARDIAC SPHINCTER** (Fig. 12.7), which anatomically is a weakly developed structure (physiologically it may effectively constrict the esophagealgastric junction). The opening from the esophagus through the cardiac sphincter is the **CARDIAC OSTIUM** (1).

The pyloric portion is composed of the pyloric antrum and pyloric canal. The **PYLORIC ANTRUM** (2) is a slightly dilated region distal to the **ANGULAR INCISURE** (3) of the stomach.

The **PYLORIC CANAL** (4) is the caudal narrow part of the pyloric portion leading from the antrum to the pylorus. The pylorus contains a strong, well-developed band of circular smooth muscle, the **PYLORIC SPHINCTER**; the **PYLORIC OSTIUM** (5) is the opening within the sphincter that connects the lumen of the pyloric canal with that of the cranial portion of the small intestine.

Folds or wrinkles present over much of the internal surface of the stomach are named **GASTRIC RUGAE** (sing. ruga; fold) (**6**).

The **DUODENUM**
(du" o-de'num or du-od'
e-num) (Fig. 12.8), the first portion
of the small intestine, is composed of a
cranial, descending, and ascending
portions. The **CRANIAL PORTION**
(1) is the initial part of the duodenum
situated between the pylorus and the
cranial bend of the duodenum (this
portion is often confused with the
pylorus).

The **CRANIAL DUODENAL
FLEXURE** (2) is the bend in the
duodenum that occurs near the level of the
9th and 10th ribs on the right side. The
cranial portion of the duodenum and
cranial duodenal flexure are relatively
fixed in position by strong attachments to
the liver.

The **DESCENDING PORTION** (3)
of the duodenum extends from the
cranial duodenal flexure along
the right side of the abdominal
cavity to the level of the tuber
coxae.

The **CAUDAL DUODENAL
FLEXURE** (4) is the bend of
the duodenum between
descending and ascending
portions; this flexure is
positioned near the right tuber
coxae.

The **ASCENDING PORTION**
(5) of the duodenum extends
from the caudal duodenal
flexure across the median
plane to an ill-defined
**DUODENOJEJUNAL
FLEXURE**.

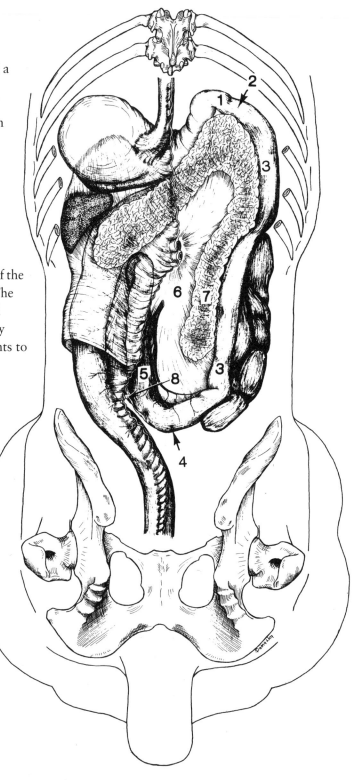

Fig.12.8. Stomach, duodenum, pancreas, and colon, dorsal view.

224

The portion of the dorsal mesentery attached to the duodenum is termed the **MESODUODENUM** (6, Fig. 12.8). The portion of the mesoduodenum that attaches the descending duodenum to the dorsal body wall also contains and supports the **RIGHT LOBE OF THE PANCREAS** (7).

The mesoduodenum of the ascending duodenum is attached to the mesocolon of the descending colon; this mesenteric attachment is called the **DUODENOCOLIC FOLD** (8).

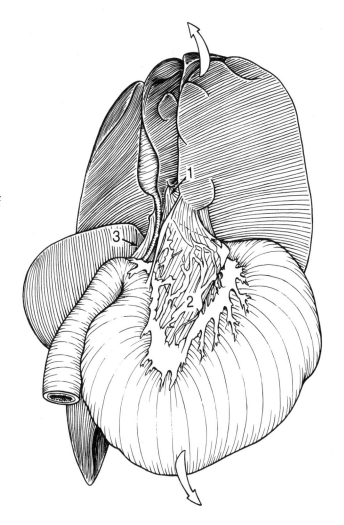

Fig.12.9. Caudal surface of the liver, parietal surface of

The **LESSER OMENTUM** (Fig. 12.9) connects the lesser curvature of the stomach and the cranial portion of the duodenum to the **PORTA** (entrance) **OF THE LIVER** (1). The portion of lesser omentum spanning the distance from stomach to liver is named the **HEPATOGASTRIC LIGAMENT** (2).

The **HEPATODUODENAL LIGAMENT** (3) is the portion of lesser omentum between the liver and the cranial portion of the duodenum. The hepatoduodenal ligament is fused with the cranial portion of the mesoduodenum.

In young dogs the **FALCIFORM HEPATIC LIGAMENT** extends in the median plane from the liver to the ventral abdominal wall; in older dogs the falciform ligament may be observed as a fatty remnant on the deep surface of the abdominal wall in the umbilical region. The **ROUND LIGAMENT OF THE LIVER**, observed in some young dogs as an atrophied remnant of the umbilical vein along the caudodorsal edge of the falciform ligament, extends from the fatty tissue near the umbilicus toward the porta of the liver. A portion of the diaphragmatic surface of the liver is fused by connective tissue to the diaphragm.

225

The **CORONARY** (crown) **HEPATIC LIGAMENT** is formed by a circular reflection of visceral peritoneum away from the liver mass onto the diaphragm as parietal peritoneum. Right and left lateral extensions (**TRIANGULAR LIGAMENTS**) of the coronary hepatic ligament are present as folds of mesentery.

From the porta of the liver (1, Fig. 12.10), ventrally and laterally, the liver is divided by deep fissures into lobes. Six lobes are present in the liver of the dog.

The **GALL BLADDER** (2) is in a fossa between the **RIGHT MEDIAL LOBE** (3) and the **QUADRATE LOBE** (4). The **LEFT MEDIAL LOBE** (5) is in contact with the left surface of the quadrate lobe; the **LEFT LATERAL LOBE** (6) is the lobe situated furthest to the left.

The **RIGHT LATERAL LOBE** (7) is positioned to the right of the right medial lobe. The sixth lobe is the **CAUDATE LOBE** (8), which is positioned dorsally on the right side. Two processes of the caudate lobe should be observed: the **CAUDATE PROCESS** (8a) is in contact with the right kidney, and the **PAPILLARY PROCESS** (8b) is in contact with the lesser curvature of the stomach.

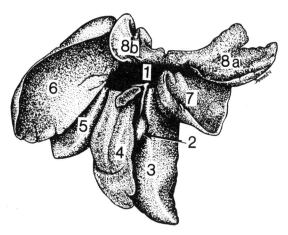

Fig.12.10. Liver, caudal view.

The gall bladder (1, Fig. 12.11) is connected to the **BILE DUCT** (2) by the **CYSTIC** (bladder) **DUCT** (3). Ducts that conduct bile from the liver, where it is formed, are named **HEPATIC DUCTS** (4). The hepatic ducts combine to form a **COMMON HEPATIC DUCT**. The bile duct is formed by the combination of the common hepatic and cystic ducts.

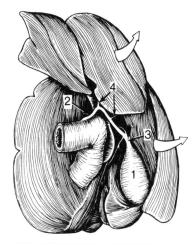

DOG IN VENTRAL RECUMBENCY

Fig.12.11. Liver, gall bladder, and biliary ducts, right caudolateral view.

In the dog some small ducts (**HEPATOCYSTIC DUCTS**) pass from the liver directly to the gall bladder. Much of the bile formed in the liver passes through the hepatic ducts and then up the cystic duct to the gall bladder for storage. When needed in the duodenum, bile is forced out of the gall bladder through the cystic duct and down the bile duct to the duodenum. The bile duct passes through the hepatoduodenal ligament to reach the cranial portion of the descending duodenum. After passing obliquely through the right dorsolateral wall of the duodenum, the bile duct discharges bile through the **MAJOR DUODENAL PAPILLA**, which is partially obscured by the mucosal surface.

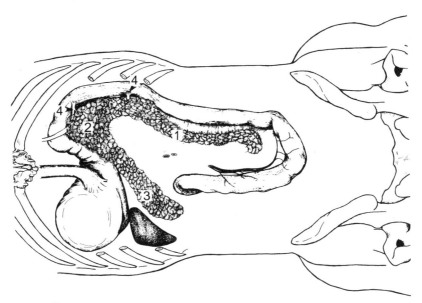

Fig.12.12. Stomach, duodenum, and pancreas, dorsal view.

The right lobe of the pancreas (1, Fig. 12.12) has already been observed in the mesoduodenum of the descending duodenum. The **BODY OF THE PANCREAS** (2) is the portion near the cranial duodenal flexure. The **LEFT LOBE OF THE PANCREAS** (3) is positioned in a deep portion of the greater omentum.

The **PANCREATIC DUCTS** (4) interconnect within the pancreatic tissue. Pancreatic juice is usually carried into the cranial portion of the descending duodenum by means of two ducts: one duct opens into the duodenum through the

major duodenal papilla with the bile duct, the other (a larger duct) opens into the duodenum through the mucosa, 1–4 inches caudal to the major papilla.

The **SLENDER** (small) **INTESTINE** is composed of **DUODENUM, JEJUNUM, and ILEUM**. The jejunum and ileum, which are situated dorsal to the greater omentum in the caudoventral portion of the abdominal cavity, are difficult to differentiate. Both the jejunum and ileum are supported by mesentery, which allows them considerable movement.

The mesenteries gather toward one area of attachment (dorsally) near the level of the 2nd lumbar vertebra (Fig. 12.13); this narrow area of attachment is the **ROOT OF THE MESENTERY** (1) through which the proximal portion of the cranial mesenteric artery passes.

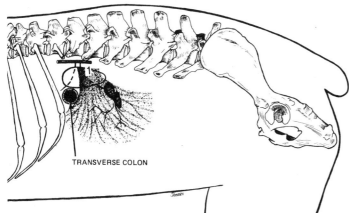

TRANSVERSE COLON

Fig.12.13. Schematic of the root of the mesentery, left lateral view.

227

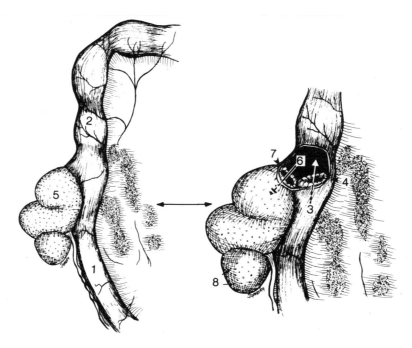

Fig.12.14. Ileocolic and cecocolic junctions, ventral view.

The terminal portion of the ileum and the first part of the large intestine (ascending colon and cecum) are on the right dorsal side of the body (Fig. 12.14). The lumen of the ileum (1) is continuous with that of the ascending colon (2) through the **ILEAL OSTIUM** (3). The circular layer of smooth muscle around the ileal orifice forms the **ILEAL SPHINCTER MUSCLE** (4).

The **CECUM** (5) is a blind-ending diverticulum off the first portion of the ascending colon. The lumen of the cecum is continuous with that of the colon through the **CECOCOLIC OSTIUM** (6); the **CECAL SPHINCTER MUSCLE** (7) encircles the cecocolic orifice.

LYMPH NODULES (8), which occur in the wall of much of the intestine, are quite noticeable in the gas-filled cecum of the dead animal.

(DIFFERENCES TO BE NOTED IN THE CAT: The cecum of the cat is a short, comma–shaped structure.)

The **THICK** (large) **INTESTINE** is composed of colon, cecum, rectum, and anal canal (Fig. 12.15).

The short **ASCENDING COLON** (1) passes cranially in the right dorsal portion of the abdominal cavity to a transverse level near the root of the mesentery (2). A bend, the **RIGHT COLIC FLEXURE** (3), marks the junction of the ascending and transverse colons.

The **TRANSVERSE COLON** (4) is transversely oriented across the dorsal portion of the abdominal cavity cranial to the root of the mesentery.

On the left side, the **LEFT COLIC FLEXURE** (5) occurs dorsally between the transverse and descending portions of the colon.

As the **DESCENDING COLON** (6) enters the pelvic canal it passes caudally, dorsal to the longitudinal axis of the trunk, as the rectum (straight) (7).

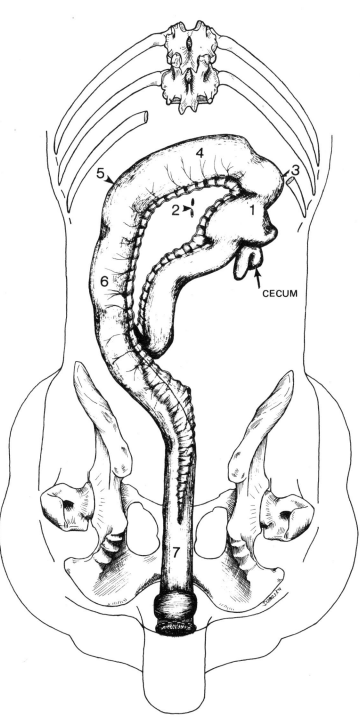

Fig.12.15. Large intestine, dorsal view.

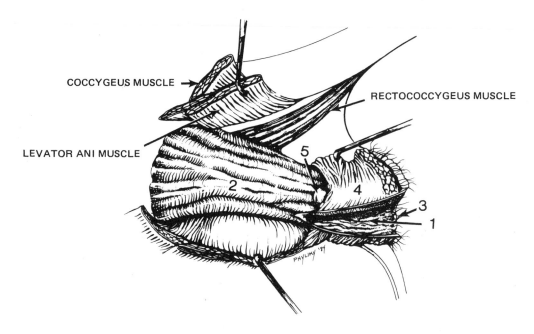

Fig.12.16. Caudal portion of the alimentary canal, left lateral view with part of the wall incised to reveal the mucosa.

The **ANAL CANAL** (1, Fig. 12.16) is the short terminal part of the large intestine extending from the rectum (2) to the **ANUS** (3). It is surrounded by sphincter muscles: the **EXTERNAL** (4) and **INTERNAL ANAL SPHINCTERS**.

The internal anal sphincter is composed of smooth muscle continuous with the smooth muscle of the rectum. The external anal sphincter is composed of striated (voluntary) muscle that encircles collectively the anal canal and the **PARANAL SINUSES** (5) of both sides (see p. 21).

The **PELVIC DIAPHRAGM** (Figs. 12.17, 12.18) is an important muscular and fascial structure in the caudal portion of the pelvic canal. Prolapse of pelvic viscera and perianal hernias are normally prevented, in part, by the presence of a strong pelvic diaphragm. The pelvic diaphragm also has an important role in terminating the act of defecation.

The two striated muscles constituting the muscular portion of the pelvic diaphragm,

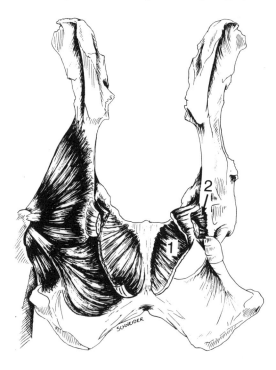

Fig. 12.17. Pelvic girdle, deep muscles of the coxal articulation, and pelvic diaphragm, dorsal view.

230

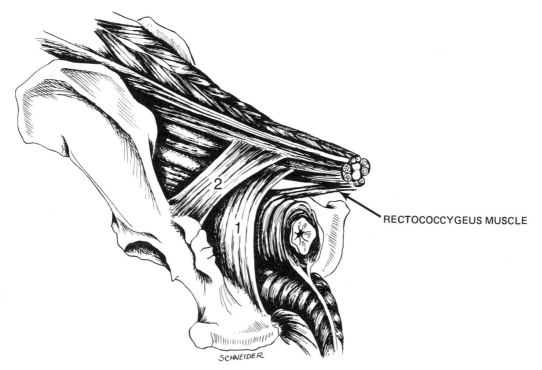

RECTOCOCCYGEUS MUSCLE

SCHNEIDER

Fig.12.18. Pelvic girdle, tail muscles,and muscles in the ischiorectal fossa, caudolateral view.

the **LEVATOR ANI** (1) and **COCCYGEUS** (kok-sij' e-us) (2), may be located by cleaning fat out of the **ISCHIORECTAL FOSSA** (see p. 131–32).

The levator ani is a broad, flat muscle that arises from the ventral floor and lateral wall of the pelvic cavity and inserts on the 4th to 7th caudal vertebrae.

The coccygeus is a shorter, stronger muscle that arises from the ischiatic spine and inserts on the 2nd to 4th caudal vertebrae; thus the thicker coccygeus is lateral and slightly cranial to the dorsal portion of the levator ani muscle.

A third muscle associated with the caudal portion of the rectum/anus is the **RECTOCOCCYGEUS MUSCLE** (1, Fig. 12.19). As a caudal continuation of the outer smooth muscle of the rectum, it passes caudodorsally from the dorsal surface of the rectum to insert on the ventral surface of the caudal vertebrae.

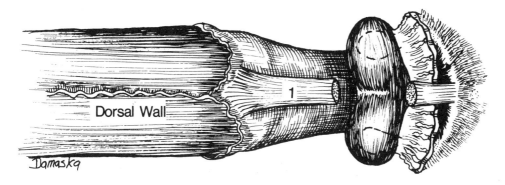

Dorsal Wall

Damaska

Fig.12.19. Rectum, anal canal, and paranal sinuses, dorsal view.

Unit VI

Urogenital System

In the two chapters that follow, you will study the organization and identity of structures of the female and male urinary and reproductive systems.

Contents:

233

Chapter 13

FEMALE REPRODUCTIVE SYSTEM

Objectives: Be able to identify the structures of the urinary and female reproductive systems and to locate their normal positions in the body.

Urinary: Kidney, Ureter, Urinary Bladder, and Urethra; Renal Hilus, Sinus, and Pelvis; Renal Capsule, Renal Cortex, and Renal Medulla; Renal Papilla and Renal Crest; Apex, Body, and Neck of Urinary Bladder; Ureteric Crest, Ureteric Ostia and Trigone of the Bladder; External Urethral Orifice

Vulva: Pudendal Labia, Rima Pudendi; Dorsal and Ventral Commisures

Vagina: Vestibule of the Vagina; Fossa and Glands of the Clitoris; Fornix of the Vagina

Uterus: Uterine Cervix and Cervical Canal and Ostia; Uterine Body, Uterine Horns, and Uterine Tubes; Mesometrium, Mesosalpinx, and Mesovarium; Intercornual Ligament; Infundibulum of Uterine Tube, Tubal Fimbriae, and Abdominal Ostium of Uterine Tube; Round Ligament of the Uterus

Ovary and Ovarian Bursa; Suspensory and Proper Ligaments of Ovary

Pelvic Cavity: Cranial and Caudal Pelvic Apertures; Pubovesicular, Vesicogenital, and Rectogenital Excavations; Pararectal Fossae

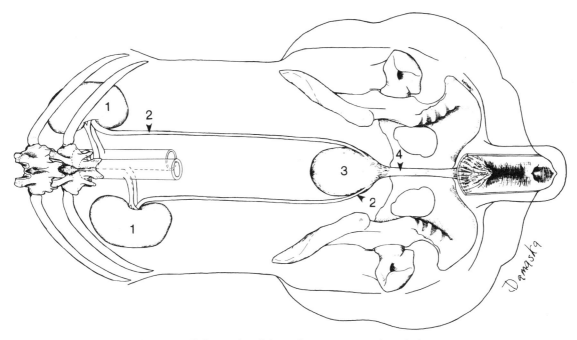

Fig.13.1. Schematic of the urinary system, dorsal view.

The urinary system (Fig. 13.1) consists of the kidneys (1), ureters (2), urinary bladder (3), and urethra (4). The right kidney is ventrolateral to the 1st through 3rd lumbar vertebrae; the position of the left kidney, more variable than the right, is ventrolateral to the 2nd through 4th lumbar vertebrae.

The **URETERS** are slender, muscular tubes that course caudally from the medial surface of the kidney to the dorsolateral surface of the urinary bladder. They are situated in the dorsal subserous fascia of the abdominal cavity to each side of the major vessels (the **ABDOMINAL AORTA** and **CAUDAL VENA CAVA**).

(DIFFERENCE TO BE NOTED IN THE CAT: Right and left kidneys are approximately at the same level, L2 through L4.)

The **KIDNEY** is a bean-shaped structure with a convex lateral margin and a concave medial margin (Fig. 13.2). Since the parietal peritoneum covers its ventral but not its dorsal surface, the

kidney is described as being retroperitoneal; one may remove a retroperitoneal kidney through a dorsolateral abdominal incision without incising the peritoneum (i.e., one does not need to enter

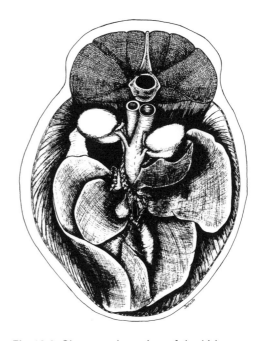

Fig.13.2. Shape and postion of the kidneys.

the peritoneal cavity). The left kidney is less firmly attached to the dorsal body wall than is the right and is thus more mobile.

A depression, or **RENAL HILUS** (1, Fig. 13.3), is in the center of the concave medial margin through which vessels and nerves pass to and from the kidney. The hilus leads into a fat-filled cavity, the **RENAL SINUS** (2), which contains fat, blood vessels, and the expanded urine-receiving portion of the ureter (**RENAL PELVIS**). A fibrous **RENAL CAPSULE** (3) covers the surface of the kidney.

The kidney (Fig. 13.4) is composed of two major portions, the **RENAL CORTEX** (1) and the **RENAL MEDULLA** (2), both of which are grossly distinguishable.

The renal cortex is a reddish brown, granular, superficial layer of the kidney situated between the renal capsule (3) and the renal medulla. It is within the renal cortex that blood under high pressure escapes as a filtrate from capillary tufts; the filtrate enters tiny tubules to be concentrated and carried toward the ureter as urine.

The renal medulla is the light-colored, finely striated deeper portion of the kidney. The striations are due to the presence of many collecting ducts that convey urine toward the renal hilus.

If a kidney is sectioned through its median plane (Fig. 13.5), a rather simple renal medulla will be observed, which has a linear **RENAL CREST** (1) projecting into the renal pelvis (2). Urine drips out into the renal pelvis from duct orifices in the **CRIBRIFORM** (krib' ri-form; forms a sieve) **AREA** of the renal crest.

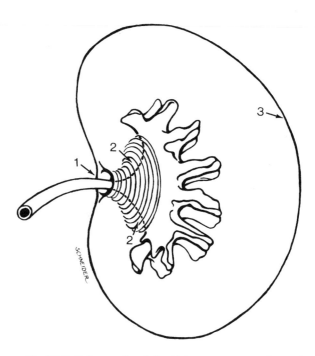

Fig.13.3. Schematic of the kidney ureter, and renal pelvis, diverticulae, and sinus.

Since the dog kidney is composed of a number of fused lobes, a sagittal section through the kidney yields an entirely different view of the medullary structure. The fusion of renal lobes is so complete that lobation is not grossly apparent either externally or in the cortex.

The medulla (3) of each lobe (in a unilobate mammalian kidney or embryologically) is shaped like a pyramid, with its base (4) against the cortex and the apex projecting into the renal pelvis. The renal papillae are fused in the dog, forming a median renal crest; however, to each side of the median plane the medulla of each lobe appears to be separate when observed in a sagittal section.

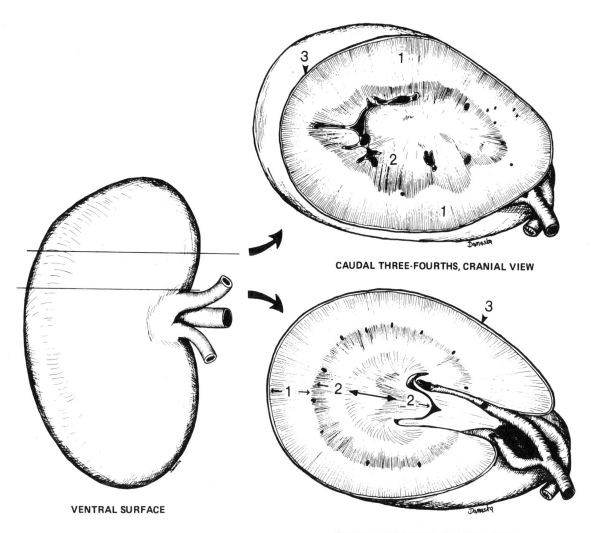

CAUDAL THREE-FOURTHS, CRANIAL VIEW

VENTRAL SURFACE

CAUDAL TWO-THIRDS, CRANIAL VIEW

Fig.13.4. Right kidney.

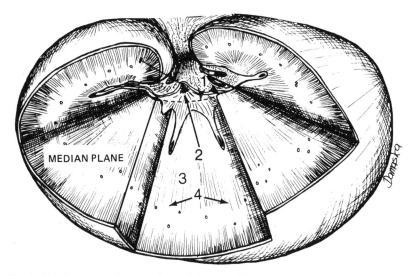

Fig.13.5. Kidney with a portion of the renal cortex and medulla removed.

239

The **URINARY BLADDER** (Fig. 13.6) is a highly distendable urine storage organ; it is situated within the pelvic cavity when empty and in the abdominal cavity when full. The regions of the urinary bladder are the **APEX** (1), **BODY** (2), and **NECK** (3).

The body is the main portion of the urinary bladder; irregular bands, resulting from smooth muscle fibers deep to the surface, may be observed grossly in the walls. The neck of the urinary bladder is continuous with the **URETHRA** (4).

The ureters (5) enter the dorsolateral surface of the urinary bladder near the neck. Because the ureters pass obliquely through the wall of the urinary bladder, the smooth muscle of the bladder acts upon them as a physiological sphincter. The **URETERIC OSTIA** (6) each open through a ridge on the dorsal internal surface of the urinary bladder; both of these ridges converge distally to form a dorsal ridge in the urethra, the **URETHRAL CREST** (7).

The **TRIGONE** (tri'gon; triangular) **OF THE BLADDER** (8) is the area between the converging ridges of tissue.

The urinary bladder is supported by two **LATERAL LIGAMENTS** (1, Fig. 13.7) and one ventral **MEDIAN LIGAMENT** (2). The median ligament represents a caudal remnant of the ventral mesentery. The **URACHUS** (u' rah-kus), a vestige of the fetal allantoic stalk, is present in the median ligament; if it remains patent (open) in the newborn pup, urine may pass from the urinary bladder out through the umbilicus.

The urethra (1, Fig. 13.8) conducts urine from the urinary bladder (2) to the **VAGINA** (3). Smooth muscle of the urinary bladder extends into the urethra, forming a

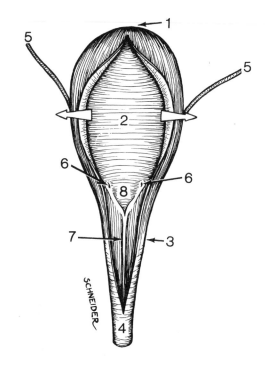

Fig.13.6. Urinary bladder with the ventral wall incised and partially reflected, ventral view.

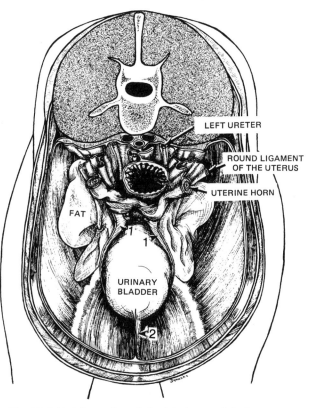

Fig.13.7. Pelvic cavity of the bitch, cranial view.

240

functional (not an anatomical) sphincter. Skeletal muscle, the **URETHRALIS**, is present in the urethral wall and forms a sphincter that is under voluntary control. The **EXTERNAL URETHRAL ORIFICE** (4) is the opening between the urethra and the vagina.

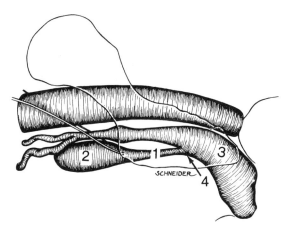

Fig.13.8. Rectum and urogenital structures,

The external genital structure of the bitch is the **VULVA** (Fig. 13.9), which consists of the **PUDENDAL** (ashamed) **LABIA** (1) and the vulvar cleft, or **RIMA PUDENDI** (2). The rima pudendi is the opening common to both urinary and genital systems. The **DORSAL** (3) and **VENTRAL** (4) **LABIAL COMMISSURES** are the fusion lines of the labia, dorsal and ventral to the rima pudendi, respectively.

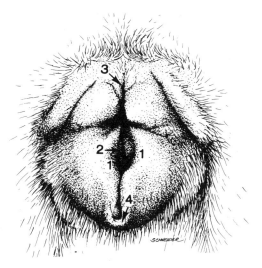

Fig.13.9. Vulva, caudal view.

An incision (episiotomy) (e-piz " e-ot' o-me; cutting the vulva) through the dorsal commissure reveals the **VESTIBULE OF THE VAGINA** (Fig. 13.10), which extends from the rima pudendi to the **URETHRAL TUBERCLE** (I).

A fossa in the ventral surface of the caudal portion of the vestibule is the **FOSSA CLITORIDIS** (2). The **GLANS OF THE CLITORIS** (3) projects caudodorsally into the fossa; the clitoris, consisting of **CRURA, BODY** and **GLANS**, is homologous to the penis of the male (see p. 260). The body and crura of the clitoris are within the wall of the vaginal vestibule. The urethral tubercle projects (slightly in nulliparous animals) into the vagina from the cranioventral surface of the vestibule; the **EXTERNAL URETHRAL ORIFICE** (4) opens into the vestibule through or under the urethral tubercle.

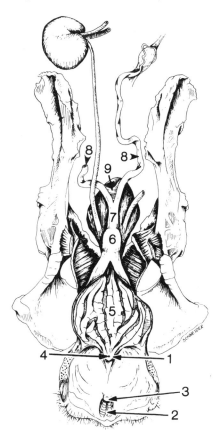

Fig.13.10. Urogenital tract of the bitch, dorsal view.

241

The **VAGINA** (5) extends cranially for a considerable distance; longitudinal and transverse folds (**RUGAE**) in the vagina allow for its expansion. The caudal portion of the uterus may be felt as a hard, muscular **UTERINE CERVIX** (6).

The **UTERUS** is composed of uterine cervix, **UTERINE BODY** (7), and **RIGHT** and **LEFT UTERINE HORNS** (8). An **INTERCORNUAL LIGAMENT** (9) connects the two cornua near their junction with the uterine body.

When catheterizing the urethra of a bitch, one needs to ensure that the catheter does not enter the blind-ending fossa clitoridis (1, Fig. 13.11).

A longitudinal dissection through the lateral surface of the vagina reveals the **FORNIX OF THE VAGINA** (1, Fig. 13.12), a space in the vagina cranioventral to the intravaginal portion of the cervix. The small passage through the uterine cervix (2) is the **UTERINE CERVICAL CANAL**; the cranial and caudal openings into the cervical canal are named **INTERNAL** (3)

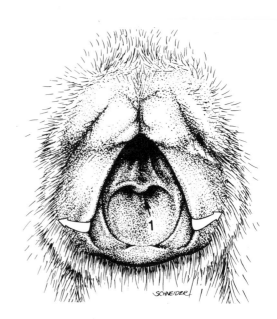

Fig.13.11. Vulva, pudendal labia retracted.

and **EXTERNAL** (4) **UTERINE OSTIA** (sing. ostium; opening). The external uterine ostium is oriented caudoventrally. A muscular ridge extends caudally from the cervix along the dorsal wall of the vagina, protruding ventrally into the vaginal lumen.

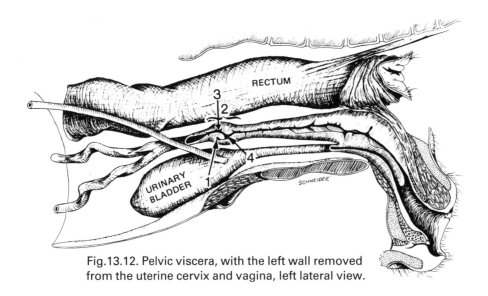

Fig.13.12. Pelvic viscera, with the left wall removed from the uterine cervix and vagina, left lateral view.

242

Two muscles of considerable importance in the bitch (Fig. 13.13) are the **CONSTRICTOR VESTIBULI** (1) and **CONSTRICTOR VULVAE** (2). These striated muscles that encircle the vestibule and vulva comprise the **BULBOSPONGIOSUS MUSCLE**.

Constriction of the penile veins by the constrictors vulvae and vestibuli enhances erection in the dog. The enlarged distal portion of the penis (glans) in turn supports vascular engorgement of the female genital structures.

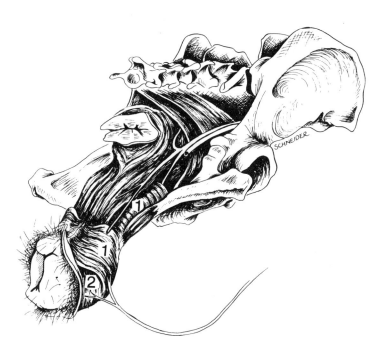

Fig.13.13. Muscles of the female perineal region and pelvic diaphragm, right caudolateral view.

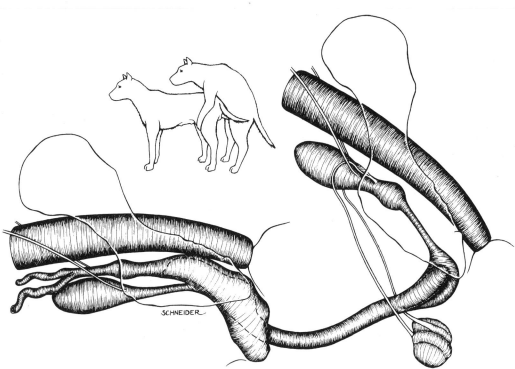

Fig.13.14. Schematic of the initial phase of coitus, lateral view.

The glans of the penis is intravaginal during coitus (Fig. 13.14). Ejaculation of sperm occurs within the first minute of coitus. Approximately 1 minute after intromission the male turns 180 degrees (Fig. 13.15) and remains "locked" from 5 to 45 minutes. During this time interval, a voluminous sperm-free seminal fluid is ejaculated. The penis displaces the vagina dorsolaterally, with the rectum displaced to the opposite side. The uterine cervix is displaced as far cranially as the lumbosacral articulation.

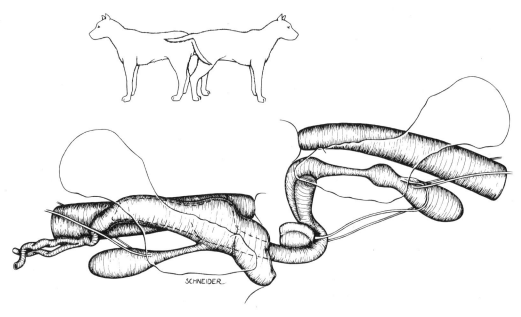

Fig.13.15. "Locking" phase of coitus.

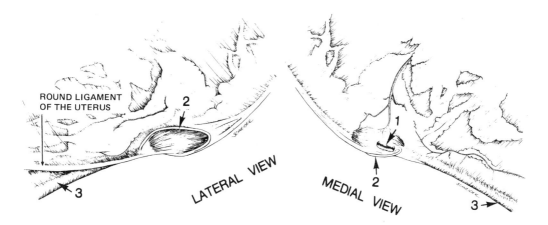

Fig.13.16. Right ovarian bursa and uterine tube.

The cranial portion of the female reproductive system is difficult to visualize because of its small size and the serous membranous sac that surrounds the ovary (Fig. 13.16).

The **OVARIAN BURSA** is a peritoneal space that partially contains the **OVARY.** A small slitlike opening (1) through the medial surface of the membranous sac connects the peritoneal cavity with the bursa.

The **UTERINE TUBE** (2) of each side winds around within the wall of the membranous sac and merges caudally with the cranial extent of the uterine horn (3). The **INFUNDIBULUM OF THE UTERINE TUBE** is a funnel-shaped dilatation of the uterine tube that opens into the ovarian bursa near the slit between bursa and peritoneal cavity.

TUBAL FIMBRIAE (sing. frimbia; fringe) are extremely small fingerlike processes on the free edge of the infundibulum that partially protrude from the bursa into the peritoneal cavity.

The **ABDOMINAL OSTIUM OF THE UTERINE TUBE** (1, Fig. 13.17) is the opening of the ovarian end of the uterine tube into the infundibulum (2). Although grossly nondiscernible, a relatively wide initial segment is the **AMPULLA** (pl. ampullae; jug) **OF THE UTERINE TUBE** (3).

The narrow portion between the ampulla and the uterine horn is the **ISTHMUS OF THE UTERINE TUBE** (4). Fertilization of the ovum occurs within the uterine tube.

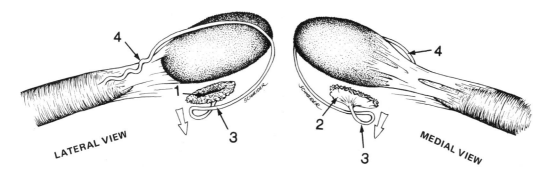

Fig.13.17. Schematic of the right ovary, uterine tube, and initial segement of the uterine horn.

245

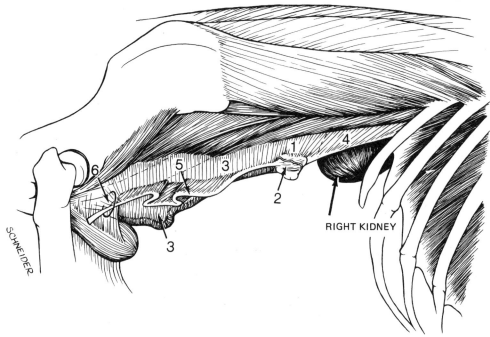

Fig.13.18. Supporting mesenteries of the ovary, uterine tube, and uterus, right lateral view.

The mesentery or peritoneal folds supporting the abdominal and pelvic portions of the female reproductive tract are fairly complex (Fig. 13.18).

The **MESOVARIUM** (1) supports the ovary from the abdominal wall; the ovarian vessels pass from the dorsal abdominal vessels in the mesovarium to reach the hilus of the ovary.

The **MESOSALPINX** (mes " o-sal' pinks) (2) is a fold of tissue arising from the lateral surface of the mesovarium; the uterine tube is contained within the mesosalpinx.

The **MESOMETRIUM** (3) is a supporting mesentery, containing smooth muscle, that attaches the uterine horn and body to the abdominal wall.

The **BROAD LIGAMENT OF THE UTERUS,** composed of the mesovarium, mesosalpinx, and mesometrium, allows considerable movement of the uterus.

The ovaries, which are located near the 3rd and 4th lumbar vertebral levels, are also attached cranially to the transversalis fascia of the dorsolateral abdominal wall and thoracic diaphragm by the **SUSPENSORY LIGAMENT OF THE OVARY** (4). This ligament limits movement of the ovaries within the abdominal cavity. The suspensory ligament is continuous caudally with the mesovarium.

The caudal extremity of the ovary is attached by the **PROPER LIGAMENT OF THE OVARY** to the cranial tip of the uterine horn. The **ROUND LIGAMENT OF THE UTERUS** (5) is a lateral fold from the mesometrium; it passes through the **INGUINAL CANAL** (6), connecting the cranial tip of the uterine horn to the superficial fascia of the vulvar area.

246

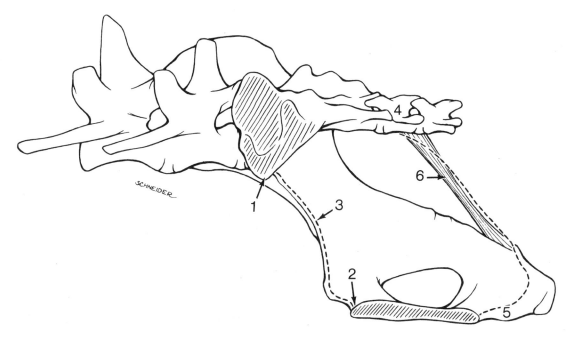

Fig.13.19. Pelvic cavity, with the left os coxae removed, left lateral view.

The **PELVIC CAVITY** (Fig. 13.19) extends between the **CRANIAL** and **CAUDAL PELVIC APERTURES**. The peritoneal membranes and space are continuous from the abdominal cavity into the pelvic cavity.

The cranial pelvic aperture is an osseous opening formed dorsally by the sacral promontory (1), ventrally by the cranial border of the pubic bones (2), and laterally by the arcuate lines (3).

The caudal pelvic aperture is an opening formed dorsally by the 1st caudal vertebra (4), ventrally by the ischiatic arch (5), and laterally by the sacrotuberous ligaments (6) and superficial gluteal muscles.

Ventrally, the parietal peritoneum extends into the pelvic cavity for a very short distance before reflecting dorsally onto the neck of the urinary bladder (Figs. 13.20, 13.21). The peritoneal recesses formed by reflections of the parietal

peritoneum onto the various pelvic viscera are termed excavations.

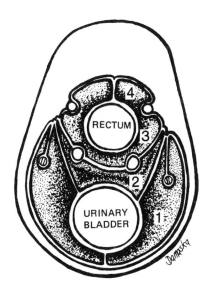

Fig.13.20. Schematic of the pelvic peritoneal recesses as observed in transverse section.

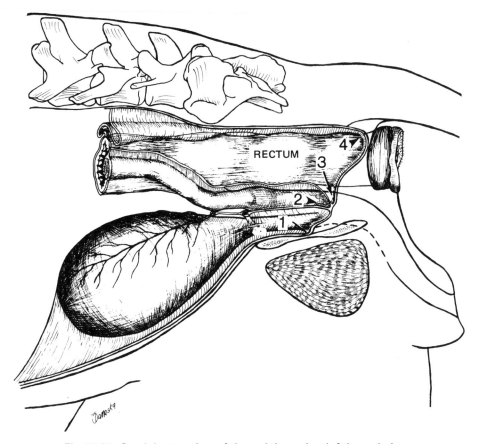

Fig.13.21. Caudal extension of the pelvic cavity, left lateral view.

Two ventral recesses, one on each side of the median ligament of the bladder, between the ventral wall of the pelvic cavity and the urinary bladder are the **PUBOVESICULAR EXCAVATIONS** (1).

The **VESICOGENITAL EXCAVATION** (2) is the space formed by the reflection of visceral peritoneum from the dorsal surface of the urethra onto the ventral surface of the vagina. A dorsal reflection from the dorsal surface of the vagina onto the ventral surface of the rectum

forms a space known as the **RECTOGENITAL EXCAVATION** (3). The portions of the rectogenital excavation situated dorsolateral to the rectum are termed the right and left **PARARECTAL FOSSAE** (4).

In terms of craniocaudal orientation, the rectogenital excavation is more caudal than the vesicogenital excavation, which in turn is more caudal than the pubovesicular excavation.

Chapter 14

MALE REPRODUCTIVE SYSTEM

Objectives: Be able to identify structures and understand the normal positions of male reproductive organs.

Urinary System: Preprostatic, Prostatic, and Post-prostatic portion of the Pelvic Urethra; Spongy portion of the Penile Urethra; External Urethral Orifice

Prepuce: External and Internal Layers; Preputial Ostium and Cavity; Suspensory Ligament of the Penis

Scrotum and contents: Scrotal Septum; Parietal and Visceral Layers of the Vaginal Tunic; Vaginal Cavity; Spermatic Cord; Cremaster Muscle; Testis; Head, Body, and Tail of Epididymis; Proper Ligament of Testis and Caudal Ligament of Epididymis; Tunica Albuginea

Vaginal and Inguinal Canals; Vaginal and Deep Inguinal Rings; Mesorchium and Mesoductus Deferens; Pampiniform Plexus and Rete Testis; Ductus Deferens

Prostate Gland; Colliculus Seminalis

Penis: Root, Body, and Crura; Retractor Penis Muscle, Ischiocavernosus, Bulbospongiosus, and Ischiourethralis Muscles; Corpus Cavernosum and Corpus Spongiosum Penis; Tunica Albuginea; Bulbus Glandis, Pars Longa Glandis, and Bulb of the Penis; Os Penis and Urethral Groove

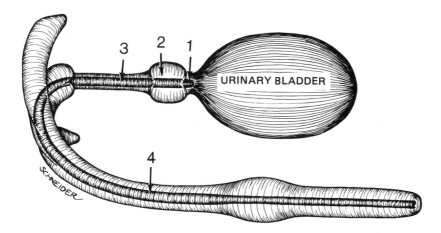

Fig.14.1. Schematic of the urinary bladder, prostate gland, urethra, and erectile portion of the penis, right ventromedial view.

The urinary system of the male is quite similar to that of the female (see pp. 237–40); the urethra (Fig. 14.1) is modified both in its pelvic and spongy portions.

The **PELVIC PORTION** is composed of preprostatic, prostatic, and postprostatic parts. The short **PREPROSTATIC PART** (1) of the urethra extends between the urinary bladder and the prostate gland; smooth muscle of the urinary bladder extends into the preprostatic urethra forming a functional internal sphincter.

The **PROSTATIC PART** (2) of the urethra is described with the prostate (p. 258).

The relatively long **POSTPROSTATIC PART** (3) is encircled by the urethralis muscle, a striated muscle. The

SPONGY PORTION (4) of the urethra is described with the penis (pp. 259–61), with which it is associated.

The organs of the male reproductive system (Fig. 14.2) include the prepuce (1), scrotum (2), testis (3), epididymis (4), spermatic cord, ductus deferens (5), prostate gland (6), urethra (7), and penis (8).

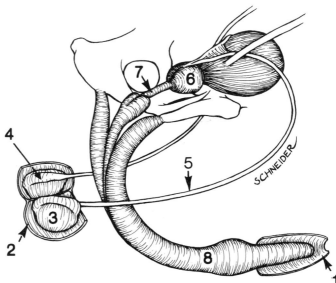

Fig.14.2. Schematic of the male genital organs, right caudolateral view.

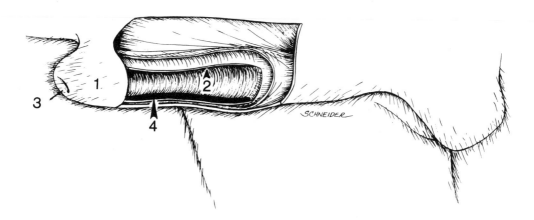

Fig.14.3. Prepuce, with part of the prepuce removed, left lateral view.

The **PREPUCE** (pre' pyoos) (Fig. 14.3) is a sheath formed of modified integument. It consists of a hairy **EXTERNAL LAYER** (1) and an **INTERNAL LAYER** (2) that meet at the **PREPUTIAL OSTIUM** (3).

The space between the internal layer and the glans penis is the **PREPUTIAL CAVITY** (4). A strong, fibrous **SUSPENSORY LIGAMENT OF THE PENIS** is present in the median plane between the abdominal wall (dorsally) and the penis (ventrally).

The **SCROTUM** (Fig. 14.4), a paired cutaneous pouch containing the **TESTIS** (pl. testes) (1), is composed of skin, **DARTOS TUNIC** (coat) (2), and fascia. The dartos tunic is a layer of smooth muscle closely adherent to the skin of the scrotum; it contracts in response to cold or mechanical stimulation.

Much of the **SCROTAL SEPTUM** (pl. septa) (3), a median partition dividing the scrotum into two compartments, is also composed of the dartos tunic.

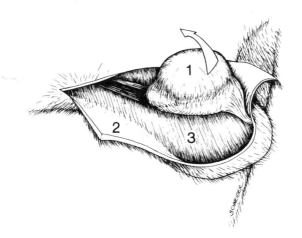

Fig.14.4. Scrotum, with the left scrotal sac incised and the left testicle reflected.

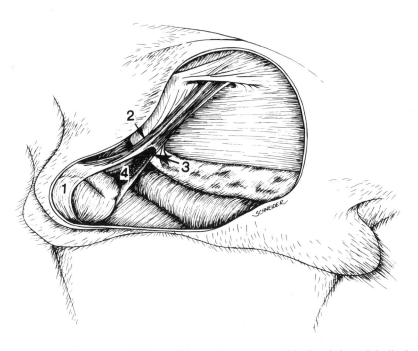

Fig.14.5. Scrotum, right testicle, and prepuce, with the right pelvic limb removed and the right vaginal tunic incised, right lateral view.

An incision through the scrotum reveals the **PARIETAL LAYER OF THE VAGINAL TUNIC** (1, Fig. 14.5). The **VAGINAL TUNIC** is continuous through the inguinal canal with the lining of the peritoneal cavity.

The **CREMASTER MUSCLE** (2), a striated muscle arising from the caudal margin of the internal abdominal oblique, inserts on the parietal layer of the vaginal tunic.

An incision through the parietal layer of the vaginal tunic reveals the **VAGINAL "CAVITY"** (3) and the **VISCERAL LAYER OF THE VAGINAL TUNIC** (4). The visceral layer of the vaginal tunic plus its contents (proximal to the testis) are termed the **SPERMATIC CORD**.

Blood vessels (1), lymph vessels, and nerve fibers from the abdominal cavity and the deferent (to carry away) ducts (2) from the pelvic cavity pass through the abdominal wall (Fig. 14.6) to reach the testes.

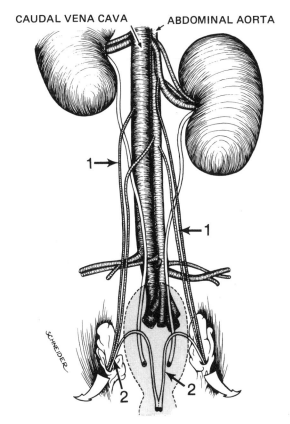

CAUDAL VENA CAVA   ABDOMINAL AORTA

Fig.14.6. Schematic of the kidneys, ureters, urinary bladder, ductus deferentes, and vaginal canals, ventral view.

253

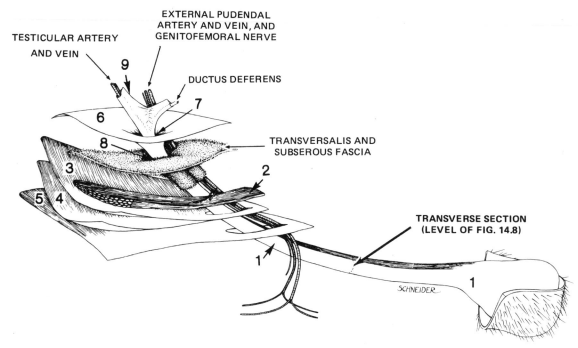

Fig.14.7. Schematic of the right vaginal and inguinal canals and the structures that pass through the inguinal canal, medial view.

The **INGUINAL CANAL** (Fig. 14.7) is a passage peripheral to the parietal layer of the vaginal tunic (1), and through or past the various layers of abdominal muscles: rectus abdominis (2), transversus abdominis (3), internal abdominal oblique (4), and external abdominal oblique (5).

The reflection of parietal peritoneum (6) into the inguinal canal forms a serous membrane ring and canal, the **VAGINAL RING** (7) and **VAGINAL CANAL.**

The reflection of fascia from the abdominal cavity into the inguinal canal, peripheral to the vaginal ring, is named the **DEEP INGUINAL RING** (8).

The **MESORCHIUM** (9, Fig. 14.7) suspends the testicular vessels from the dorsolateral wall in the abdominal cavity; in the vaginal tunic the mesorchium (1, Fig. 14.8) suspends the testicular vessels from the parietal vaginal tunic (2). The venous plexus formed by the

TESTICULAR VEIN is called the **PAMPINIFORM PLEXUS** (3); this plexus has a role in heat exchange between the warm blood of the testicular artery and the cooler blood of the plexus. The **MESODUCTUS DEFERENS** (4) is a fold of tissue in the vaginal sac that supports the **DUCTUS DEFERENS** (5).

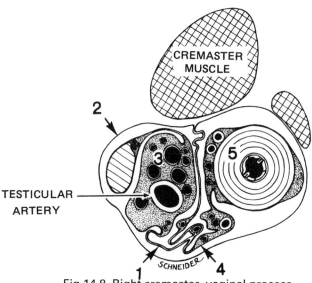

Fig.14.8. Right cremaster, vaginal process, testicular vessels, and ductus deferens, transverse section.

The lumen within that portion of the parietal vaginal tunic in the inguinal canal is the vaginal canal; the vaginal canal is patent and continues craniodorsally with the peritoneal cavity and caudally with the vaginal cavity. **A SCROTAL HERNIA** is a protrusion of an abdominal organ or tissue through the vaginal ring into the vaginal cavity, resulting in an elongated enlargement of the scrotal area.

An **INGUINAL HERNIA** is a fold of mesentery or intestine that protrudes into the inguinal canal peripheral to the vaginal canal; an inguinal hernia forms a soft enlargement in the subcutaneous tissue to one side of the penis.

The **TUNICA ALBUGINEA** (al " bu-jin ' e-ah), the outermost white, tough covering of the testis (of the ovary as well), and the visceral vaginal tunic are firmly bound to each other and are grossly indistinguishable as separate structures.

A connective tissue mass within the testis, the **MEDIASTINUM TESTIS**, is connected to the peripheral tunica albuginea by connective tissue septa; these septa separate the testis into conical lobules. Each lobule of the testis is oriented with its apex toward the mediastinum testis and its base toward the tunica albuginea. **SEMINIFEROUS TUBULES** and interstitial cells are present within the lobules.

Branches of the **TESTICULAR ARTERY** reach the lobules of the testis by passing through the mediastinum. The **RETE** (rete, pl. retia; net) **TESTIS** is a network of interconnecting tubules within the mediastinum testis that collects the spermatozoa from the seminiferous tubules and conducts them toward the epididymis.

The testes are abdominally located in the newborn pup; they are near the deep inguinal ring at approximately 55–60 days of fetal development and pass through the inguinal canal at approximately 10–15 days of postnatal age.

The **EPIDIDYMIS** (pl. epididymides) (Fig. 14.9) is a highly convoluted tube that collects

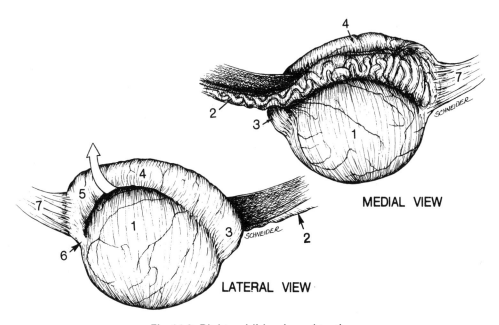

Fig.14.9. Right epididymis and testis.

255

spermatozoa from the testis (1), stores them and then passes them on to the ductus deferens (2). The **HEAD OF THE EPIDIDYMIS** (3) is the portion of the epididymis at the cranial pole of the testis. The spermatozoa pass from the testis to the head of the epididymis.

The **BODY OF THE EPIDIDYMIS** (4), the major portion of the epididymis, is situated on the dorsal border of the testis between the head and **TAIL OF THE EPIDIDYMIS** (5), which is the portion situated on the caudal extremity of the testis. The tail of the epididymis is continuous with the ductus deferens.

The caudal border of the testis is attached to the epididymis by the **PROPER LIGAMENT OF THE TESTIS** (6). The **CAUDAL LIGAMENT OF THE EPIDIDYMIS** (7), a homolog of the round ligament of the uterus of the bitch, is often very difficult to identify; it attaches the tail of the epididymis to the parietal layer of the vaginal tunic (caudal margin of the mesorchium).

The ductus deferens (1, Fig. 14.10) conveys spermatozoa from the epididymis to the urethra (2). It arises from the tail of the epididymis, passes cranially within the spermatic cord, enters the abdominal cavity through the inguinal canal, loops around the ventral surface of the ureter (3), and enters the dorsal surface of the prostatic portion of the urethra.

Although grossly nondiscernible, the slightly enlarged prostatic end of the ductus deferens (external to the prostate) is the **AMPULLA OF THE DUCTUS DEFERENS** (4).

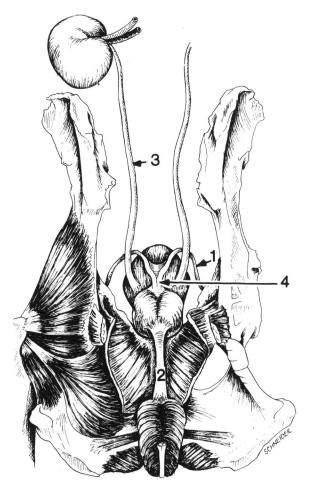

Fig.14.10. Male urogenital organs, with the epaxial structures and alimentary canal removed, dorsal view.

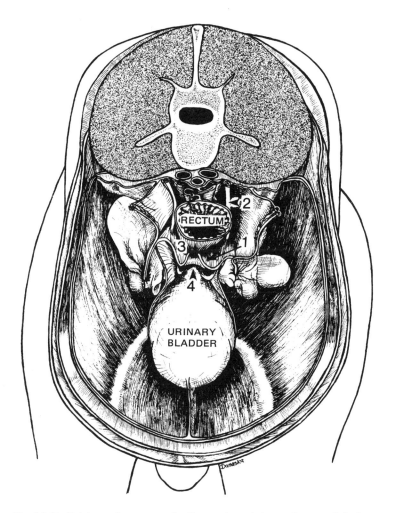

Fig.14.11. Folds and recesses in the male pelvic cavity, cranial view.

The paired ducti deferentes are suspended by a horizontal fold of peritoneum (1, Fig. 14.11) near their junction with the urethra. The caudal portions of the ureters (2) are also contained within this thin membranous fold. The rectogenital excavation (3) is dorsal and the vesicogenital excavation (4) ventral to this transverse fold (see p. 248).

257

The **PROSTATE** (pros' tate) **GLAND** (Fig. 14.12) is both around and scattered within the tissue of the pelvic urethra. The **BODY OF THE PROSTATE GLAND** (1) is divided by a median groove in the dog into right and left lobes surrounding the urethra.

The prostate is an accessory genital organ that produces a milky alkaline fluid; this fluid neutralizes urethral acidity, aids in the activation of sperm, forms the bulk of the seminal fluid, and accounts for the characteristic odor of semen.

The internal dorsal surface of the pelvic portion of the urethra has a longitudinal ridge of mucosa. This ridge, the urethral crest (1, Fig. 14.13), terminates as the **COLLICULUS** (ko-lik' u-lus; small elevation) **SEMINALIS** (2), a mucosal elevation in the prostatic portion of the urethra.

The urethral openings of the ductus deferens are in the colliculus seminalis. A number of small prostatic ductules open into the urethra on each side of the colliculus seminalis (if the prostate gland is squeezed, prostatic secretions may be observed entering the urethra).

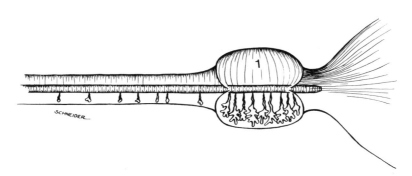

Fig. 14.12. Schematic of the urethra and prostate gland, dorsal view

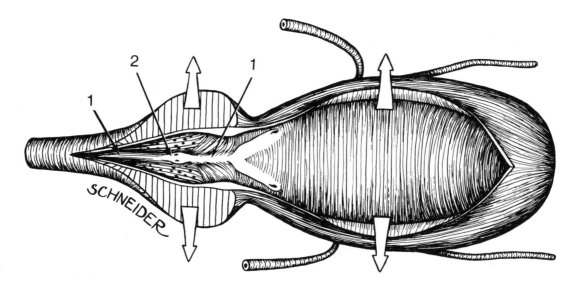

Fig. 14.13. Urinary bladder, ureters, ductus deferentes, prostate, and pelvic urethra, with a portion of the ventral wall of the urinary bladder and urethra removed, ventral view.

The **PENIS** is composed of erectile, muscular, vascular, and nervous tissue.

Paired (although seemingly single) **RETRACTOR PENIS MUSCLES** (1, Fig. 14.14) arise from the caudal vertebrae, pass around each side of the anal canal, and extend along the caudal and ventromedial surfaces of the penis to terminate near the glans penis (2). The retractor penis muscle is composed primarily of smooth muscle.

The skeletal muscles of the penis include the **ISCHIOCAVERNOSUS** (is ke-o-kav' er-no sus) (3), **BULBOSPONGIOSUS** (4), and ischiourethralis. The ischiocaverno sus muscle arises from the ischiatic tuberosity and terminates on the proximal ventral surface of the **CORPUS CAVERNOSUM PENIS** (5).

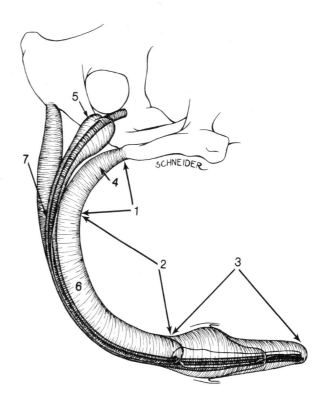

Fig.14.15. Schematic of the penis, right caudolateral view.

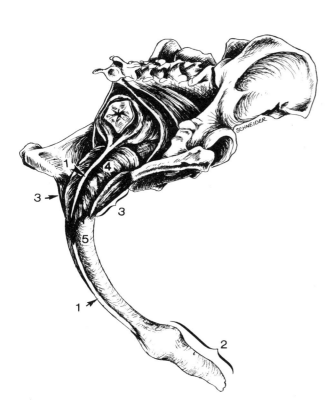

Fig.14.14. Penis, right caudolateral view.

The bulbospongiosus muscle is situated between the ischiocavernosus muscles of each side and deep to the retractor penis muscle; it partially encircles the urethra and the erectile **CORPUS** (pl. corpora; body) **SPONGIOSUM PENIS** in the proximal portion of the penis.

The penis (Fig. 14.15) is described as consisting of erectile tissue that is subdivided into **ROOT** (1), **BODY** (2), and **GLANS** (3), with the root of the penis consisting of the **CRURA OF THE PENIS** (4) and the **BULB OF THE PENIS** (5).

The crura of the penis attaches proximally to the ischiatic tuberosity and continues distally as the **CORPORA CAVERNOSA PENIS** (6). Each corpus cavernosum penis arches cranioventrally and converges with its member of the opposite side, forming the bulk of the body of the penis, ending at the proximal portion of the glans penis. The tough white connective tissue around the erectile tissue is the **TUNICA ALBUGINEA** of the corpus cavernosum. The bulb of the penis, a bibbed structure in the caudoventral portion of the pelvic cavity, is continuous distally in the penis as the slender erectile corpus spongiosum penis (7). The corpus spongiosum in the body of the penis is positioned ventromedial to the paired corpus cavernosum and contains the spongy portion of the urethra.

The glans penis (Fig. 14.16) is composed primarily of erectile tissue that is continuous with the corpus spongiosum penis.The large

BULBUS GLANDIS (1) forms the proximal portion of the glans. It is this erectile tissue that is locked in the vagina of the bitch during coitus caused by vascular engorgement of the bulbus glandis and contraction of constrictor muscles of the vagina and vestibule; see p. 244.

The external distal portion of the glans is formed by the **PARS LONGA GLANDIS** (2); vascular sinuses in the pars longa glandis are connected with both the bulbus glandis and the corpus spongiosum penis. Within the glans penis, the corpus spongiosum penis (which surrounds the penile urethra) lies in a groove in the **OS PENIS** (3). The os penis, which provides support for the

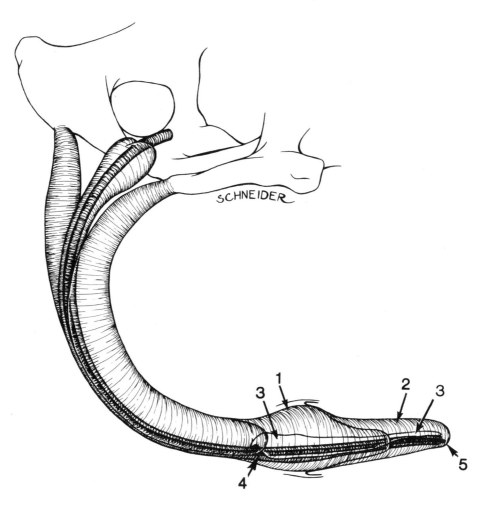

Fig.14.16. Schematic of the penis, right caudolateral view.

glans, is the distal continuation of the corpus cavernosum penis.

The **URETHRAL GROOVE** (4), in the ventral surface of the os penis, prevents urethral expansion; urinary **CALCULI** (sing. calculus) often lodge in the urethra at the caudal (proximal) end of the os penis. The external urethral orifice (5) is in the distal ventral surface of the glans penis.

The paired **ISCHIOURETHRALIS MUSCLES** (1, Fig. 14.17) arise from the ischiatic tuberosities and insert on a fibrous ring, ventral to the bulb of the penis and dorsal to the ischiatic symphysis. Contraction of the ischiourethralis muscles results in a reduction of venous blood flow from the penis through the fibrous ring. This reduction in quantity of blood flowing from the penis is a major factor in the erection mechanism.

(DIFFERENCES TO BE NOTED IN THE CAT: The preprostatic part of the urethra is relatively long as compared to the dog. BULBOURETHRAL GLANDS are present adjacent to the bulb of the feline penis, deep to striated muscle. This muscle, a craniodorsal part of the bulbospongiosus, is continuous with the urethralis muscle. The flaccid penis is directed caudoventrally, a position that often leads to incorrect sexing by the cat owner. Small keratinized spines are present on the surface of the feline glans penis.)

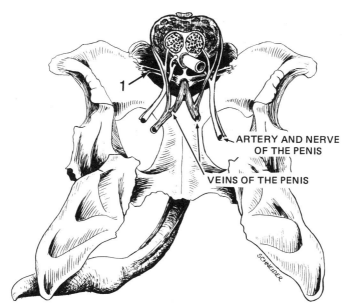

Fig.14.17. Ossa coxarum and root of the penis with associated vessels, with muscles and cavernous tissue of the penis sectioned transversely, dorsal view.

Unit VII

Cardiovascular System

In the seven chapters that follow, you will study the heart and the major vessels of the body.

Contents:

Chapter 15
CARDIOVASCULAR SYSTEM—HEART & PERICARDIUM

Objectives: Examine the structure of the heart and pericardium and understand the path by which blood passes from the body to the heart, through the lungs, back to the heart, and out to body tissues. Understand the structure and location of valves.

Pericardium: Parietal and Visceral Pericardium and Pericardial Cavity; Epicardium, Phrenicopericardiac Ligament

Heart: Right and Left Atria; Right and Left Ventricles; Base and Apex; Right and Left Ventricular Margins; Coronary Groove; Paraconal and Subsinuosal Interventricular Grooves; Right and Left Atrioventricular Valves and Ostia; Interatrial and Interventricular Septa

Major Vessels: Conus Arteriosus and Pulmonary Trunk; Right and Left Pulmonary Arteries and Veins; Ascending Aorta; Cranial and Caudal Venae Cavae; Right Azygous Vein

Right Atrium: Right Auricle; Ostia of Cranial and Caudal Venae Cavae; Coronary Sinus; Intervenous Tubercle and Fossa Ovalis; Pectinate Muscles and Terminal Crest; Endocardium

Atrioventricular Valves: Parietal and Septal Cusps; Chordae Tendinae and Papillary Muscles

Right Ventricle: Trabeculae Carneae and Trabeculae Septomarginalis

Pulmonary and Aortic Valves: Semilunar Valvules

Aortic Sinus and Right and Left Coronary Arteries: Paraconal Interventricular and Circumflex Branches of Left Coronary Artery

Great Cardiac Vein, Ligamentum Arteriosum, Brachiocephalic Trunk and Left Subclavian Artery

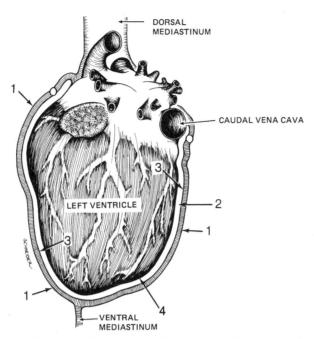

Fig.15.1. Heart with the parietal pericardium and mediastinum schematically represented, caudal view.

The thoracic cavity contains the two pleural cavities and a third serous membrane-lined space, the **PERICARDIAL CAVITY**. The portion of the mediastinum superficial to the heart (Fig. 15.1) is lined by **PERICARDIAL MEDIASTINAL PLEURA** (1).

The **PERICARDIUM**, composed of fibrous and serous layers and of the pericardial cavity (2), is situated within the mediastinum.

The **PARIETAL PERICARDIUM** (3) forms the superficial wall of the pericardium and is composed of an external fibrous layer and an internal serous layer.

An extension of the fibrous pericardium connects the pericardium to the diaphragm; this strong connective tissue band is the **PHRENICOPERICARDIAC** (phrenic: frenik; diaphragm) **LIGAMENT**.

The deep wall of the pericardial cavity is formed by a visceral layer of serous pericardium, or **EPICARDIUM** (4), tightly bound to heart muscle. The pericardial cavity normally contains only a thin film of fluid positioned between parietal and visceral layers of serous pericardium.

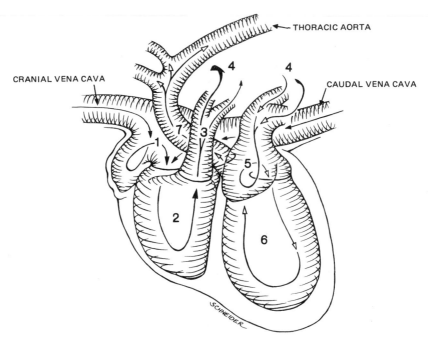

Fig.15.2. Schematic of the blood pathway through the heart.

The **HEART** is a four-chambered muscular structure positioned between venous and arterial systems (Fig. 15.2).

Venous blood from the entire body (except for the lungs and some of the heart) enters the **RIGHT ATRIUM** (1) and then flows sequentially through the **RIGHT VENTRICLE** (2), **PULMONARY TRUNK** (3), pulmonary arteries/capillary bed/pulmonary veins (4), **LEFT ATRIUM** (5), **LEFT VENTRICLE** (6), and **ASCENDING AORTA** (7) and into all of the body (except for the alveoli).

The flattened **BASE OF THE HEART** (1, Fig. 15.3) is the wide craniodorsal portion of the heart through which major vessels enter and leave.

The **APEX OF THE HEART** (2) is directed caudoventrally. The cranial portion of the base of the heart is situated at the approximate level of the 3rd rib; the apex is located near the 6th rib and slightly to the left of the median plane. The major portion of the heart is formed by the muscular right (3) and left (4) ventricles, each of which face both right and left thoracic walls since they are positioned more cranioventrally (right ventricle) and caudodorsally (left ventricle) than "right" and "left."

The **RIGHT VENTRICULAR MARGIN** (5) forms the convex cranioventral surface of the heart, which is positioned nearly parallel to the curvature of the sternum.

The **LEFT VENTRICULAR MARGIN** (6), which slopes nearly vertically from the base of the heart dorsally to the apex ventrally, forms the caudodorsal surface of the heart.

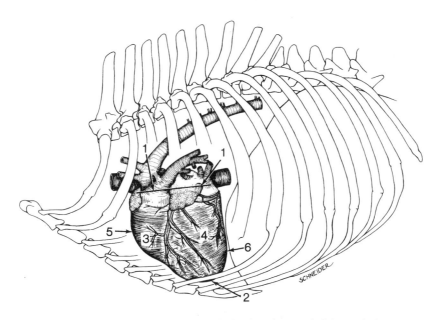

Fig.15.3. Heart and major vessels in the thorax, left lateral view.

The tricipital margin of the brachium (see p. 63) overlies the transverse level of the 5th to 6th ribs (Fig. 15.4); therefore, all but the apex and caudal surface of the heart is medial or deep to the thoracic limb. When palpating the heart, maximum detection of the beat usually may be located at the left fifth intercostal space.

The location for detection of sounds created by the four valves of the heart and the major vessels (shortly to be described) are as follows: left atrioventricular valve—left fifth intercostal space at the level of the costochondral junction; aortic valve—left fourth intercostal space, ventral to a dorsal plane through the humeral articulation; right atrioventricular valve—right third or fourth intercostal space, near the dorsal plane of the costochondral junction; and the pulmonary valve—left third intercostal space, ventrally near the sternum.

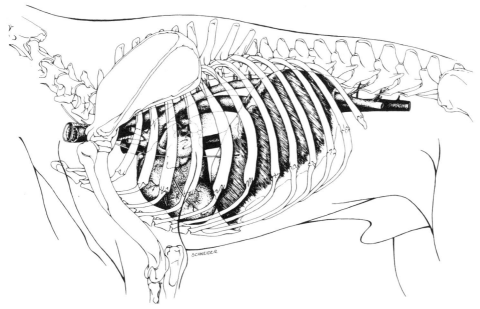

Fig.15.4. Position of the heart in the thorax, relative to the thoracic limb.

269

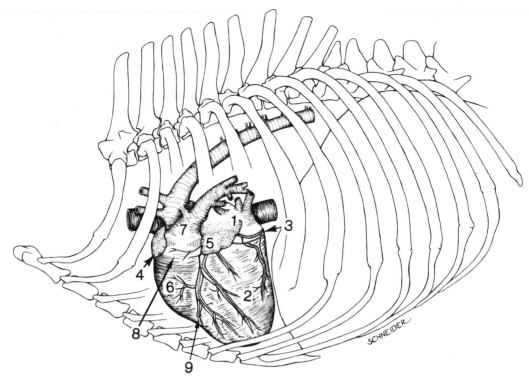

Fig.15.5. Auricular surface of the heart.

The earlike appendages of both right and left atria are directed toward the left side of the thoracic cavity (Fig.15.5). The appendages are termed AURICLES; thus the left side of the heart is described as the **AURICULAR SURFACE.**

The left atrium (1) is separated from the left ventricle (2) on the auricular surface of the heart by the **CORONARY GROOVE (3).**

The tips of right (4) and left (5) auricles are directed toward each other across the junction between right ventricle (6) and pulmonary trunk (7). This funnel-shaped junction is the **CONUS ARTERIOSUS (8).**

The pulmonary trunk branches into **RIGHT** and **LEFT PULMONARY ARTERIES,** which supply the lobes of right and left lung, respectively.

The fatty streak oriented from heart base to near the apex on the auricular surface is the **PARACONAL INTERVENTRICULAR GROOVE (9),** which contains a large branch of the left coronary artery and the great cardiac vein.

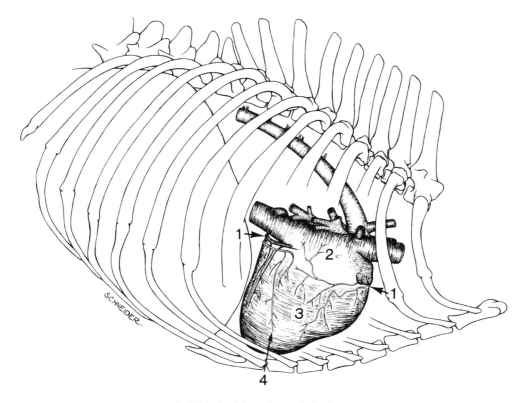

Fig.15.6. Atrial surface of the heart.

The **ATRIAL SURFACE OF THE HEART** (Fig. 15.6) is the surface related to the right ribs. The large coronary groove (1), a fat-filled area situated transversely with respect to the heart, marks the separation of the right atrium (a' tre-um, pl. atria; hall) (2), dorsocranially, from the ventricles (3), caudoventrally. The coronary groove, which contains the proximal portion of the coronary vessels, may be followed around the dorsocaudal aspect of the heart to the left side.

Two or more fatty streaks, containing vessels, are on the ventricular portion of the atrial surface.

One fatty streak on the right caudodorsal aspect of the heart superficial to the interventricular septum is the **SUBSINUOSAL INTERVENTRICULAR GROOVE** (4).

Thus a cardiac puncture from either right or left side may enter the somewhat flabby-walled right ventricle or the thick-walled, muscular left ventricle. A cardiac puncture also may enter the interventricular septum, with possible damage to coronary vessels that travel over the surface of the heart in grooves overlying the partition. A number of vascular branches also course over the surface of the ventricles at sites other than in the grooves overlying the septum.

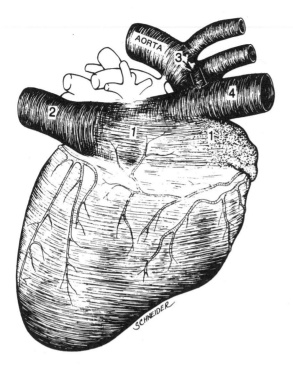

Fig.15.7. Major venous drainage into the right atrium, right lateral view.

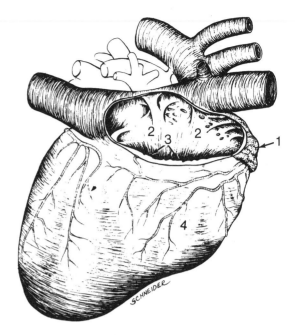

Fig.15.8. Right atrium, with much of its lateral wall removed.

Four major veins drain blood into the right atrium (1, Fig. 15.7): three vessels from the body and one from the heart (for cardiac drainage see pp. 273, 279).

The **CAUDAL VENA CAVA** (pl. venae cavae) (2) extends cranially from the dorsal portion of the abdominal cavity through the vena caval foramen of the thoracic diaphragm into the thoracic cavity; it discharges venous blood into the caudal portion of the right atrium.

The **RIGHT AZYGOUS VEIN** (3), which collects venous blood from the vertebral canal and much of the thoracic and abdominal walls, crosses the right surface of the trachea cranioventrally and discharges venous blood into the right atrium or into the **CRANIAL VENA CAVA** (4).

The cranial vena cava discharges venous blood, collected primarily from the head, neck, and thoracic limbs, into the cranial portion of the right atrium.

Due to subatmospheric pressures in the pleural and pericardial cavities, the atria, with intraluminal pressures similar to atmospheric pressure, are expanded, allowing venous blood to flow into them with little resistance. The right atrium by muscular contraction forces blood into the right ventricle; the blood is unable to back up into the major veins because blood pressure in the atrium is lower than that in the venae cavae.

The right atrium (Fig. 15.8) is composed of the small earlike **RIGHT AURICLE** (1) and the large **SINUS VENARUM CAVARUM** (2). An opening, the **RIGHT ATRIOVENTRICULAR OSTIUM** (3) discharges blood into the right ventricle (4).

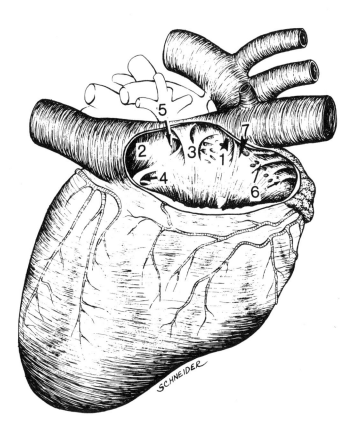

Fig.15.9. Medial wall of the right atrium and the
ostia, which open into the atrium, right lateral view.

The right atrium receives blood from three or four veins (Fig. 15.9). The **OSTIA OF THE CRANIAL** (1) and **CAUDAL** (2) **VENAE CAVAE** are at cranial and caudal ends of the right atrium. Blood coming into the atrium from the two venae cavae is directed ventrally by the **INTERVENOUS TUBERCLE** (3), which is situated on the medial wall of the atrium parallel with the long axis of the heart.

The third point of venous discharge into the right atrium is the **CORONARY SINUS** (4), through which the great cardiac vein discharges blood collected from veins draining the surface of the heart. The coronary sinus is ventral to the ostium of the caudal vena cava.

A small depression, the **FOSSA OVALIS** (5), is immediately caudal to the intervenous tubercle; this oval fossa is the remnant of the embryological opening (**FORAMEN OVALE**) between right and left atria. This foramen normally closes within a few weeks of postnatal life.

Muscular bands on the internal surface of the right auricle are termed **PECTINATE** (comblike) **MUSCLES** (6); most of the pectinate muscles attach to the **TERMINAL CREST** (7), a ridge of muscle ventral to the ostium of the cranial vena cava.

The **ENDOCARDIUM** is the thin glistening membrane that forms the inner or luminal surface of the four chambers of the heart.

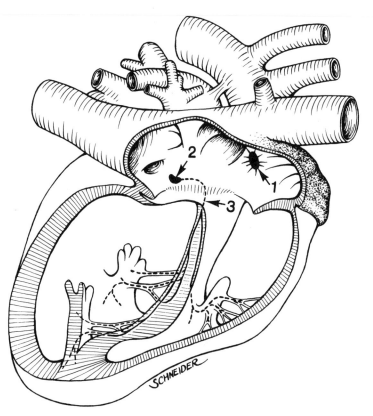

Fig.15.10. Schematic of the conductive system of the heart, with much of the atrial surface removed, right lateral view.

The **SINUATRIAL (SA) NODE** (1, Fig. 15.10), or center from which each intrinsic beat of the heart originates, is in the terminal crest; the SA node cannot be observed grossly.

The **ATRIOVENTRICULAR (AV) NODE** (2), also not grossly discernible, is in the medial wall of the right atrium (**INTERATRIAL SEPTUM**), cranial and ventral to the coronary sinus.

From the AV node a conducting system of modified muscle fibers, the **ATRIOVENTRICULAR FASCICULUS** (3), courses distally through the interatrial septum, branches, and spreads distally near the

luminal surface of the interventricular septum. Parasympathetic nerve fibers to the heart terminate primarily in the atria (many terminate on the SA and AV nodes), whereas sympathetic fibers terminate at many points distally in the ventricles.

Right (1, Fig. 15.11) and left (2) atria, the pulmonary trunk (3), and the ascending aorta (4) attach to a delicate "cardiac skeleton" that separates the preceding structures from right (5) and left (6) ventricles. This skeleton is composed in part of fibrous rings of collagenous tissue upon which four sets of valves attach.

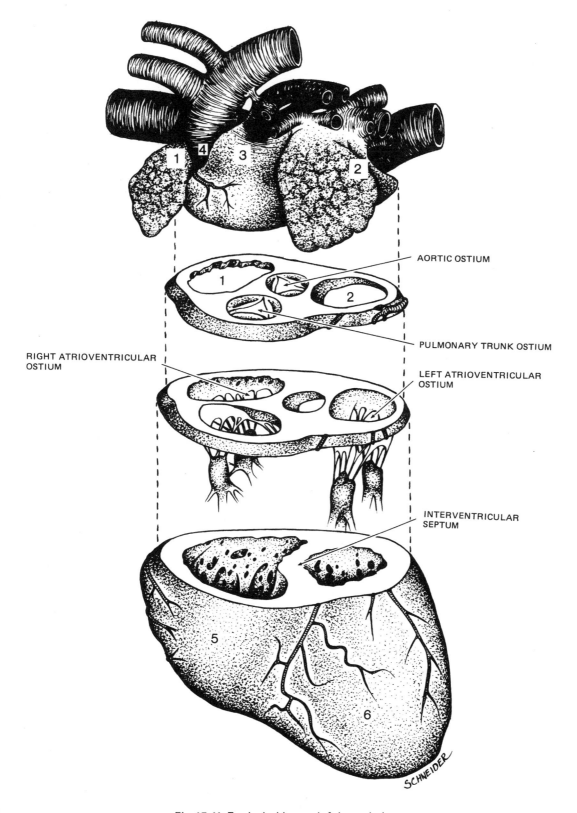

AORTIC OSTIUM

PULMONARY TRUNK OSTIUM

RIGHT ATRIOVENTRICULAR
OSTIUM

LEFT ATRIOVENTRICULAR
OSTIUM

INTERVENTRICULAR
SEPTUM

Fig. 15.11. Exploded heart, left lateral view.

The right atrioventricular ostium is bounded by the **RIGHT ATRIOVENTRICULAR VALVE,** which consists of two wide, thin flaps of tissue held open under tension by thin strands of tissue (Fig. 15.12).

The flaps, or cusps, are named according to origin from the fibrous skeleton as parietal or septal. The **PARIETAL CUSP** (1) arises from the external atrial-ventricular wall; the **SEPTAL CUSP** (2) arises from the junction of interatrial and interventricular septa.

Cone-shaped muscular projections from the **INTERVENTRICULAR SEPTUM,** called **PAPILLARY MUSCLES** (3), give origin to the fibromuscular **CHORDAE TENDINEAE** (4).

Muscular ridges on the luminal surface of the ventricle are named **TRABECULAE CARNEAE** (kar'ne; fleshy) (5). A relatively thin fibrous cord spanning the lumen of the right ventricle from the septum to the parietal wall, termed the **TRABECULA SEPTOMARGINALIS** (6), serves both to provide support for the parietal wall and as a pathway of conducting fibers (part of the atrioventricular fasciculus) (pl. fasciculi; small bundle).

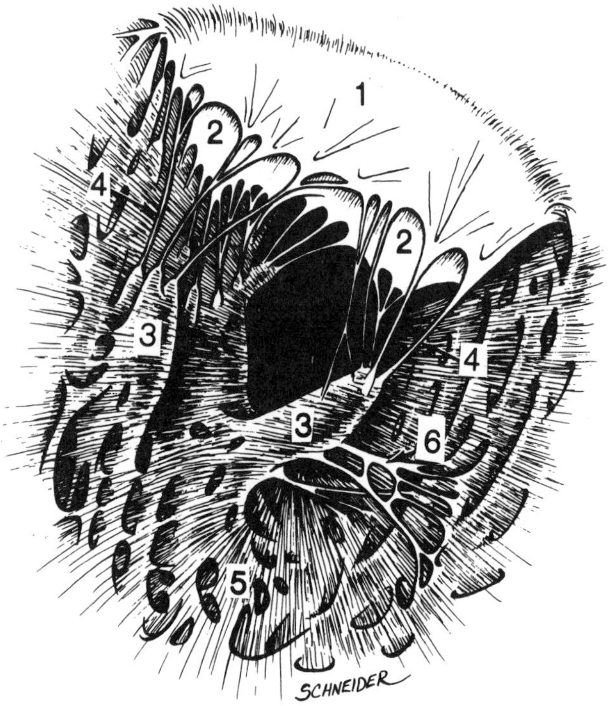

The funnel-shaped conus arteriosus (1, Fig. 15.13) portion of the right ventricle leads to the **PULMONARY TRUNK OSTIUM,** which is closed during part of the cardiac cycle by three **SEMILUNAR** (half moon) **VALVULES** (**RIGHT, LEFT,** and **INTERMEDIATE**) that form the **PULMONARY TRUNK VALVE** (2).

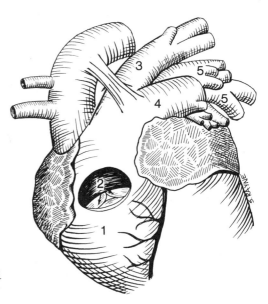

Fig.15.13. Conus arteriosus and pulmonary vessels, left dorsolateral view.

Fig.15.12. Right atrioventricular valve and internal surface of the right ventricle, viewed from the right.

The semilunar valvules are shaped like pockets, with the open portion of each pocket directed toward the distal end of the pulmonary trunk; backflow of blood opens the free margins of the three pockets against each other, closing off reentry of blood into the right ventricle.

276

Nonoxygenated blood is carried from the pulmonary trunk through right (3) and left (4) pulmonary arteries to right and left lungs. Oxygenated blood returns from both right and left lungs through five or six **PULMONARY VEINS** (5) into the left atrium.

In the left atrium the portion of the interatrial septum that overlies the fossa ovalis (see p. 273) may bear a small flap of tissue, the valvule of the foramen ovale. The left atrium pumps blood through the **LEFT ATRIOVENTRICULAR OSTIUM** into the left ventricle.

The left atrioventricular ostium (1, Fig. 15.14) is bounded by the **PARIETAL** (2) and **SEPTAL** (3) **CUSPS OF** the **LEFT ATRIOVENTRICULAR VALVE.** Unlike the right ventricle, in the left ventricle the papillary muscles (4) arise from the outer or parietal wall.

The **AORTIC OSTIUM** (5) is located near the center of the base of the heart. The **AORTIC VALVE** (6), which consists of three semilunar valvules (right, left, and septal), protects the aortic ostium from backflow of blood.

The dorsal portion of the interventricular septum, medial to the septal cusp of the right and left atrioventricular valves, is quite thin and membranous. Embryologically, this is the last portion of the interventricular septum to form; failure to close properly produces an interventricular foramen.

The ascending aorta (1, Fig. 15.15) arises from the left ventricle (2) medial (deep) to the pulmonary trunk (3) on the left and medial (deep) to the right atrium (4) and cranial vena cava (5) on the right.

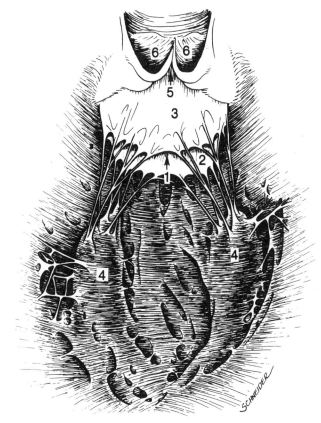

Fig.15.14. Left atrioventricular valve, parietal wall of the left ventricle, viewed from septal wall.

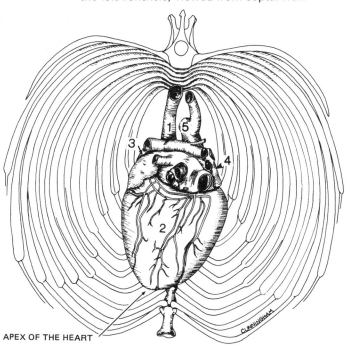

APEX OF THE HEART

Fig.15.15. Heart and thoracic cage, caudal view.

The aorta is descriptively divided into ascending aorta (1, Fig. 15.16), **AORTIC ARCH** (2), and **DESCENDING (THORACIC and ABDOMINAL) AORTA** (3). The slightly expanded origin (**AORTIC BULB**) of the ascending aorta and its cavity (**AORTIC SINUS**) gives rise to the first aortic branches, the RIGHT (4) and **LEFT** (5) **CORONARY ARTERIES.**

The next branch of the aorta arises from the aortic arch and passes cranially and to the right, across the ventral surface of the trachea.

This large branch is the **BRACHIOCEPHALIC TRUNK** (6), which supplies blood to the head through both **RIGHT** and **LEFT COMMON CAROTID ARTERIES** and to the neck, right thoracic limb, and cranial part of the thorax via the **RIGHT SUBCLAVIAN ARTERY**. The next arterial branch off the aortic arch is the **LEFT SUBCLAVIAN ARTERY** (7).

The right coronary artery (1, Fig. 15.17) originates from the aortic sinus (2) distal to the right septal valvule and carries blood through

the coronary groove of the atrial surface of the heart. Branches of the right coronary artery course distally over the surface of the right ventricle. The left coronary artery (3) carries blood from behind (caudolateral to) the left semilunar cusp to the coronary groove of the caudal auricular surface (partially covered by the left auricle).

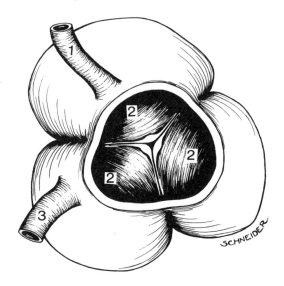

Fig.15.17. Aortic bulb, sinus, and valves, observed through transected ascending aorta.

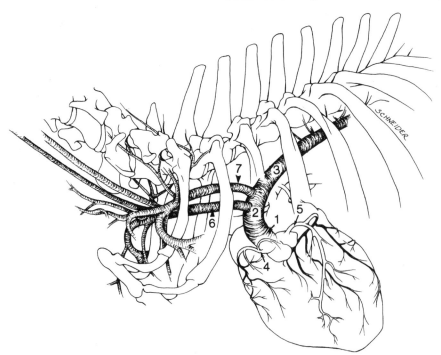

Fig.15.16. Branches of the ascending aorta and aortic arch, left lateral view.

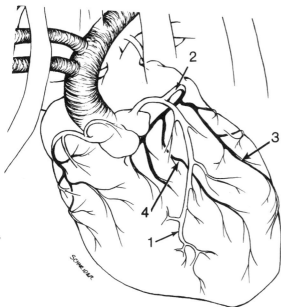

Fig.15.18. Schematic of the heart and coronary arteries, left lateral view.

A **PARACONAL INTERVENTRICULAR BRANCH** (1, Fig. 15.18) of the left coronary artery carries blood through the paraconal interventricular groove. Another large branch, the **CIRCUMFLEX BRANCH** (2), continues toward the right side around the caudodorsal surface of the heart in the coronary groove.

An **INTERMEDIATE BRANCH** (3) and a **SUBSINUOSAL INTERVENTRICULAR BRANCH** (4) course over the surface of the heart between the subsinuosal and paraconal interventricular grooves and in the subsinuosal interventricular groove, respectively.

The **GREAT CARDIAC VEIN** (1, Fig. 15.19) arises in the paraconal interventricular groove, courses around the caudodorsal surface of the heart in the coronary groove in association with the circumflex branch of the left coronary artery. It opens into the caudal portion of the right atrium ventral to the ostium of the caudal vena cava as the coronary sinus (2).

A fibrous band of tissue, the **LIGAMENTUM ARTERIOSUM** (1, Fig. 15.20) arises from the pulmonary trunk (2) near the bifurcation of the trunk into right and left pulmonary arteries, and passes to the aortic arch distal to the origin of the left subclavian artery (3). The ligamentum arteriosum is an embryonic vestige of the **DUCTUS ARTERIOSUS,** which acted to shunt blood from the pulmonary trunk to the aortic arch, thus bypassing the nonfunctional lungs of the fetus.

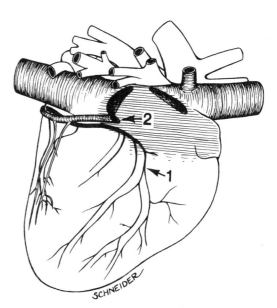

Fig.15.19. Path of the great cardiac vein, right lateral view.

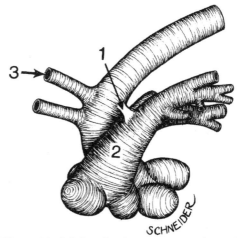

Fig.15.20. Origin of pulmonary vessels, and aorta, left lateral view.

279

Chapter 16

CARDIOVASCULAR SYSTEM—TRUNK VESSELS

Objectives: To identify major veins and arteries within the neck, thorax, and abdomen.

Veins: Right and Left External and Internal Jugular Veins; Right and Left Superficial Cervical and Cephalic Veins; Right and Left Subclavian Veins; Right and Left Brachiocephalic Veins; Right and Left Internal Thoracic and Costocervical Veins; Right Azygous Vein; Cranial and Caudal Venae Cavae

Arteries branching from:

Thoracic Aorta: Left and Right Coronary Arteries; Brachiocephalic Trunk, Left Subclavian Artery, Dorsal Intercostal Arteries, and Left and Right Costoabdominal Arteries

Brachiocephalic Trunk: Left Common Carotid, Right Common Carotid, and Right Subclavian Arteries

Right and Left Common Carotids: Cranial Thyroid Artery

Right and Left Subclavian Arteries: Internal Thoracic Artery, Vertebral Artery, Costocervical Trunk, Superficial Cervical Artery, and Axillary Artery

Right and Left Costocervical Trunks: Dorsal Scapular, Deep Cervical, and Thoracic Vertebral Arteries

Right and Left Internal Thoracic: Ventral Intercostal Arteries; Cranial Epigastric Arteries

Left and Right Carotid Sheathes, Bronchoesophageal Artery

Abdominal Aaorta: Right and Left Lumbar Arteries, Right and Left Phrenicoabdominal Arteries, Right and Left Renal Arteries, Right and Left Ovarian (Testicular) Arteries, Right and Left Deep Circumflex Iliac Arteries, Right and Left External Iliac Arteries, Right and Left Internal Iliac Arteries, Median Sacral Artery, Celiac Artery, Cranial Mesenteric Artery, Caudal Mesenteric Artery

Phrenicoabdominal Artery: Caudal Phrenic and Cranial Abdominal Arteries

Right and Left Uterine Arteries: Uterine Branch

Right and Left External Iliac Arteries: Right and Left Deep Femoral Arteries

Hepatic Portal and Hepatic Veins

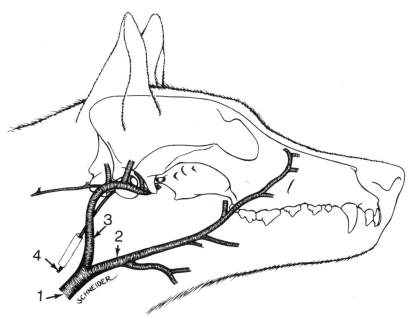

Fig.16.1. Schematic of the venous drainage from the head, right lateral view.

Most of the blood from the head (Fig. 16.1) drains caudally through the **EXTERNAL JUGULAR VEIN** (1). The **LINGUOFACIAL VEIN** (2), draining much of the surface of the head, and the **MAXILLARY VEIN** (3), draining much of the deeper portions of the head, join at the level of the 1st cervical vertebra to form the external jugular vein. The **INTERNAL JUGULAR VEIN** (4) drains some blood from the head through the carotid sheath.

In the caudal portion of the neck (Fig. 16.2), the external jugular vein (1) receives blood from the **OMOBRACHIAL VEIN** (2), a small superficial vein that drains blood from the thoracic limb (see p. 302). Near the level of the 1st rib, in the jugular fossa, the external jugular vein receives blood from the **SUPERFICIAL CERVICAL** (3), **CEPHALIC** (4), and internal jugular (5) veins.

The confluences of external jugular and **SUBCLAVIAN** (6) **VEINS** of right and left sides forms the **RIGHT** and **LEFT BRACHIOCEPHALIC VEINS** (7).

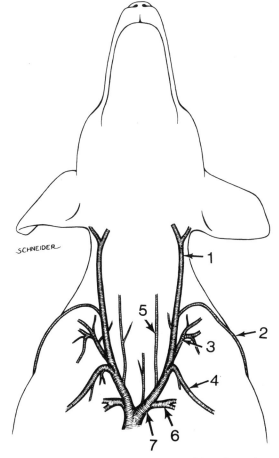

Fig.16.2. Branches of the external jugular vein, ventral view.

283

THE **CRANIAL VENA CAVA** (1, Fig. 16.3), which is formed near the cranial thoracic aperture by the confluence of right (2) and left (3) brachiocephalic veins, receives venous blood draining through **INTERNAL THORACIC** (4), **COSTOCERVICAL** (5), and **RIGHT AZYGOUS** (az' i-gus; unpaired) (6) **VEINS.**

The first four branches of the aorta (Fig. 16.4) have been described on page 278. They are the right (1) and left (2) coronary arteries off the ascending aorta and the brachiocephalic trunk (3) and left subclavian artery (4) off the aortic arch.

The three main branches of the brachiocephalic trunk are the **LEFT COMMON CAROTID** (5), **RIGHT COMMON CAROTID** (6), and **RIGHT SUBCLAVIAN** (7) **ARTERIES.**

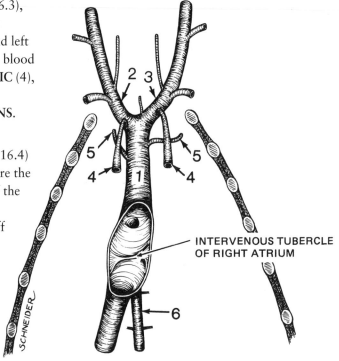

INTERVENOUS TUBERCLE OF RIGHT ATRIUM

Fig.16.3. Cranial vena cava and its tributaries, ventral view.

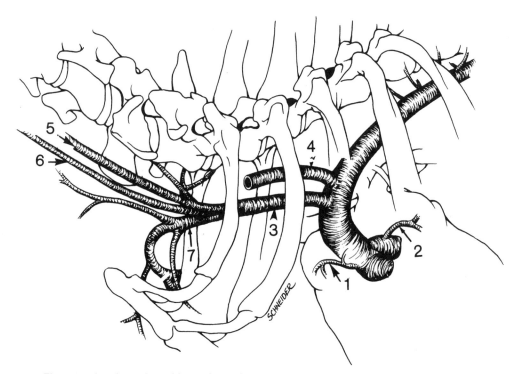

Fig.16.4. Aortic arch and branches of the brachiocephalic trunk, left lateral view.

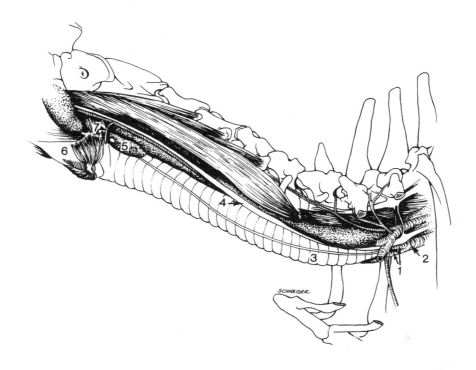

Fig.16.5. Deep structures of the neck, left ventrolateral view.

Both right and left (1, Fig. 16.5) common carotids arise from the brachiocephalic trunk (2) near the ventrolateral surface of the trachea (3).

Each common carotid artery courses through the neck with the vagosympathetic trunk (4) and the internal jugular vein in the carotid sheath (see p. 29). Each common carotid artery supplies blood to the **THYROID GLAND** (5), the larynx (6), and the cervical portion of the trachea and esophagus by way of the **CRANIAL THYROID ARTERY** (7).

In the cervical region (Fig. 16.6) the **RIGHT CAROTID SHEATH** (1) is positioned between the longus capitis muscle(2) dorsolaterally and the trachea (3) ventromedially. The **LEFT CAROTID SHEATH** (4) is positioned between the esophagus (5) dorsomedially and the longus capitis muscle dorsolaterally. Both right and left subclavian arteries have

similar branches although their origins are different; the right subclavian artery is a branch of the brachiocephalic trunk and the left subclavian originates from the aortic arch.

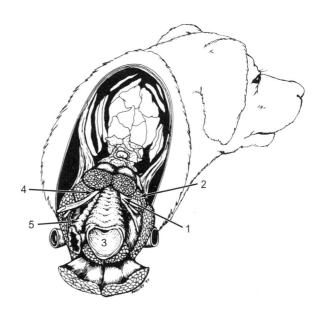

Fig.16.6. Positions of the carotid sheaths.

285

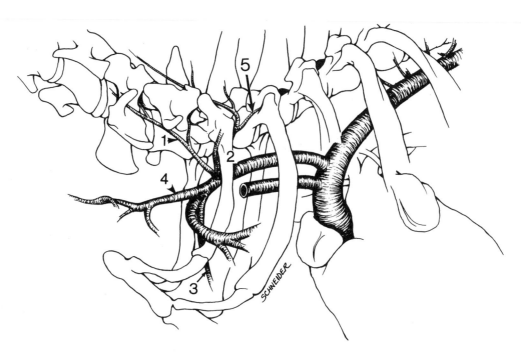

Fig.16.7. Branches of the left subclavian artery, left lateral view.

The branches of each subclavian artery (Fig. 16.7) are vertebral artery (1), costocervical trunk (2), internal thoracic artery (3), and superficial cervical artery (4). All four arteries arise within the thoracic cavity near the level of the first intercostal space; the subclavian artery continues distally past the 1st rib as the axillary artery.

The **VERTEBRAL ARTERY** (1) passes dorsocranially into the neck between the longus colli and scalenus muscles. It passes through the transverse foramina of the cervical vertebrae in association with the sympathetic vertebral nerve.

Branches of the vertebral artery pass through each intervertebral foramen and the lateral vertebral foramen, supplying blood to the meninges and blood vessels of the vertebral canal.

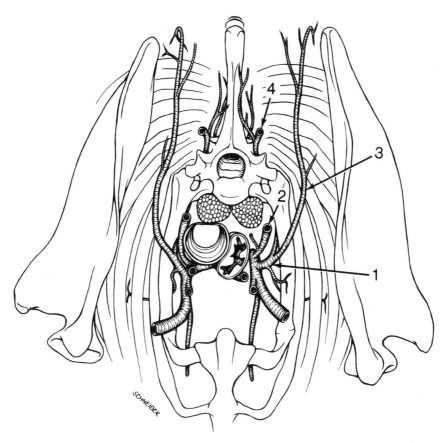

Fig.16.8. Bony thorax, illustrating the branches of the costocervical trunks, cranial view.

The **COSTOCERVICAL TRUNKS** (1, Fig. 16.8) course dorsally, lateral to the esophagus on the left side of the body, lateral to the trachea on the right side of the body, and lateral to the vertebral artery (2) near its origin on both sides.

A cranial branch, the **DORSAL SCAPULAR ARTERY** (3), arises from the costocervical trunk, passes dorsally cranial to the 1st rib, and supplies blood to the serratus ventralis muscle.

The other main branch of the costocervical trunk is a vessel that passes between the first two ribs and supplies blood to deep epaxial musculature via the **DEEP CERVICAL ARTERY** (4) and to the dorsal portion of the first several intercostal spaces via the **THORACIC VERTEBRAL ARTERY** (5, Fig. 16.7; 1, Fig. 16.9).

287

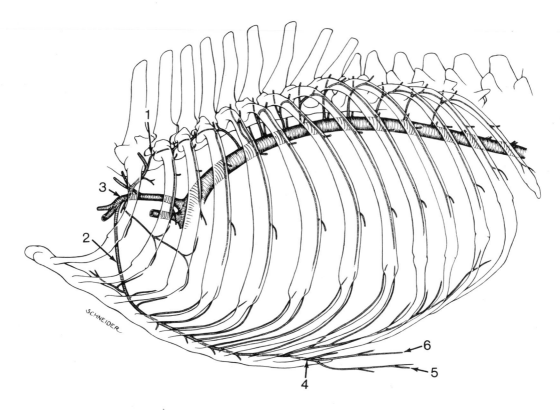

Fig.16.9. Bony thorax and branches of the thoracic aorta, left lateral view.

The **INTERNAL THORACIC ARTERY** (2, Fig. 16.9) courses caudoventrally from the subclavian artery (3), passing caudally between the transversus thoracis muscle and the costal cartilages.

Branches of the internal thoracic artery supply the mediastinum, **THYMUS**, cranial portion of the phrenic nerve (**PERICARDIACOPHRENIC ARTERY**), ventral intercostal spaces (**VENTRAL INTERCOSTAL BRANCHES**), pectoral muscles, thoracic mammary glands, and ventral portion of the thoracic diaphragm.

Near the eighth intercostal space, the internal thoracic artery passes through the diaphragm as the **CRANIAL EPIGASTRIC** (upon the belly) **ARTERY** (4), which divides at the level of the xiphoid process into two parallel, caudally coursing vessels, the **CRANIAL SUPERFICIAL** (5) and **CRANIAL DEEP** (6) **EPIGASTRIC ARTERIES**. The cranial deep epigastric is usually larger and may be observed on the deep surface of the rectus abdominis muscle. The cranial superficial epigastric is situated in the superficial fascia and may be quite large in the lactating bitch.

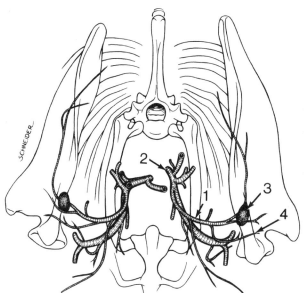

A **LATERAL THORACIC ARTERY** (4) courses caudally with the lateral thoracic nerve to supply axillary lymph nodes and latissimus dorsi, deep pectoral, and cutaneus trunci muscles.

The arterial branches of the axillary and its continuation, the **BRACHIAL ARTERY,** are described with vessels of the thoracic limb (see pp. 303–306).

Fig.16.10. Bony thorax, illustrating the branches of the brachio-cephalic trunk and subclavian, and axillary

The **SUPERFICIAL CERVICAL ARTERY** (1, Fig. 16.10) arises from the subclavian artery (2) near the 1st rib and courses into the region of the cranial extrinsic limb muscles. Branches of the superficial cervical may be observed in the region of the superficial cervical lymph nodes (3) deep to the omotransversarius muscle, and in the area of the scapular notch (4), with the suprascapular nerve.

The **AXILLARY ARTERY** (1, Fig. 16.11) is the continuation of the subclavian artery (2) past the cranial surface of the 1st rib into the axilla (with the brachial plexus).

A small **EXTERNAL THORACIC ARTERY** (3) is from the axillary artery and supplies the pectoral muscles.

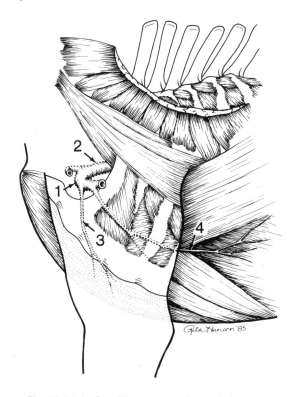

Fig.16.11. Left axillary artery, lateral view.

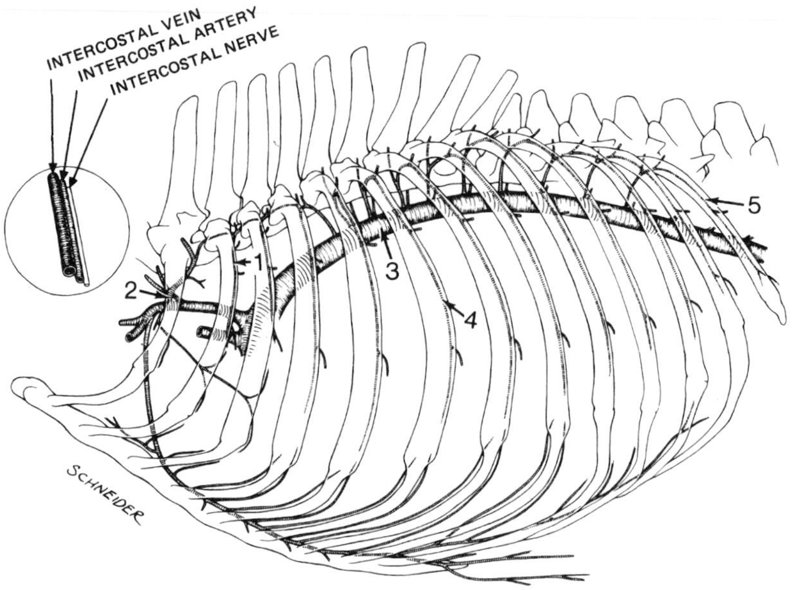

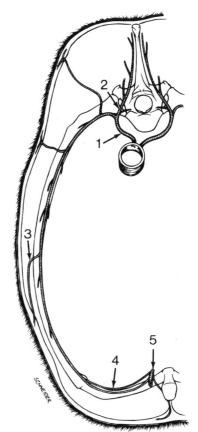

Fig.16.12. Bony thorax and arteries supplying the thoracic wall, left lateral view.

The first several intercostal spaces receive small **DORSAL INTERCOSTAL ARTERIES** (1, Fig. 16.12) from a branch of the costocervical trunk (2). The thoracic portion of the descending aorta (3) provides paired dorsal segmental branches to the caudal nine intercostal spaces and a branch to the portion of the body wall caudal to the 13th rib.

The paired segmental arteries to the intercostal spaces are the dorsal intercostal arteries (4); the vessel caudal to the 13th rib is named, like the accompanying nerve, the **DORSAL COSTOABDOMINAL ARTERY** (5).

The dorsal intercostal arteries (1, Fig. 16.13) pass into the intercostal spaces and supply dorsal branches (2) to the vessels of the vertebral canal and to muscles and skin of the epaxial area; and lateral cutaneous branches (3), which appear superficially along the ventral border of the latissimus dorsi muscle (some of these lateral cutaneous branches supply the mammae).

The dorsal intercostal arteries course along the caudal surface of each rib, superficial to the parietal pleura, and anastomose with the ventral intercostal branches (4) of the internal thoracic artery (5), forming a collateral circulation.

Fig.16.13. Branches of the inter-costal arteries, caudal view.

290

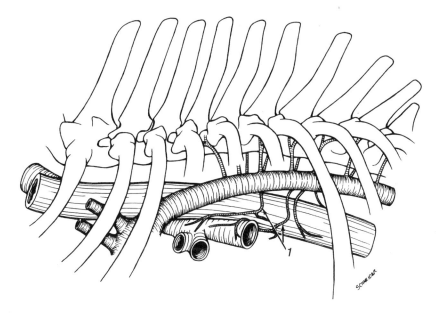

Fig.16.14. Bronchoesophageal arteries, left lateral view.

The small **BRONCHO-ESOPHAGEAL ARTERY** (1, Fig. 16.14) is one or more vessels that may arise from the right 4th to 6th dorsal intercostal arteries or from the thoracic aorta. Although the bronchoesophageal artery usually arises from a right intercostal vessel, it crosses the left surface of the esophagus. This artery provides the main blood supply to the conducting airways of the lungs as well as esophageal branches to the thoracic portion of the esophagus.

The abdominal portion of the descending aorta, termed the **ABDOMINAL AORTA** (1, Fig. 16.15), supplies seven segmental, paired **LUMBAR ARTERIES** (2). Each lumbar artery supplies blood to a vertebra, to the vertebral canal and spinal cord, and to the muscles and skin of the epaxial area. Within the abdominal cavity, three unpaired arteries branch from the ventral surface of the aorta and supply viscera. The most cranial of the three arises at the level of the 1st lumbar vertebra near

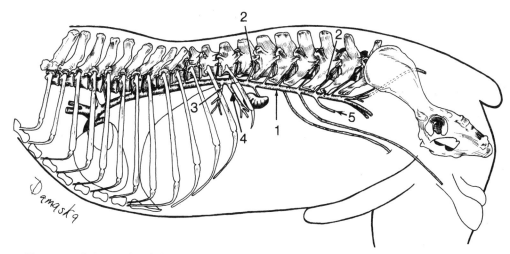

Fig.16.15. Schematic of the body, illustrating the parietal and visceral branches of the abdominal aorta, left lateral view.

the aortic hiatus; this is the **CELIAC** (se' le-ak; belly) **ARTERY** (3), which supplies blood to the stomach, liver, and spleen (as well as other structures; see p. 345).

The next caudal unpaired visceral branch is the **CRANIAL MESENTERIC ARTERY** (4), which also branches ventrally from the aorta at the level of the 1st lumbar vertebra; the celiac and cranial mesenteric arteries arise close together but diverge as the celiac artery passes cranioventrally and the cranial mesenteric artery passes caudoventrally.

The cranial mesenteric artery supplies blood to the pancreas, duodenum, jejunum, ileum, cecum, and a portion of the colon.

The third unpaired visceral artery, the **CAUDAL MESENTERIC ARTERY** (5), arises from the aorta at the level, approximately, of the 5th to 6th lumbar vertebrae. It supplies blood to the caudal portion of the colon and to the cranial portion of the rectum.

A large, paired parietal branch, the **PHRENICOABDOMINAL ARTERY** (1, Fig. 16.16), arises from the aorta caudal to the origin of the cranial mesenteric artery (2). Small branches supply the **ADRENAL GLAND** (3). It then divides, forming a **CAUDAL PHRENIC ARTERY** (4) and a **CRANIAL ABDOMINAL ARTERY** (5).

Each caudal phrenic artery courses cranially, supplies blood to the thoracic diaphragm, and anastomoses with phrenic branches of the last several intercostal arteries (collateral circulation).

The cranial abdominal artery supplies the abdominal wall of the middle abdominal region, anastomosing with the phrenic vessels cranially, with the epigastric vessels ventrally, and with the deep circumflex iliac artery caudally.

Paired **RENAL ARTERIES** (6) arise from the aorta near the level of the 3rd lumbar vertebra; the origin of the right renal artery is cranial to that of the left. Two left renal arteries may be observed in some animals. Adrenal branches usually arise from each renal artery and pass cranially to the adrenal gland.

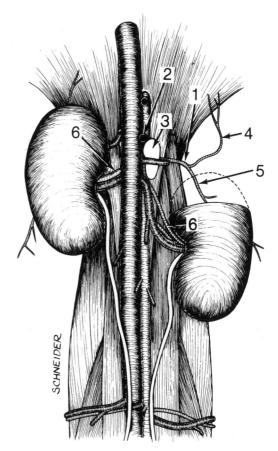

Fig.16.16. Parietal branches and the severed stumps of visceral branches of the abdominal aorta, ventral view.

The renal arteries usually divide into **DORSAL** (1, Fig. 16.17) and **VENTRAL** (2) **BRANCHES** prior to entering the kidney. The dorsal and ventral branches divide into **INTERLOBAR ARTERIES** (3), which course between renal pyramids to the corticomedullary junction.

Each interlobar artery branches into a number of **ARCUATE ARTERIES** (4), which spread out over the renal medulla between cortical and medullary tissue.

INTERLOBULAR ARTERIES arise from the arcuate vessels and pass at right angles toward the periphery of the cortex, which they supply with blood to be filtered.

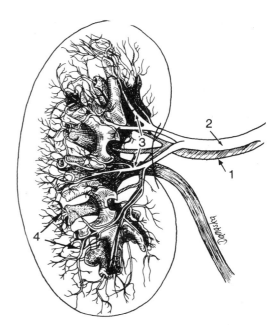

Fig.16.17. Schematic of the arterial supply to the right kidney, ventral view.

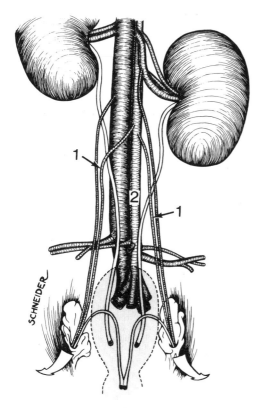

Fig.16.18. Intraabdominal course of the testicular arteries and veins, ventral view.

In the dog paired **TESTICULAR ARTERIES** (1, Fig. 16.18) arise from the aorta (2) at about the 5th lumbar vertebra; the origin of the right testicular artery usually is cranial to that of the left. The testicular arteries pass through the inguinal canal and supply the testis with blood.

The paired **OVARIAN ARTERIES** (1, Fig. 16.19) of the bitch arise from the aorta (2) similarly to the testicular arteries of the male. The ovarian artery and its branches are usually very tortuous; these vessels supply blood to the ovary, wall of the ovarian bursa (3), and uterine tube. A small **UTERINE BRANCH** of the ovarian artery forms an anastomosis with the uterine artery, thus supplying some of the uterus with blood.

The paired **DEEP CIRCUMFLEX ILIAC ARTERY** (1, Fig. 16.20) arises from the aorta (2) at the approximate level of the 6th lumbar vertebra. Its origin is usually slightly caudal to that of the unpaired caudal mesenteric artery. The deep circumflex iliac artery, which may be observed superficially with branches of the lateral cutaneus femoral nerve (see pp. 399, 440), is the main blood supply for the caudodorsal portion of the abdominal wall and much of the skin of the craniolateral femoral region.

The paired **EXTERNAL ILIAC ARTERY** (3) is a large branch of the abdominal aorta that arises near the level of the 6th or 7th lumbar vertebra and exits from the abdominal cavity through the **VASCULAR LACUNA**. The vascular lacuna of each side is a gap between the inguinal arch and the ilium. Major branches include the **DEEP FEMORAL** (4) and **FEMORAL** (5) **ARTERIES.**

The abdominal aorta terminates as the internal iliac and median sacral arteries. The **INTERNAL ILIAC ARTERY** (6) provides blood to pelvic viscera (and some abdominal structures), to gluteal and caudal thigh muscles, and to the tail.

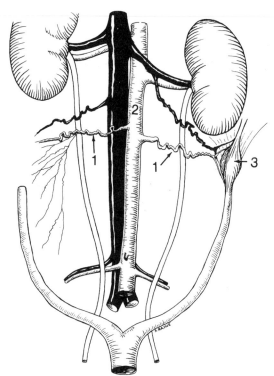

Fig.16.19. Ovarian arteries and veins, ventral view.

The **MEDIAN SACRAL ARTERY** (7) continues into the tail as the **MEDIAN CAUDAL ARTERY**.

The distal continuation of the external iliac (1, Fig. 16.21) through the vascular lacuna (2) is the femoral artery (3), which supplies blood to much of the pelvic limb.

The deep femoral artery (4) branches caudally away from the external iliac within the abdominal cavity; the **PUDENDOEPIGASTRIC TRUNK**, a ventral branch of the deep femoral artery, in turn provides caudal deep epigastric and external pudendal arterial branches. (In cases where the caudal deep epigastric and external pudendal arteries arise separately, a pudendoepigastric trunk is not present.)

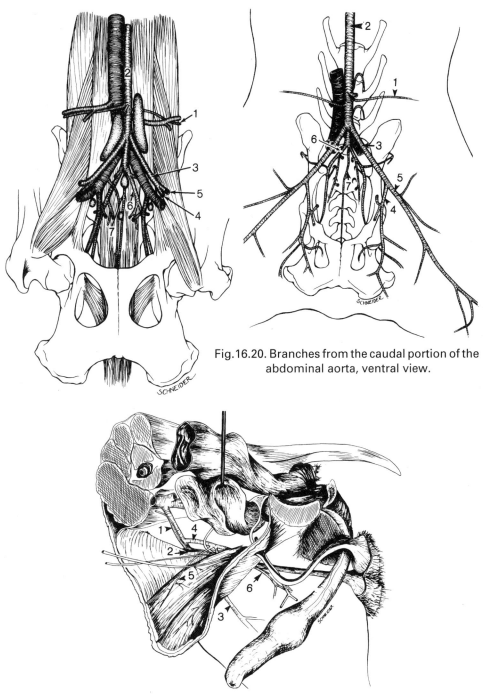

Fig.16.20. Branches from the caudal portion of the abdominal aorta, ventral view.

Fig.16.21. External iliac artery and its branches; right pelvic limb, medial view.

The **CAUDAL DEEP EPIGASTRIC ARTERY** (5) courses cranially on the deep surface of the rectus abdominis muscle; it forms an anastomosis with the cranial deep epigastric artery (collateral circulation). The **EXTERNAL PUDENDAL ARTERY** (6) leaves the abdominal cavity through the caudal portion of the inguinal canal.

Near the superficial inguinal lymph node (1, Fig. 16.22) the external pudendal artery (2) branches into **CAUDAL SUPERFICIAL EPIGASTRIC** (3) and **VENTRAL LABIAL** (bitch) or **VENTRAL SCROTAL** (4) (dog) **ARTERIES.** The caudal superficial epigastric artery courses cranially in the superficial fascia to supply blood to the caudal mammary glands (bitch) or preputial region (dog).

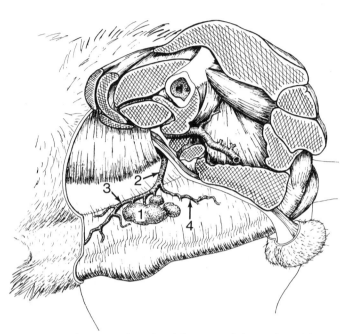

Fig.16.22. Left external pudendal artery of the male, with the left pelvic limb transected and removed, lateral view.

The continuation of the deep femoral artery (1, Fig. 16.23) through the vascular lacuna (2) is the **MEDIAL CIRCUMFLEX FEMORAL ARTERY** (3), which supplies blood to the adductor muscles (4) and to the nutrient foramen of the femoral bone.

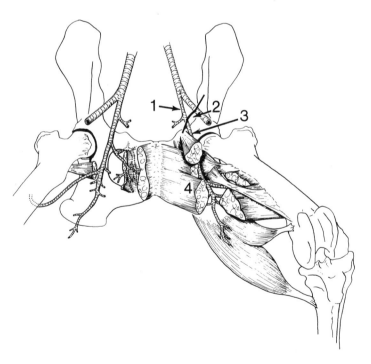

Fig.16.23. Course and distribution of the deep femoral artery and its continuation and the medial circumflex femoral artery, ventral view.

The caudal vena cava (1, Fig. 16.24) collects venous blood from the caudal portion of the trunk through veins that parallel the pathway of arteries; the names of the veins are similar to those arteries with which they course. It should be noted that the **LEFT OVARIAN** (2) or **LEFT TESTICULAR VEIN** usually drains into the **LEFT RENAL VEIN** (3).

The venous blood of the hepatic portal system (Fig. 16.25) is quite separate from that of the caudal vena cava; blood collects into larger veins from capillaries in the pancreas, spleen, stomach, and small and large intestines and then passes through the **HEPATIC PORTAL VEIN** (1) into sinusoid capillaries of the liver.

Blood is then collected from the sinusoids into terminal branches of a number of **HEPATIC VEINS** (2), which drain from the liver into the caudal vena cava (3) at a level near the vena caval foramen of the thoracic diaphragm. The branches of the hepatic portal vein are described with the visceral vasculature (see pp. 349–50).

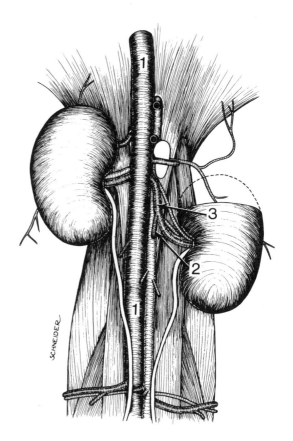

Fig.16.24. Caudal vena cava and it's abdominal tributaries, ventral view.

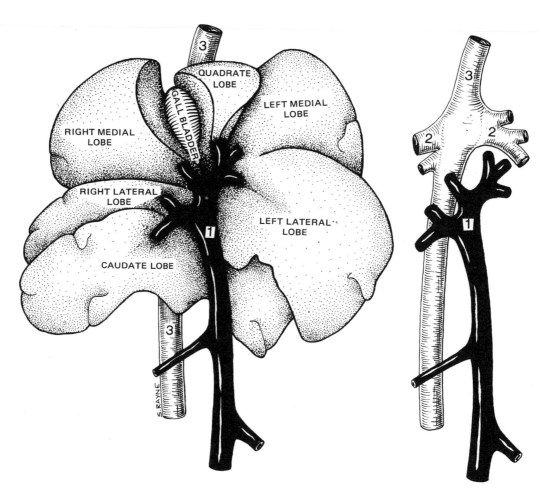

Fig.16.25. Hepatic portal and hepatic veins, ventral view.

Chapter 17

CARDIOVASCULAR SYSTEM—THORACIC LIMB

Objectives: To identify major veins and arteries within the thoracic limb.

Veins: Cephalic and Accessory Cephalic Veins; Median Cubital, Axillobrachial, and Median Cubital Veins

Arteries branching from:

Axillary Artery: External Thoracic and Lateral Thoracic Arteries; Subscapular and Brachial Arteries

Subscapular Artery: Thoracodorsal and Caudal Circumflex Scapular Arteries

Brachial Artery: Cranial Circumflex Humeral, Deep Brachial, Bicipital, Superficial Brachial, Median Cubital, Collateral Ulnar, Common Interosseous, and Median Arteries

Superficial Brachial Artery: Cranial Superficial Antebrachial Artery and its lateral and medial branches

Common Interosseous Artery: Cranial and Caudal Interosseous Arteries

Median Artery: Recurrent Ulnar, Deep Antebrachial, and Radial Arteries

Arteries within the Manus:

Dorsal Common Digital Arteries, Dorsal Metacarpal Arteries

Palmar Common Digita Arteries, Palmar Metacarpal Arteries

Axial and Abaxial Proper Digital Arteries

Hepatic Portal and Hepatic Veins

The venous system of the thoracic limb consists of two sets of vessels, one deep and one superficial. The deep set consists of veins that accompany arteries and are named accordingly.

The superficial set (Fig. 17.1) consists of the cephalic (1), accessory cephalic (2), omobrachial (3), and axillobrachial (4) veins. The **CEPHALIC VEIN** (1) collects venous blood from the palmar surface of the manus, then passes dorsoproximally across the medial surface of the distal antebrachium to reach a position on the cranial surface of the antebrachium. The **ACCESSORY CEPHALIC VEIN** (2) arises in the dorsal metacarpal region and joins the cephalic vein on the distal cranial surface of the antebrachium.

The cephalic and deeper brachial veins are interconnected at the level of the cubital articulation by the **MEDIAN CUBITAL VEIN** (5). Occlusion of the cephalic vein proximal to the median cubital vein (preliminary to venous injection) may not produce stasis of blood and vessel distension unless the median cubital vein is also occluded.

In the proximal brachial region the **CEPHALIC VEIN** (1, Fig. 17.2) passes from the superficial craniolateral surface of the triceps muscle (2) across the cranial border of the brachium, deep to the cleidobrachialis muscle (3), and joins the external jugular vein.

The **AXILLOBRACHIAL VEIN** (4) is a large vessel that continues to course proximally from the cephalic vein on the lateral proximal surface of the brachium, then passes deep through the muscle mass caudal to the humeral articulation. The axillobrachial vein joins the axillary vein in

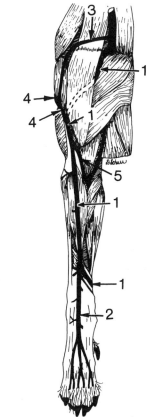

Fig.17.1. Veins of the right thoracic limb, cranial view.

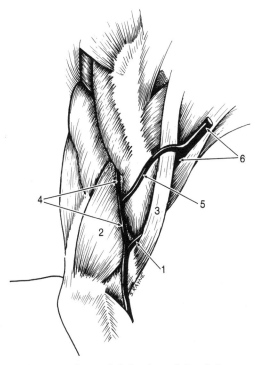

Fig.17.2. Superficial veins of the right brachium, lateral view.

the axilla. A branch of the axillobrachial vein that courses cranioproximally across the superficial surface of the cleidocervicalis is the **OMOBRACHIAL VEIN** (5), which discharges blood into the external jugular vein (6).

The **SUBCLAVIAN ARTERY** (Fig. 17.3) is called the **AXILLARY ARTERY** when it exits from the thoracic cavity and enters the axillary space past the cranial surface of the 1st rib. The **SUPERFICIAL CERVICAL ARTERY** (1) arises from the subclavian artery near the 1st rib. Two proximal branches off the axillary artery are the external and lateral thoracic arteries.

The **EXTERNAL THORACIC ARTERY** (2) courses with the cranial pectoral nerves and supplies blood to the superficial pectoral muscles.

The **LATERAL THORACIC ARTERY** (3), which courses caudally with the lateral thoracic nerve, supplies blood to the axillary lymph nodes and the latissimus dorsi, deep pectoral, and cutaneus trunci muscles as well as the skin of the lateral thoracic region.

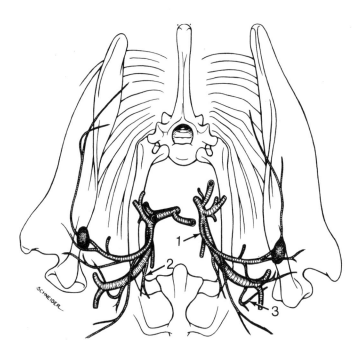

Fig.17.3. Branches of the brachiocephalic trunk, subclavian, and axillary arteries, cranial view.

The axillary artery (1, Fig. 17.4) terminates as the **SUBSCAPULAR** (2) and **BRACHIAL** (3) **ARTERIES**. The brachial artery is located along the medial surface of the brachium, cranial to the brachial vein.

The subscapular artery passes caudolaterally with the axillary nerve through the intermuscular septum between the teres major and subscapularis muscles; it provides a number of branches at the level of the humeral articulation, then courses caudodorsally along the caudal border of the scapula. Branches of the subscapular and superficial cervical arteries supply muscles, tendons, and joint capsule of the humeral articulation.

The branches of the subscapular artery are the caudal circumflex humeral (4), thoracodorsal (5), circumflex scapular (6), and, in some dogs, the cranial circumflex humeral (7) arteries.

The **THORACODORSAL ARTERY** (5) arises from the caudomedial surface of the subscapular and courses caudally with the thoracodorsal nerve to the latissimus dorsi muscle. Small branches off the subscapular artery arborize around both medial and lateral surfaces of the scapula, providing nutrient arteries to the scapula, and forming collateral circulation with branches of the superficial cervical artery.

Arising from either the subscapular or the brachial artery, the small **CRANIAL CIRCUMFLEX HUMERAL ARTERY** (7) passes cranially on the proximal medial surface of the brachium, courses deep to the biceps brachii muscle, and forms a collateral circulation with the caudal circumflex humeral artery and a branch of the superficial cervical artery.

Fig.17.4. Schematic of the tributaries of the left brachium, as observed through the sternum and ribs, medial view.

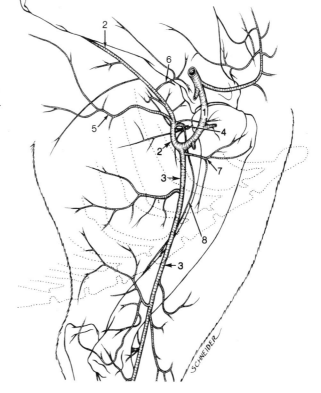

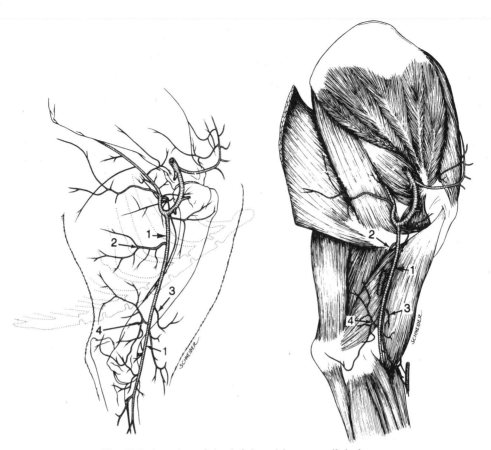

Fig.17.5. Arteries of the left brachium, medial view.

The **CAUDAL CIRCUMFLEX HUMERAL** (4) branch of the subscapular courses caudolaterally, supplying blood to the triceps brachii and deltoideus muscles; a descending branch, the **COLLATERAL RADIAL ARTERY** (8), accompanies the radial nerve to the level of the cubital articulation. The collateral radial artery provides the nutrient arterial branch to the humerus.

The brachial artery (1, Fig. 17.5) courses through the brachium on the medial surface of the medial head of the triceps brachii muscle between the musculocutaneus nerve (cranially) and the median and ulnar nerves (caudally).

A **DEEP BRACHIAL ARTERY** (2) separates from the caudal surface of the brachial artery in the proximal portion of the brachium and supplies blood to the triceps brachii muscle.

A small **BICIPITAL ARTERY** (3), which courses craniodistally from the brachial artery in the distal portion of the brachium, supplies the biceps brachii muscle. A branch of the brachial artery that courses caudodistally across the medial surface of the distal brachium, between the ulnar and the caudal cutaneous antebrachial nerves, is the **COLLATERAL ULNAR ARTERY** (4).

A small arterial branch arises from the cranial surface of the brachial artery (Fig. 17.6) near the level of the cubital articulation and courses craniodistally across the surface of the biceps brachii muscle to reach the cranial antebrachial region. This small artery is named the **SUPERFICIAL BRACHIAL ARTERY** (1) in the brachium and the **CRANIAL SUPERFICIAL ANTEBRACHIAL ARTERY** in the antebrachium.

The cranial superficial antebrachial artery courses through the antebrachium as lateral (2) and medial (3) branches, one on each side of the cephalic vein, to supply blood to the dorsum of the paw. **DORSAL COMMON** and **DORSAL PROPER DIGITAL ARTERIES** receive blood via branches of the cranial superficial antebrachial artery (see p. 307).

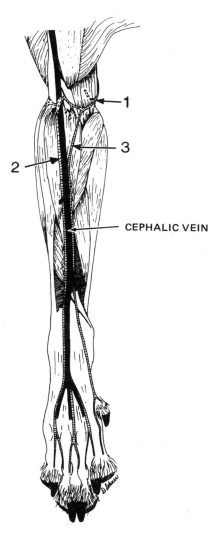

Fig. 17.6. Superficial brachial artery and its branches: cranial view of the antebrachium and dorsal view of the manus.

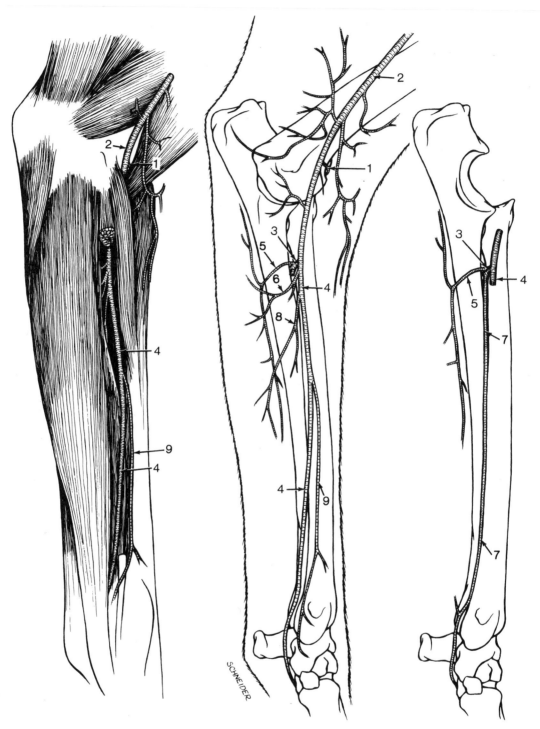

Fig.17.7. Arteries of the left antebrachium, medial view.

The **TRANSVERSE CUBITAL ARTERY** (1, Fig. 17.7) arises from the craniolateral surface of the brachial artery (2) near the deep surface of the distal end of the biceps brachii muscle.

The brachial artery courses deep to the pronator teres muscle to reach the antebrachium, where it terminates as it divides into two branches, the **COMMON INTEROSSEOUS ARTERY** (3) and the **MEDIAN ARTERY** (4).

The common interosseous artery is a very short vessel that passes caudolaterally deep into the interosseous space between radius and ulna. The **ULNAR ARTERY** (5) is a branch of the common interosseous that courses caudodistally across the medial surface of the ulna. The ulnar artery and nerve course distally between the deep digital flexor and flexor carpi ulnaris muscles.

A **RECURRENT ULNAR ARTERY** (6), which may arise from the brachial, common interosseous, or ulnar artery, courses caudoproximally and forms an anastomosis with the collateral ulnar artery (collateral circulation).

The common interosseous artery courses into the interosseous space where it divides into cranial and caudal interosseous arteries.

The **CRANIAL INTEROSSEOUS ARTERY** passes laterally between the radius and ulna; the **CAUDAL INTEROSSEOUS ARTERY** (7) courses distally in the interosseous space, lateral to the pronator quadratus muscle.

NUTRIENT ARTERIES to the radius and ulna arise from the common interosseous artery or one of its branches.

The median artery continues distally through the antebrachium in association with the median nerve. The **DEEP ANTEBRACHIAL ARTERY** (8) is a caudal branch to the flexor muscles. The **RADIAL ARTERY** (9) branches from the median artery craniodistally near the distal portion of the antebrachium.

(DIFFERENCES TO BE NOTED IN THE CAT: The brachial artery passes through the supracondylar foramen of the distal brachium. The common interosseous artery and omobrachial vein are usually not present.)

The cranial superficial antebrachial, median, radial, caudal interosseous, and ulnar arteries enter the carpus and contribute to the blood supply of the digits.

Vessels of the metacarpus are located at four levels: dorsal superficial, dorsal deep, palmar superficial, and palmar deep.

Superficial vessels of the metacarpus are named **COMMON DIGITAL** arteries and veins; deep vessels are named **METACARPAL** arteries and veins.

The dorsal arterial plan (Fig. 17.8) is as follows: the superficial **DORSAL COMMON DIGITAL ARTERIES I–IV** (1–4) supplied by medial (5) and lateral (6) branches of the cranial superficial antebrachial artery; and the deep **DORSAL METACARPAL ARTERIES II, III,** and **IV**

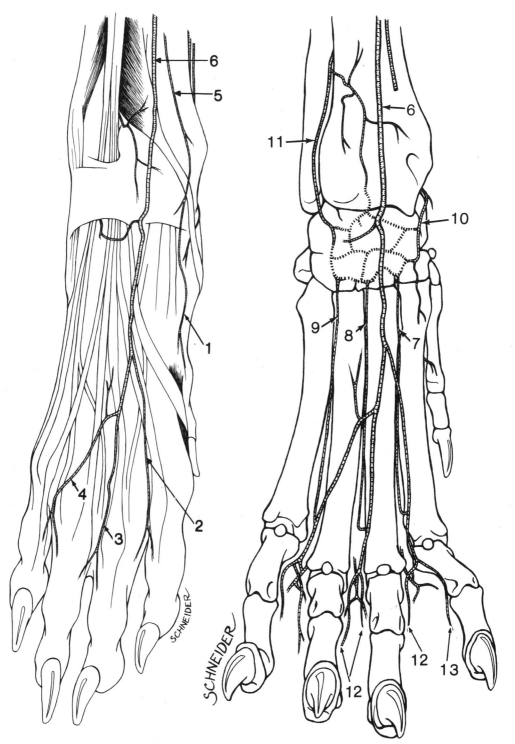

Fig.17.8. Dorsal arteries of the right manus, dorsal view.

(7–9) supplied by the radial artery (10) and a branch of the caudal interosseous artery (11).

The designation of common digital or metacarpal arteries as I, II, III, or IV is made according to whether the artery is situated within the 1st, 2nd, 3rd, or 4th intermetacarpal space. Each metacarpal artery unites with the correspondingly numbered common digital artery in the distal portion of the metacarpus.

Each of the four vessels thus formed interconnects with a palmar vessel and divides into two digital arteries.

These dorsal digital arteries are named **DORSAL AXIAL** (12) or **ABAXIAL** (13) **PROPER DIGITAL ARTERY II–IV** according to digit number and whether it is on the side of the digit

closest (axial) or farthest (abaxial) from the axis of the foot (see p. 8).

The palmar arterial plan (Fig. 17.9) is as follows: the superficial **PALMAR COMMON DIGITAL ARTERIES I-IV** (1–4) supplied by the median artery (5), with some collateral flow from the caudal interosseous artery; and the deep **PALMAR METACARPAL ARTERIES II–IV** (6–8), which receive blood from both the radial (9) and caudal interosseous (10) arteries. Palmar common digital and palmar metacarpal arteries of each intermetacarpal space join in the distal metacarpus.

Each vessel thus formed has an arterial branch interconnecting with the corresponding dorsal vessel and divides into **PALMAR AXIAL** and **ABAXIAL PROPER DIGITAL ARTERIES.**

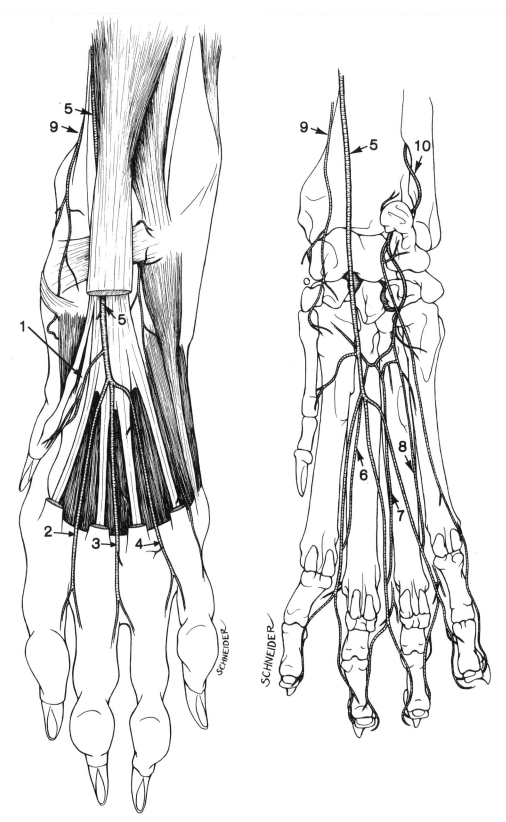

Fig.17.9. Palmar arteries of the right manus.

Chapter 18

CARDIOVASCULAR SYSTEM—PELVIC LIMB

Objectives: To identify major veins and arteries within the pelvic limb.

Veins: Medial and Lateral Saphenous Veins, Distal Caudal Femoral and Femoral Veins

Medial Circumflex Femoral Artery

Arteries branching from:

Femoral Artery: Superficial Circumflex Iliac and Lateral Circumflex Femoral Arteries; Proximal, Middle, and Distal Caudal Femoral Arteries; Descending Genicular and Saphenous Arteries, Popliteal Artery; Cranial and Caudal Tibial Arteries

Saphenous Artery: Cranial, Intermediate, and Caudal Branches

Cranial Tibial Artery: Dorsal Pedal Artery and its Arcuate branch

Caudal Gluteal Artery: Iliolumbar, Caudal Gluteal, Lateral Caudal, and Dorsal Perineal Arteries

Arteries in the Pes:

Proximal Perforating Artery II

Dorsal Common Digital and Dorsal Metatarsal Arteries

Plantar Common Digital and Plantar Metatarsal Arteries

The superficial set of pelvic limb veins (Fig. 18.1) includes a medial and a lateral saphenous vein. The **MEDIAL SAPHENOUS VEIN** (1), which is formed distally by cranial (2) and caudal (3) branches, accompanies the saphenous artery and nerve in the crus; the medial saphenous vein joins the **FEMORAL VEIN** (4) in the distal medial femoral region. The **LATERAL SAPHENOUS VEIN** (5), which is formed distally by cranial and caudal branches, discharges into the **DISTAL CAUDAL FEMORAL VEIN** (6) of the popliteal region.

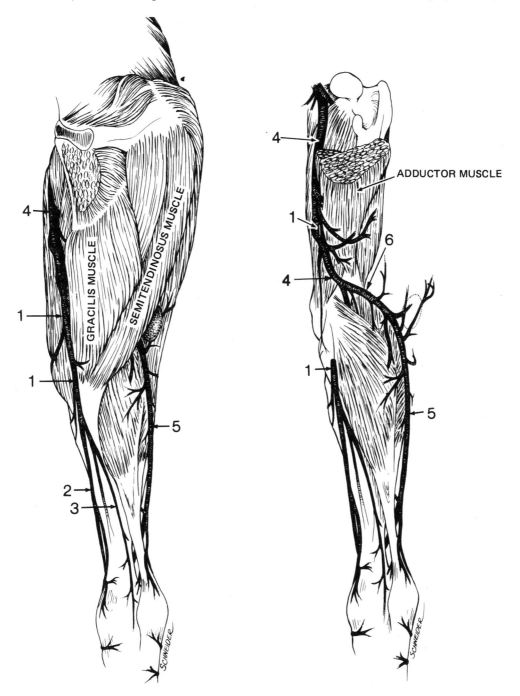

Fig.18.1. Veins of the right pelvic limb, caudomedial view.

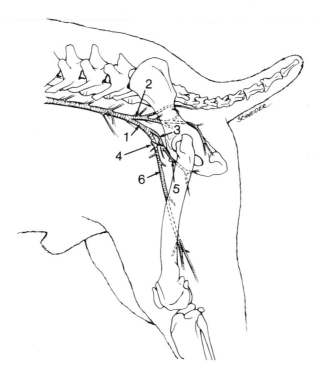

Fig.18.2. Schematic of the arteries that supply the left pelvic limb, lateral view.

The pelvic limb receives blood via branches of both the **EXTERNAL** (1, Fig. 18.2) and **INTERNAL** (2) **ILIAC ARTERIES.** Of these two vessels, the external iliac provides most of the pelvic limb with blood.

The **DEEP FEMORAL ARTERY** (3), which arises from the external iliac within the abdominal cavity (see p. 294), passes out into the medial femoral muscles through the caudal portion of the vascular lacuna (4); the continuation of the deep femoral artery peripheral to the vascular lacuna is named the

MEDIAL CIRCUMFLEX FEMORAL ARTERY (5).

The medial circumflex femoral artery passes through fascia between the vastus medialis and pectineus muscles to supply the muscles of the area, the nutrient foramen of the femoral bone, and the articular capsule of the coxal articulation. The external iliac artery also passes from the abdominal cavity through the vascular lacuna, after which it is named the **FEMORAL ARTERY** (6).

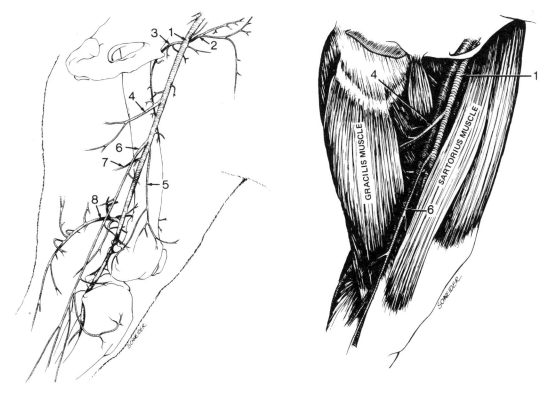

Fig.18.3. Arteries of the left pelvic limb, medial view.

Proximally in the femoral triangle (Fig. 18.3; see also p. 99), the femoral artery (1) may be felt for the purpose of taking a pulse. The following branches to the pelvic limb arise from the femoral artery (listed from proximal to distal according to origin): superficial circumflex iliac (2), lateral circumflex femoral (3), proximal caudal femoral (4), descending genicular (5), saphenous (6), middle caudal femoral (7), and distal caudal femoral (8) arteries.

The **SUPERFICIAL CIRCUMFLEX ILIAC ARTERY** (2) branches from the lateral surface of the femoral artery in the proximal portion of the femoral triangle either separately from or in common with the **LATERAL CIRCUMFLEX FEMORAL ARTERY** (3).

The **PROXIMAL CAUDAL FEMORAL ARTERY** (4) is one of three caudally coursing muscular branches (proximal, middle, and distal); as it crosses the distal superficial surface of the pectineus muscle to supply blood to the adductor magnus et brevis and gracilis muscles, it is vulnerable to injury during surgery in the femoral triangle.

The terminal branches of the superficial circumflex iliac artery anastomose with those of the deep circumflex iliac artery; the terminal branches of the lateral and medial circumflex femoral arteries likewise form a collateral circulation. Branches of the superficial circumflex iliac artery supply blood to the sartorius, tensor fasciae latae, and rectus femoris muscles.

Branches of the lateral circumflex femoral supply blood to the quadriceps femoris muscle, the articular capsule of the coxal articulation, and muscles of the gluteal region.

315

The small **DESCENDING GENICULAR** (1, Fig. 18.4) and **SAPHENOUS** (sah-fe'nus) (2) **ARTERIES** usually arise from the femoral artery (3) either as a common trunk or close together. The descending genicular artery supplies blood to the cranial and medial genicular regions.

The saphenous artery courses with the saphenous nerve distally across the superficial surface of the genu, near the fascial cleft separating the sartorius and gracilis muscles. The positional relationship of nerve and vessels is the same here as in many other parts of the body, i.e., nerve-artery-vein (NAV).

The saphenous artery divides into cranial and caudal branches on the medial surface of the proximal portion of the crus. The **CRANIAL**

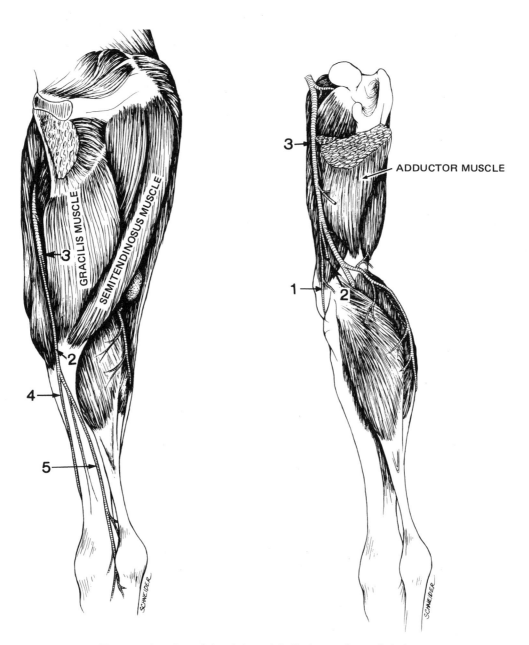

Fig.18.4. Arteries of the right pelvic limb, caudomedial view.

BRANCH (4) courses craniodistally to the flexor surface of the tarsus and supplies blood to the dorsal superficial surface of the pes (DORSAL COMMON DIGITAL ARTERIES I–IV).

The CAUDAL BRANCH (5) courses distally along the fascial cleft separating the medial surface of the gastrocnemius muscle from the medial head of the deep digital flexor muscle; at the level of the tarsus, the caudal saphenous branch divides into medial and lateral plantar arteries.

The MEDIAL PLANTAR ARTERY supplies blood to the superficial set of plantar vessels (PLANTAR COMMON DIGITAL ARTERIES II–IV).

The LATERAL PLANTAR ARTERY supplies some of the blood to the deep metatarsal vessels (PLANTAR METATARSAL ARTERIES II–IV).

The MIDDLE CAUDAL FEMORAL ARTERY (1, Fig. 18.5) arises from the caudolateral surface of the femoral artery (2) in the distal portion of the femoral region; it courses caudally and supplies the adductor magnus et brevis and semimembranosus muscles with blood. The middle caudal femoral vessel is usually smaller than the proximal caudal femoral artery (3) with which it forms a collateral circulation.

The DISTAL CAUDAL FEMORAL ARTERY (4) arises from the femoral artery immediately proximal to where the continuation of the femoral artery (as the popliteal artery) passes distally between the lateral and medial heads of the gastrocnemius muscle. The large distal caudal femoral artery courses caudally and breaks up into a number of branches that supply the popliteal lymph node, muscles crossing the flexor surface of the genu, and the skin of the area.

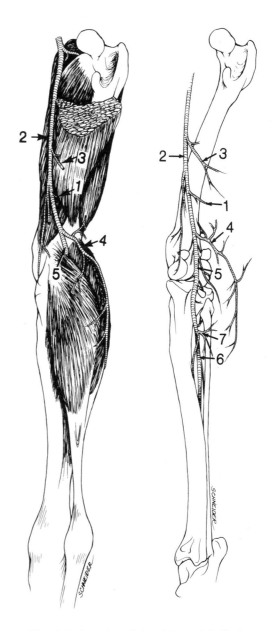

Fig.18.5. Arteries of the right pelvic limb, caudomedial view.

Terminal branches of the distal caudal femoral artery form collateral circulations with the middle caudal femoral, proximal caudal femoral, medial circumflex femoral, and caudal gluteal arteries.

The **POPLITEAL ARTERY** (5) is the distal continuation of the femoral artery through the fascia separating lateral and medial heads of the gastrocnemius muscle. It perforates the deep digital flexor muscle and enters the interosseous space between the tibia and fibula, where it divides, forming the **CRANIAL TIBIAL ARTERY** (6) and the very small **CAUDAL TIBIAL ARTERY** (7).

Small branches of the popliteal artery supply the articular capsule of the genual articulation, the cruciate and collateral ligaments, and muscles of the area.

The caudal tibial artery supplies blood to the deep digital flexor muscle.

The cranial tibial artery, the larger of the two terminal branches of the popliteal artery, passes craniodistally through the interosseous space deep to the proximal portion of the fibularis longus muscle. It courses through the crus, with the deep fibular nerve, deep to the fascial cleft separating cranial tibial and long digital extensor muscles. The cranial tibial artery supplies branches to the nutrient foramina of the tibia and fibula, flexor muscles of the tarsus, and extensor muscles of the digits.

The cranial tibial artery (1, Fig. 18.6) on the distal cranial surface of the crus passes deep to the crural extensor retinaculum (2); the

continuation of the cranial tibial artery in the flexor angle of the tarsus is named the **DORSAL PEDAL ARTERY** (3). This short artery terminates as two branches, which supply blood to deep vessels of both dorsal and plantar surfaces of the pes.

The **ARCUATE ARTERY** (4), passes laterally, giving off **DORSAL METATARSAL ARTERIES III** and **IV** (5, 6). The **DORSAL METATARSAL ARTERY II** (7) is a distal continuation of the dorsal pedal artery.

The **PROXIMAL PERFORATING BRANCH II** (8), a branch of the dorsal metatarsal artery II, passes between metatarsal bones II and III to reach the deep plantar surface of the pes. It unites with deep branches of the caudal saphenous arterial branch. The proximal perforating branch II is of nearly the same diameter as the dorsal pedal artery.

Near the level of the distal metatarsal region, the dorsal metatarsal arteries and the dorsal common digital arteries (9) unite to supply blood to the digits via **AXIAL** and **ABAXIAL DORSAL PROPER DIGITAL ARTERIES** (10). The dorsal metatarsal arteries are supplied with blood via the dorsal pedal artery; the dorsal common digital arteries are supplied via the cranial branch of the saphenous artery.

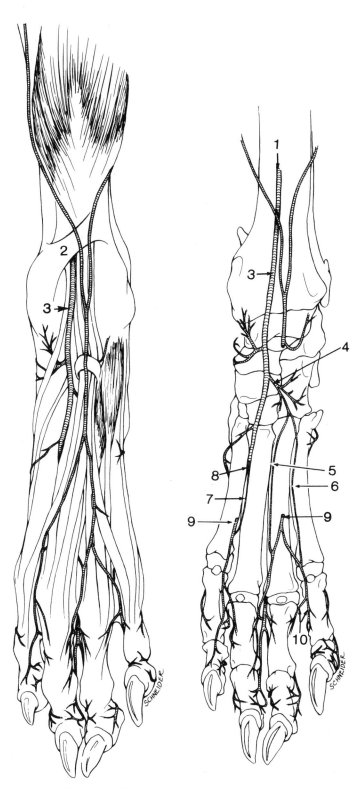

Fig.18.6. Dorsal arteries of the left pes, dorsal view.

The plantar vessels derive blood from the caudal branch of the saphenous artery (1, Fig. 18.7) and the proximal perforating branch II (2). The superficially positioned plantar common digital arteries II–IV (3) are branches of the medial plantar artery (4). The deeply positioned plantar metatarsal arteries II–IV (5) transport blood supplied primarily by the proximal perforating branch II but also by the lateral plantar artery (6) (see p. 317).

The internal iliac artery (1, Fig. 18.8) supplies blood to the pelvic viscera and to structures of the gluteal, ischiorectal, perineal, and caudal femoral regions. The visceral branches of the internal iliac, i.e., the **UMBILICAL** (2) and **INTERNAL PUDENDAL** (3) **ARTERIES,** are described in the chapter on the pelvis and tail (see pp. 325).

The **CAUDAL GLUTEAL ARTERY** (4) arises as one of two terminal branches of the internal iliac artery, ventral to the sacroiliac articulation, and passes caudally out of the pelvic cavity in association with the ischiatic nerve. The other terminal branch of the internal iliac artery, the internal pudendal artery, is ventromedial to the caudal gluteal artery.

Branches of the caudal gluteal artery in the dog are the iliolumbar, cranial gluteal, lateral caudal, and dorsal perineal arteries. The **ILIOLUMBAR ARTERY** (5) branches laterally away from the caudal gluteal artery and crosses the ventral surface of the ilium to reach the gluteal muscles. It supplies blood to the psoas minor, iliopsoas, sartorius, tensor fasciae latae, and middle gluteus muscles.

The **CRANIAL GLUTEAL ARTERY** (6) branches laterally from the caudal gluteal artery and courses past the dorsal surface of the major

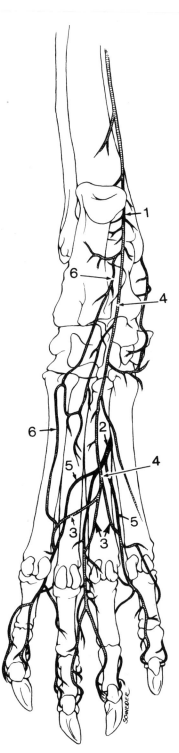

Fig.18.7. Plantar arteries of the left pes, plantar view.

ischiatic notch with the cranial gluteal nerve. It supplies blood to the middle gluteus muscle and forms a collateral flow with the iliolumbar artery.

The **LATERAL CAUDAL ARTERY** (7) arises dorsomedially from the caudal gluteal artery and courses caudally past the deep surface of the superficial gluteus muscle to enter and supply the tail.

The **DORSAL PERINEAL ARTERY** (8) arises from the caudal gluteal artery within the ischiorectal fossa (near the origin of the lateral

caudal artery) and passes caudally, where it supplies blood to the skin and fascia of the perineal region.

The caudal gluteal artery courses caudodistally through the lesser ischiatic notch, deep to the sacrotuberous ligament, to supply blood to the proximal portion of the caudal thigh muscles. Branches of the caudal gluteal artery may be observed with muscular branches of the ischiatic nerve.

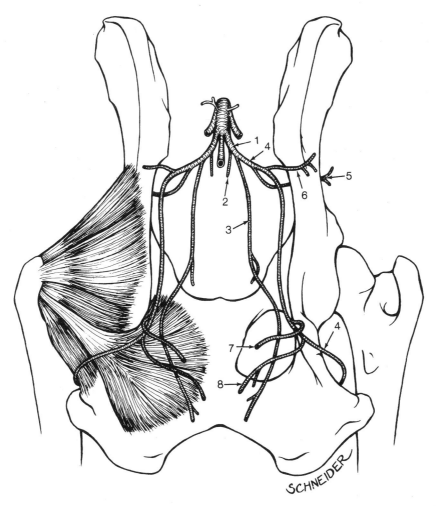

Fig.18.8. Branches of the internal iliac and caudal gluteal arteries, dorsal view.

Chapter 19

CARDIOVASCULAR SYSTEM—PELVIS & TAIL

Objectives: To identify major veins and arteries within the pelvic cavity and tail region.

Branches of arteries:

Median Sacral Artery: Dorsal Sacral Arteries, Median Caudal Artery

Right and Left Internal Iliac Arteries: Umbilical Artery, Caudal Gluteal Arteries, and Internal Pudendal Arteries

Right and Left Internal Pudendal Arteries: Uterine/Prostatic artery; Ventral Perineal Artery; Artery of the Clitoris/Penis

Right and Left Uterine/Prostatic Arteries: Caudal Vesicular Artery; Urethral Artery, Ureteric Artery, Middle Rectal Artery, Uterine Artery/Artery of the Ductus Deferens

Right and Left Artery of the Clitoris/Penis: Artery of the Bulb of the Penis, Deep Artery of the Penis, Dorsal Artery of the Penis

Most of the vasculature of the pelvis is described on pages 294 and 320 with vessels of the trunk and pelvic limb.

The **MEDIAN SACRAL ARTERY** (1, Fig. 19.1) supplies **SACRAL BRANCHES** that enter the ventral sacral foramina and continues caudally along the ventral surface of the tail as the **MEDIAN CAUDAL ARTERY**. The median caudal artery and the bilaterally paired **LATERAL CAUDAL ARTERIES** (2), branches of the caudal gluteal arteries, are the three major sources of blood to the tail.

A small **UMBILICAL ARTERY** (3) arises from the **INTERNAL ILIAC ARTERY** (4), near the division of the aorta, into paired internal iliac arteries and the median sacral artery. The umbilical artery courses ventrally along the lateral surface of the urinary bladder to supply some blood to the apex of the urinary bladder. The bilaterally paired umbilical arteries are remnants of vessels present during fetal life that carried blood to the placenta.

The two major branches of the internal iliac are the dorsolaterally situated **CAUDAL GLUTEAL**

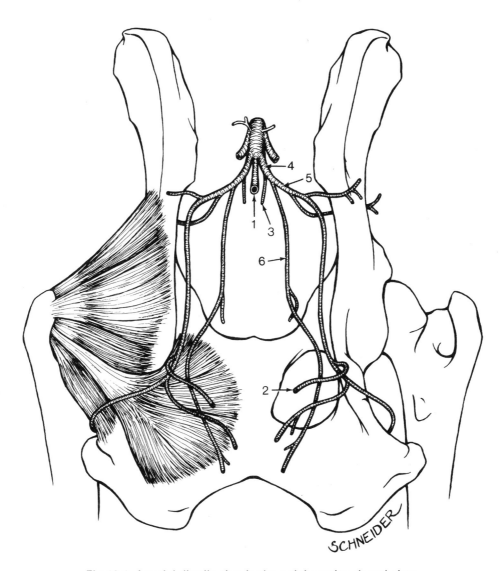

Fig.19.1. Arterial distribution in the pelvic cavity, dorsal view.

ARTERY (5) and the smaller, more ventromedially positioned **INTERNAL PUDENDAL ARTERY** (6). The branches of the caudal gluteal, described on page 310, are the iliolumbar, cranial gluteal, lateral caudal, and dorsal perineal arteries.

The internal pudendal artery (1) is the major artery to the pelvic viscera and external genitalia (Figs. 19.2, 19.3). It courses caudally along the dorsolateral surface of the rectum (2). The first major branch, the **VAGINAL** (3, Fig. 19.2) or **PROSTATIC** (3, Fig. 19.3) **ARTERY**, courses caudoventrally to the pelvic viscera. Near the anus (in the ischiorectal fossa), the terminal portion of the internal pudendal artery divides into the **VENTRAL PERINEAL ARTERY** (4) and an **ARTERY OF THE CLITORIS** (5, Fig. 19.2) or **ARTERY OF THE PENIS** (5, Fig. 19.3).

In the bitch (Fig. 19.2) the vaginal artery (3) courses caudally to the vagina. The **UTERINE ARTERY** (6), a cranioventral branch of the vaginal artery that courses along in the mesometrium, supplies blood to the uterus. The cranial portion of the uterine artery forms an anastomosis with a branch of the ovarian artery (see p. 294). The **CAUDAL VESICULAR ARTERY** (7) is a branch of the uterine artery that supplies blood to the urinary bladder; a **URETHRAL BRANCH** (8) supplies blood to the urethra; another small artery, the **URETERIC BRANCH** (9), passes cranially with the ureter. The **MIDDLE RECTAL ARTERY** (10) branches dorsally from the vaginal artery and supplies blood to the rectum.

(DIFFERENCE TO BE NOTED IN THE CAT: The uterine artery is close to the uterus in its mesometrial border.)

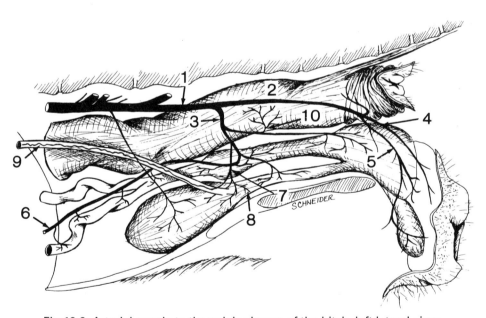

Fig.19.2. Arterial supply to the pelvic viscera of the bitch, left lateral view.

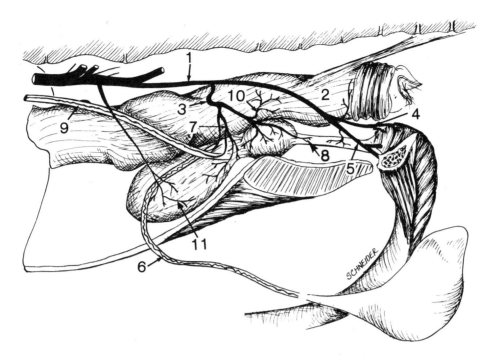

Fig.19.3. Arterial supply to the pelvic viscera of the dog, left lateral view.

In the dog (Fig. 19.3) the prostatic artery (3) courses caudoventrally to the prostate gland. A ventral branch from the prostatic artery near its origin, the **ARTERY OF THE DUCTUS DEFERENS** (6), supplies blood to the ductus deferens. This artery supplies collateral flow with the testicular artery to the epididymis (collateral circulation).

The **CAUDAL VESICULAR ARTERY** (7), a branch of the artery of the ductus deferens, is larger than the continuation of the parent artery. It supplies blood to the urinary bladder and forms a collateral circulation with the small cranial vesicular branch (11) of the umbilical artery. **URETERIC** (9) and **URETHRAL BRANCHES** of the caudal vesicular artery supply the ureter and urethra, respectively.

The **MIDDLE RECTAL ARTERY** (10) is a caudodorsal branch of the prostatic artery that supplies blood to the rectum.

The **URETHRAL BRANCH** (8) is a small vessel to the urethra that separates from the terminal portion of the prostatic artery.

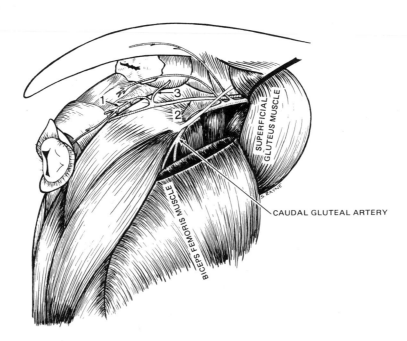

Fig.19.4. Arteries of the right ischiorectal fossa, caudolateral view.

The ventral perineal artery (1, Fig. 19.4) arises from the internal pudendal artery (2) near the anus and supplies blood to the rectum via the **CAUDAL RECTAL ARTERY** (3), and the skin of the perineum and scrotum (**DORSAL SCROTAL BRANCH**) or vulva (**DORSAL LABIAL BRANCH**).

Paired **VENTRAL SCROTAL** or **LABIAL VESSELS** carrying blood supplied by the external pudendal artery (see p. 296) form a collateral circulation with the dorsal scrotal or labial vessels.

The blood supply to the penis (Fig. 19.5) is carried via the artery of the penis (1), a branch of the internal pudendal artery. The artery divides into three branches near the proximal portion of the penis.

The **ARTERY OF THE BULB OF THE PENIS** (2) enters and supplies the corpus spongiosum penis and penile urethra.

The **DEEP ARTERY OF THE PENIS** (3) supplies the corpus cavernosum penis. The **DORSAL ARTERY OF THE PENIS** (4) passes distally along the dorsal surface of the penis to supply the bulbus glandis, pars longa glandis, and prepuce.

The **DORSAL VEIN OF THE PENIS** passes through a fibrous ring situated cranioventral to the bulb of the penis; a muscle, the ischiourethralis, arises from the ischiatic tuberosity of each side and inserts on this fibrous ring. Contraction of the paired ischiourethralis muscle results in occlusion of the dorsal vein of the penis and in engorgement of erectile tissue.

The artery of the clitoris (1, Fig. 19.6) supplies the clitoris with blood via three vessels.

328

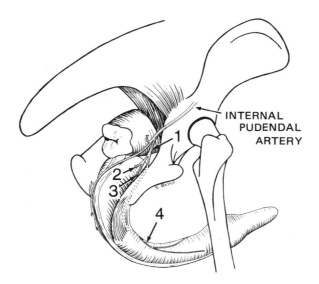

Fig.19.5. Arteries of the penis, right caudolateral view.

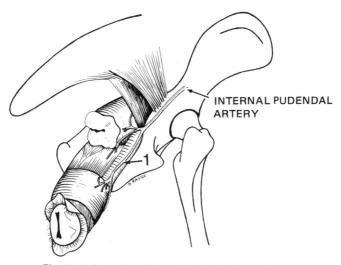

Fig.19.6. Arteries of the clitoris, right caudolateral
view.

Chapter 20

CARDIOVASCULAR SYSTEM—HEAD

Objectives: To identify major veins and arteries in the head.

Extracranial Veins:

Branches of the Left and Right Facial Veins: Angularis Oculi, Dorsal Nasal, Lateral Nasal, Superior Labial, Deep Facial, and Linguofacial

Branches of the Right and Left Linguofacial Veins: Facial and Lingual Veins

Branches of the Right and Left External Jugular Veins: Maxillary and Linguofacial Veins

Extracranial Arteries:

Branches of the Right and Left Common Carotid Arteries: Cranial Thyroid, Internal Carotid (Carotid Sinus), and External Carotid Arteries

Branches of the Right and Left External Carotid Arteries: Occipital, Ascending Pharyngeal, Lingual, Facial, Caudal Auricular, Superficial Temporal, and Maxillary Arteries

Branches of the Right and Left Caudal Auricular Arteries: Lateral, Intermediate, and Medial Auricular Arteries

Branches of the Right and Left Maxillary Arteries: Inferior Alveolar, Caudal Deep Temporal, Middle Meningeal, External Ophthalmic, Minor Palatine, Descending Palatine, Malar, and Infraorbital Arteries

Branches of the Right and Left Infraorbital Arteries: Superior Alveolar and Lateral Nasal Arteries

Intracranial Arteries:

Right and Left Internal Carotid Arteries; Right and Left Vertebral Arteries; Ventral Spinal and Basilar Arteries; Right and Left Caudal Communicating Arteries; Cerebral Arterial Circle; Right and Left Rostral, Middle, and Caudal Meningeal Arteries; Right and Left Rostral, Middle, and Caudal Cerebral Arteries

Intracranial Veins:

Right and Left Maxillary, Internal Jugular, Vertebral, and Ventral Internal Vertebral Plexus; Dorsal Sagittal Sinus; Right and Left Transverse, Temporal, and Sigmoid Sinuses; Cavernous Sinus

EXTRACRANIAL VESSELS

A number of veins are situated superficially on the head of the dog (Fig. 20.1). Some of these vessels are observable on the live animal. The **ANGULARIS OCULI VEIN** (1) drains blood from the nose to the **DORSAL EXTERNAL OPHTHALMIC VEIN** of the deep orbital region (or vice versa, since it lacks valves).

The **DORSAL NASAL VEIN** (2) of the dorsolateral surface of the nose joins with the angularis oculi vein to form the **FACIAL VEIN** (3), which drains caudoventrally over the surface of the face, deep to the levator nasolabialis muscle.

A second nasal vein, the **LATERAL NASAL VEIN** (4), may be present and joins the facial vein caudoventral to the angularis oculi-dorsal nasal venous junction.

The **SUPERIOR LABIAL VEIN** (5), which drains blood from the dorsal lip, joins the facial vein dorsal to the commissure (angle) of the lips.

A deep vein that may not be easily observed is the **DEEP FACIAL VEIN** (6). It courses dorsomedially past the cranioventral portion of the zygomatic arch to connect the facial vein with the **VENTRAL EXTERNAL OPHTHALMIC VEIN** in the orbital or pterygopalatine fossa area.

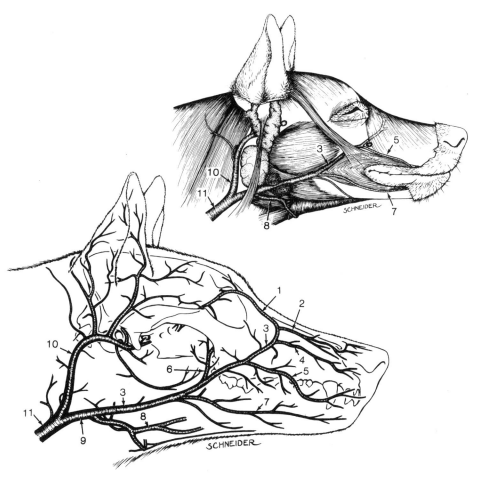

Fig.20.1. Veins of the head, right lateral view.

333

The **INFERIOR LABIAL VEIN** (7), superficial to and parallel with the mandible, drains into the facial vein at a point caudoventral to the oral commissure.

The **LINGUAL VEIN** (8) blood from the tongue, passes caudally out of the intermandibular space through the caudal portion of the mylohyoideus muscle; the lingual veins of each side are interconnected by a venous arch superficial to the basihyoid bone.

The lingual vein joins with the facial vein to form the **LINGUOFACIAL VEIN** (9) at a point ventral to the mandibular salivary glands and caudal to the mandibular lymph nodes. At the transverse level of the caudal border of the larynx, the linguofacial vein joins with the caudoventrally coursing **MAXILLARY VEIN** (10) forming the **EXTERNAL JUGULAR VEIN** (11). The maxillary vein drains the cranium, orbit, and temporal and auricular regions.

The **CRANIAL THYROID ARTERY** (1, Fig. 20.2), a branch of the **COMMON CAROTID ARTERY** (2), originates dorsolateral to the second to third tracheal ring. A **CAUDAL LARYNGEAL BRANCH** (3) of the cranial thyroid artery courses with the caudal laryngeal nerve to the larynx. The medial retropharyngeal lymph node is dorsolateral to the carotid origin of the cranial thyroid artery.

The common carotid artery courses rostrally past the deep surface of the mandibular salivary gland and branches, at a position dorsomedial to the rostral portion of the medial retropharyngeal lymph node, into the **INTERNAL CAROTID** (4) and **EXTERNAL CAROTID** (5) **ARTERIES.**

The **OCCIPITAL ARTERY** (6) branches off the external carotid artery immediately distal to the origin of the internal carotid artery.

The internal carotid artery may be distinguished from the occipital artery by the presence of a bulbous enlargement, the **CAROTID SINUS** (7), at the origin of the internal carotid, and the course of the internal carotid toward the tympanooccipital fissure (the occipital artery courses more caudodorsally, supplying branches to the deep cervical and occipital regions).

Branches of the internal carotid artery form a portion of the cerebral arterial circle at the base of the brain; the cerebral arterial circle provides a major portion of the intracranial blood supply (see pp. 340–41).

The **CRANIAL LARYNGEAL ARTERY** (8) branches ventrally from the external carotid artery, accompanying the cranial laryngeal nerve between hyopharyngeal and thyropharyngeal muscles, to supply blood to the larynx and pharynx.

A small **ASCENDING PHARYNGEAL ARTERY** (9) branches rostrodorsally from the external carotid artery near the origin of the larger occipital artery; it provides a collateral blood supply to the cerebral arterial circle by anastomosing with the internal carotid artery near the foramen lacerum.

The **LINGUAL ARTERY** (10) branches off the ventral surface of the external carotid artery and courses rostrally past the medial surface of the digastricus muscle. It supplies a branch to the palatine tonsil and enters the tongue through the genioglossus muscle in association with the hypoglossal nerve (cranial nerve XII).

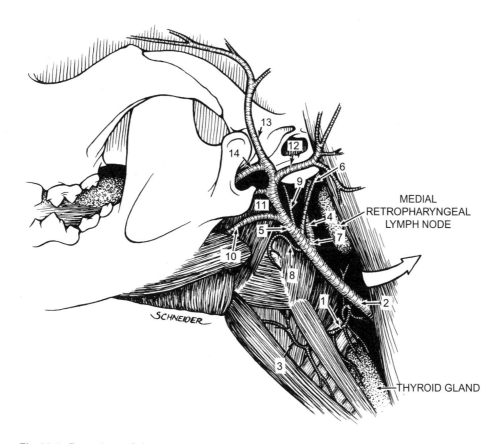

Fig.20.2. Branches of the common carotid and external carotid arteries, left lateral view.

The **FACIAL ARTERY** (11) separates from the rostral surface of the external carotid artery (5) at a level caudal to the mandibular angle, deep to the digastricus muscle and superficial to the styloglossus muscle. A relatively large branch of the facial artery supplies the mandibular and sublingual salivary glands with blood.

A branch of the facial artery, the **SUBLINGUAL ARTERY**, passes medial to the insertion of the digastricus muscle and courses rostrally along the medial surface of the body of the mandible in association with the mylohyoid nerve (a branch of cranial nerve V3). The facial artery courses rostrolaterally through the fascial cleft between the digastricus and masseter muscles to supply blood to the cheek and to the superior and inferior lips.

The **EXTERNAL CAROTID ARTERY** (5) courses dorsomedially toward the lateral surface of the tympanic bulla, gives origin dorsally to the **CAUDAL AURICULAR** (12) and **SUPERFICIAL TEMPORAL** (13) **ARTERIES** (caudal and rostral to the base of the ear, respectively), and continues rostrally as the **MAXILLARY ARTERY** (14).

The superficial temporal artery branches from the external carotid at the rostroventral border of the annular cartilage of the ear, courses dorsally past the caudal surface of the zygomatic arch, and supplies blood to the parotid salivary gland; the masseter, temporalis, and rostral auricular muscles; and the palpebrae.

335

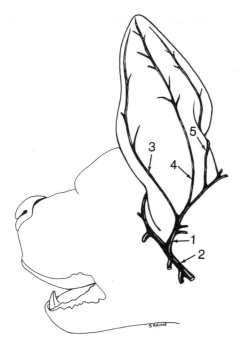

Fig.20.3. Branches of the left caudal auricular artery.

The caudal auricular artery (1, Fig. 20.3), a branch of the external carotid artery (2), courses caudally over the origin of the digastricus muscle, deep to the parotid salivary gland. In some dogs this artery's origin may be from the dorsal surface of the external carotid near the origin of the facial artery.

The caudal auricular artery supplies the convex surface of the ear via **LATERAL** (3), **INTERMEDIATE** (4), and **MEDIAL** (5) **AURICULAR BRANCHES**.

The **MAXILLARY ARTERY** (1, Fig. 20.4) passes rostromedially by curving ventrally around the temporomandibular joint toward the caudal alar foramen.

A branch of the maxillary, the **INFERIOR ALVEOLAR ARTERY** (2), passes into the mandibular foramen of the mandible and supplies blood to the roots of the mandibular teeth. By following the maxillary artery deeply toward the skull, several arterial branches may be observed.

A large **CAUDAL DEEP TEMPORAL ARTERY** (3) arises and passes dorsally supplying the temporalis and masseter muscles. A small branch may arise from the maxillary artery and enter the temporal bone of the skull to supply the middle ear.

A small **MIDDLE MENINGEAL ARTERY** (4) arises from the deep surface of the maxillary artery and enters the oval foramen; it supplies blood to much of the dura mater of the cranial meninges.

The maxillary artery enters the caudal alar foramen, courses through the alar canal, and exits rostrally from the rostral alar foramen. The maxillary artery emerges from the rostral alar foramen with the maxillary nerve.

The first major branch (or two branches) of the portion rostral to the alar canal is the **EXTERNAL OPHTHALMIC** (of-thal'mic; eye) **ARTERY** (5). Branches of this artery anastomose with the internal carotid, middle meningeal, **INTERNAL OPHTHALMIC**, and **INTERNAL ETHMOIDAL ARTERIES** (some of these arteries are described with the intracranial vessels).

The anastomotic branch with the internal ophthalmic artery is a major source of blood to the eye; two **LONG POSTERIOR CILIARY ARTERIES** reach the bulb of the eye, supplying seven or eight **RETINAL ARTERIES** to the retina, **SHORT POSTERIOR CILIARY ARTERIES** to the choroid, and **EPISCLERAL ARTERIES** to the sclera.

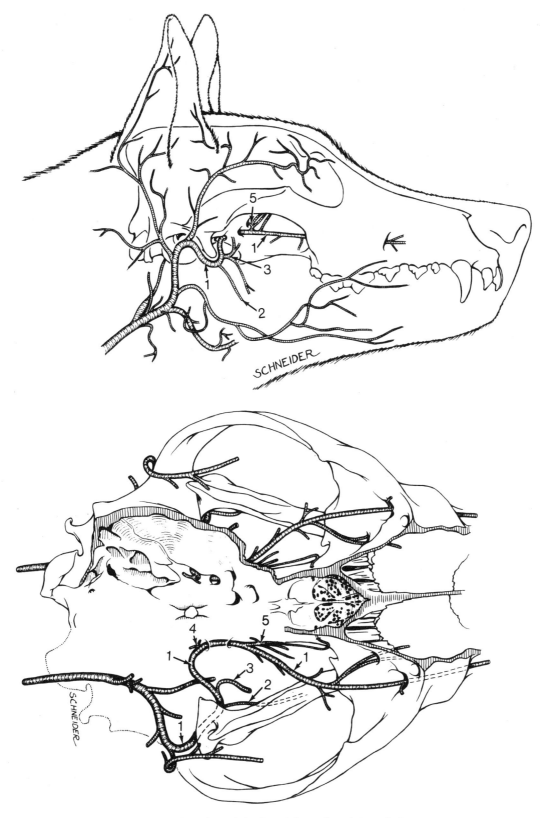

Fig.20.4. Arteries of the head, lateral and dorsal views.

The maxillary artery (1, Fig. 20.5) courses rostrally between the medial surface of the zygomatic salivary gland and the superficial surface of the medial pterygoid muscle.

A small ventral branch, the **MINOR PALATINE ARTERY** (2), courses ventrally over the palatine bone and supplies the soft palate.

The **DESCENDING PALATINE ARTERY** (3) branches off the medial surface of the maxillary artery at a transverse level deep to the zygomatic salivary gland. The descending palatine artery divides rostrally into the sphenopalatine and major palatine arteries.

The **SPHENOPALATINE ARTERY** (4) enters the sphenopalatine foramen, with the caudal nasal nerve, and supplies blood to much of the rostral portion of the nasal cavity.

The **MAJOR PALATINE ARTERY** (5) enters the caudal palatine foramen, with the major palatine nerve, and supplies blood to the hard palate. A branch of the major palatine artery passes rostrally into the nasal cavity through the palatine fissure and forms an anastomosis with a branch of the sphenopalatine artery.

The **MALAR ARTERY** (6) is a dorsal branch of the maxillary artery that arises near the maxillary foramen; it supplies blood to the lower and medial portions of the eyelids. The nasolacrimal duct and the conjunctiva also receive blood via the malar artery.

The continuation of the maxillary artery into the maxillary foramen is the **INFRAORBITAL ARTERY** (7). A number of small dental branches separate ventrally from the maxillary artery and enter small foramina of the maxillary bone; these dental branches, plus other branches arising from the infraorbital artery within the infraorbital canal, supply blood to teeth of the upper jaw.

The infraorbital artery and nerve course through the infraorbital canal and exit rostrally through the infraorbital foramen. The branches of the infraorbital artery that course over the surface of the nose, deep to the levator nasolabialis, are the **LATERAL NASAL ARTERIES**; branches of the lateral nasal arteries anastomose with branches of the malar, facial, major palatine, and sphenopalatine arteries.

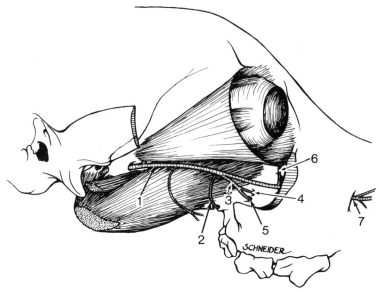

Fig.20.5. Branches of the maxillary artery in the pterygopalatine fossa, right lateral view.

INTRACRANIAL VESSELS

The blood supply to the brain of the dog is through a number of arterial channels (Fig. 20.6). The bilaterally paired **VERTEBRAL ARTERIES** (1) and **INTERNAL CAROTID ARTERIES** (2) provide the main source of blood to the brain.

A vascular connection between the extracranial external ophthalmic artery (3) and the intracranial portion of the internal carotid artery provides an alternative blood pathway. There are other arterial connections between extracranial and intracranial vessels, which are not described here.

The bilaterally paired vertebral arteries enter the vertebral canal, via the lateral vertebral foramina of the atlas, where they join with the **VENTRAL SPINAL ARTERY** (4), forming the **BASILAR ARTERY** (5). The single basilar artery passes rostrally along the ventral surface of the medulla oblongata to the junction with the bilaterally paired **CAUDAL COMMUNICATING ARTERY** (6). A number of paired arteries arise from the basilar artery and course laterally to supply structures of that portion of the brain caudal to the cerebrum.

The meninges of the brain are supplied with blood from **ROSTRAL, MIDDLE,** and **CAUDAL MENINGEAL ARTERIES** (which

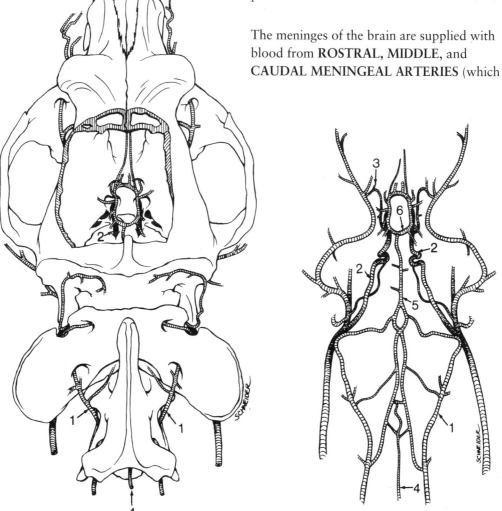

Fig.20.6. Arterial supply to the brain and meninges, dorsal view.

arise from branches of the ophthalmic, maxillary, and occipital arteries, respectively).

The middle meningeal artery, which is frequently injured in humans, supplies the meninges of most of the lateral surface of the cerebrum.

The cerebrum receives blood via the **CEREBRAL ARTERIAL CIRCLE**, an arterial circle around the hypophysis (pituitary) at the base of the brain (Fig. 20.7). It is formed primarily by two branches of the internal carotid artery (1) and the basilar artery (2). The rostral portion of the cerebral arterial circle is formed by the bilaterally paired **ROSTRAL CEREBRAL ARTERIES** (3), which curve around the cranial surface of the cerebrum within the longitudinal fissure.

The rostral cerebral arteries supply blood to the medial portion of right and left cerebral hemispheres.

The caudal portion of the cerebral arterial circle is formed by the right and left caudal communicating arteries (4), which anastomose with the single basilar artery situated in the median plane.

The **MIDDLE CEREBRAL ARTERY** (5) arises from the lateral surface of the internal carotid artery at the internal carotid-cerebral arterial circle junction. It supplies much of the lateral surface of the cerebrum.

The **CAUDAL CEREBRAL ARTERY** (6) arises from the lateral surface of the caudal communicating artery and courses caudolaterally to enter the groove between the cerebrum and cerebellum. The caudal cerebral artery of each side reaches the dorsal surface of the neural tissue, which connects right and left cerebral hemispheres, in the longitudinal fissure. Terminal branches of rostral and caudal cerebral arteries anastomose.

(DIFFERENCES TO BE NOTED IN THE CAT: A RETE MIRABILE, or plexus of arteries, arises from the maxillary artery in the deep orbital region adjacent to the round foramen and orbital fissure. The extracranial portion of the internal carotid artery is vestigial in the adult cat. The occipital and ascending pharyngeal arteries, which supply blood to the cerebral arterial circle, are innervated by glossopharyngeal nerve fibers.)

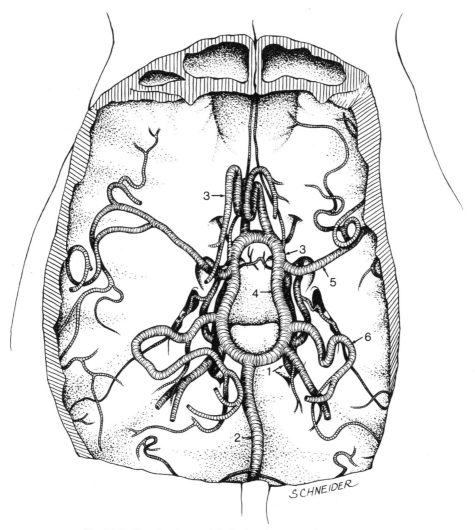

Fig.20.7. Cerebral arterial circle, dorsum of skull removed.

A number of large venous channels that do not contain valves are present in the cranium and vertebral column; a number of these venous sinuses are located in the outermost meningeal layer, the dura mater.

The deep venous sinuses of the head receive blood from the brain, cranium, and scalp and carry it via other venous sinuses and/or veins to the **MAXILLARY, INTERNAL JUGULAR,** and **VERTEBRAL VEINS** and to the **VENTRAL INTERNAL VERTEBRAL PLEXUS.**

Vertebral venous plexuses are paired vessels along the floor of the vertebral canal, superficial to the dura mater. Only a few of the venous sinuses are described here.

The venous blood of the dorsal surface of the cerebrum is collected into the **DORSAL SAGITTAL SINUS** (1, Fig.20.8), which is in the long dural fold (the falx cerebri) in the longitudinal cerebral fissure. Blood from the dorsal sagittal sinus drains caudally into the bilaterally paired **TRANSVERSE SINUSES** (2) through the foramen of the dorsal sagittal sinus.

The transverse sinus of each side carries the venous blood to the caudodorsal border of the petrous temporal bone, where it divides into a lateral **TEMPORAL SINUS** (3) and a medial **SIGMOID SINUS** (4).

Blood from the temporal sinus exits from the skull through the retroarticular foramen to reach the maxillary vein. The sigmoid sinus supplies blood to the ventral internal vertebral plexus through the condyloid canal and to the vertebral and internal jugular veins through the tympanooccipital fissure.

The **CAVERNOUS SINUS** (5), a venous pool in the floor of the rostral portion of the cranial cavity, encircles the hypophysis and may have a major role in brain temperature regulation. The venous plexuses of the orbits (external ophthalmic veins) are connected to the cavernous sinus, which in turn is connected to the sigmoid sinus.

The terminal portion of the internal carotid artery, a portion of the middle meningeal artery, and the anastomotic branch of the external ophthalmic artery of each side pass through the cavernous sinus, where an efficient heat exchange is thought to take place between venous and arterial blood systems.

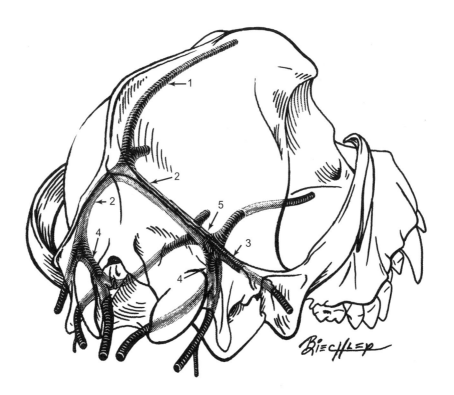

Fig.20.8. Venous sinuses within the skull.

Chapter 21

CARDIOVASCULAR SYSTEM—VISCERA

Objectives: To identify major branches of the celiac, cranial mesenteric, and caudal mesenteric arteries that supply the abdominal viscera. To understand that venous flow from the abdominal viscera is to the liver through the hepatic protal system.

Branches of arteries:

Celiac Artery: Left Gastric, Hepatic, and Splenic Arteries

Hepatic Artery: Right Gastric Artery, Gastroduodenal Artery

Gastroduodenal Artery: Right Gastroomental and Cranial Pancreaticoduodenal Arteries

Splenic Artery: Pancreatic Arteries, Short Straight Splenic Arteries, Short Gastric Arteries, and Left Gastroomental Artery

Cranial Mesenteric Artery: Caudal Pancreaticoduodenal, Common Colic, Jejunal and Ileal Arteries

Common Colic Arteries: Middle Colic, Right Colic, and Ileocolic Arteries

Caudal Mesenteric Artery: Left Colic and Cranial Rectal Arteries

Hepatic Portal System:

Branches of the Hepatic Portal Vein: Gastroduodenal, Splenic, Cranial Mesenteric, and Caudal Mesenteric Veins

Branches of the Gastroduodenal Vein: Right Gastric, Right Gastroomental, and Cranial Pancreaticoduodenal Veins

Branches of the Cranial Mesenteric Vein: Caudal Pancreaticoduodenal, Jejunal, Ileal, and Common Colic Veins

Branches of the Caudal Mesenteric Vein: Left Colic and Cranial Rectal Veins

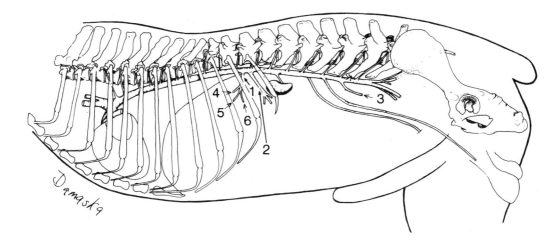

Fig.21.1. Aortic branches to the abdominal viscera, left lateral view.

The thoracic viscera exclusive of the lungs (thymus, trachea and bronchi, esophagus, pericardium, mediastinal lymph nodes) receive blood through small arteries that are branches of the internal thoracic arteries, thoracic aorta, or dorsal intercostals (see pp. 288, 290).

Blood vessels to the abdominal viscera course from the abdominal aorta through the dorsal mesentery. Most of the abdominal viscera is supplied with blood by three large, unpaired arteries (Fig. 21.1): the **CELIAC** (1), **CRANIAL MESENTERIC** (2), and **CAUDAL MESENTERIC** (3) **ARTERIES**.

Other blood vessels supply the adrenal glands, kidneys, ovaries or testes (see pp. 292–94), and that portion of the pelvic viscera extending cranially into the abdominal cavity (see p. 328).

In the following discussion of the digestive tube the terms cranial and caudal may not imply position relative to the long axis of the body; they may instead imply position relative to the long axis of the digestive tube as though it were stretched out as a straight tube, with the esophagus cranially positioned and the rectum caudally positioned.

Two of the three unpaired visceral arteries, the celiac and cranial mesenteric arteries, arise from the aorta and pass ventrally through the **ROOT OF THE MESENTERY**. The unpaired celiac artery branches to form three major vessels: left gastric (4), hepatic (5), and splenic (6) arteries (the left gastric and splenic arteries may share a short common trunk).

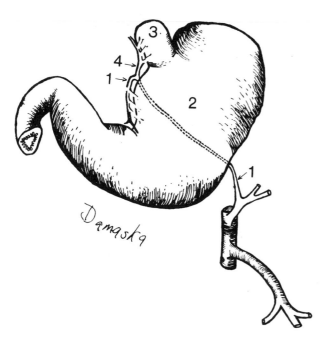

Fig.21.2. Schematic of the left gastric artery, ventral view.

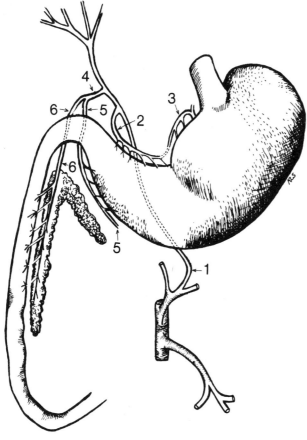

Fig.21.3. Schematic of the hepatic artery, ventral view.

The **LEFT GASTRIC ARTERY** (1, Fig. 21.2) courses cranially to the stomach (2) where it supplies the cranial portion of the stomach and the esophagus (3).

Distal to the point where the **ESOPHAGEAL BRANCHES** (4) are given off, the left gastric artery courses caudally along the lesser curvature of the stomach, supplying blood to both surfaces (right or visceral and left or parietal). The lesser curvature of the stomach is embryologically the ventral surface.

The **HEPATIC ARTERY** (1, Fig. 21.3) courses craniolaterally, dorsal to the digestive tube, and supplies blood to the liver via several hepatic branches: right lateral, right middle, and left hepatic branches. The left hepatic branch divides to form left medial and left lateral branches; the cystic artery arises from the left medial branch of the left hepatic branch shortly before the latter enters the liver.

In the portion of the ventral mesentery situated between the liver and the caudal portion of the stomach, the small **RIGHT GASTRIC ARTERY** (2) branches off the hepatic artery, or off a right hepatic branch, and supplies blood to the caudal portion of the lesser curvature of the stomach. The terminal branches of the right and left (3) gastric arteries anastomose along the lesser curvature of the stomach.

The **GASTRODUODENAL ARTERY** (4) is a short branch of the hepatic artery that courses caudally toward the duodenum; after giving off a small **RIGHT GASTROOMENTAL** (gastroepiploic) **ARTERY** (5), the gastroduodenal artery is called the **CRANIAL PANCREATICODUODENAL ARTERY** (6). The right gastroomental artery supplies blood to the caudal portion of the stomach along the greater curvature (the dorsal margin, embryologically) of the stomach. The cranial pancreaticoduodenal artery supplies blood to the body and right lobe of the pancreas and to a cranial segment of the duodenum.

The **SPLENIC ARTERY** (1, Fig. 21.4) arises from the celiac artery (2) and supplies blood to the spleen (3). **PANCREATIC BRANCHES** (4) of the splenic artery enter the left lobe of the pancreas (5).

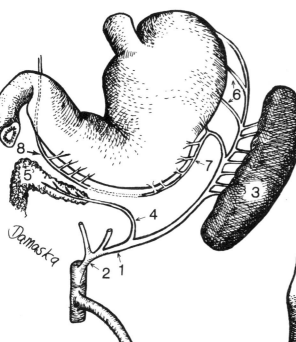

Fig.21.4. Schematic of the splenic artery, ventral view.

Several **SHORT GASTRIC ARTERIES** (6) branch from the terminal portion of the splenic artery and supply the greater curvature of the stomach.

A branch, the **LEFT GASTROOMENTAL ARTERY** (7), passes craniolaterally to the greater curvature of the stomach, then crosses

caudally along the greater curvature to form an anastomosis with the right gastroomental artery (8).

The unpaired cranial mesenteric artery (1, Fig. 21.5) passes ventrally to supply blood to most of the slender (small) intestine and to much of the thick (large) intestine.

The first two branches of the cranial mesenteric are the **CAUDAL PANCREATICODUODENAL ARTERY** (2) and the **COMMON COLIC TRUNK** (3). The caudal pancreaticoduodenal artery supplies blood to the descending portion of the duodenum (4), which is on the right side of the abdominal cavity; the right lobe of the pancreas (5); and the ascending duodenum (6). The terminal branches of the caudal and cranial pancreaticoduodenal vessels anastomose.

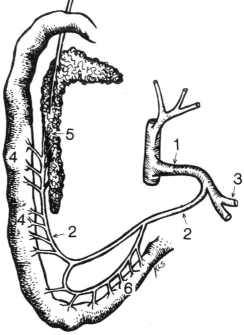

Fig.21.5. Schematic of the caudal pancreaticoduodenal artery, ventral view.

The common colic trunk supplies vascular branches to the ileum, cecum, and much of the colon (Fig. 21.6). The major branches off the common colic trunk (1) are the middle colic, right colic, and ileocolic arteries.

A great amount of variation occurs in the pattern and number of these vessels; however, by naming them according to distribution, no great difficulty should be encountered. The **MIDDLE COLIC ARTERY** (2) supplies the area of the left colic flexure (3), present craniodorsally in the left side of the abdominal cavity.

The **RIGHT COLIC ARTERY** (4) supplies blood to the region of the right colic flexure (5), present craniodorsally in the right side of the abdominal cavity. Arching branches of the right and middle colic arteries supply the portion of colon between right and left colic flexures (the transverse colon); these arcuate branches anastomose.

The **ILEOCOLIC ARTERY** (6) supplies blood to the terminal portion of the ileum, to the cecum, and to the most cranial portion (initial segment) of the colon.

The ileocolic artery (1, Fig. 21.7) divides into the colic branch, the cecal artery, and the mesenteric ileal branch. The **COLIC BRANCH** (2) supplies blood to the ascending colon, i.e., the cranial portion between the ileum (3) and the right colic flexure (4). The terminal branches of the colic branch and those of the right colic artery (5) anastomose.

The **CECAL ARTERY** (6) crosses the right (dorsal) surface of the cecum (7) and provides most of the cecal blood supply; an **ANTIMESENTERIC ILEAL BRANCH** (8) courses along the distal (caudal) portion of the ileum on the opposite surface from the dorsal mesentery. The **MESENTERIC ILEAL BRANCH** (9) passes through the mesenteric attachment of the caudal portion of the ileum.

A small **CECAL BRANCH** (10) arises from the mesenteric ileal branch and courses to the cecum.

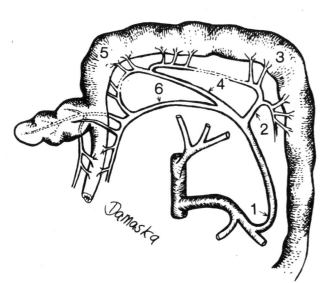

Fig.21.6. Schematic of the branches of the common colic trunk, ventral view.

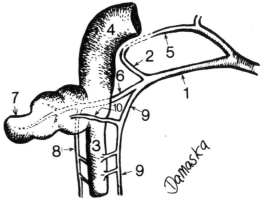

Fig.21.7. Schematic of the branches of the ileocolic artery, ventral view.

A series of **JEJUNAL** and **ILEAL ARTERIES**
(1, Fig. 21.8) arise from the cranial mesenteric
artery (2); these arteries supply the remainder of
the slender intestine. Note that these arteries of the
intestines branch in the mesentery as they approach
the intestine; they join with adjacent branches of
other arteries to form arcades. Straight branches
from the arcuate vessels that pass to the intestine
are termed **VASA** (sing. vas; vessel) **RECTA** (3).

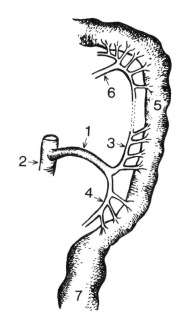

Fig.21.9. Schematic of the caudal
mesenteric artery, ventral view.

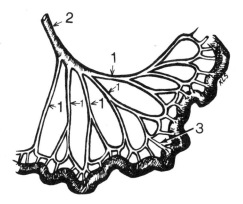

Fig.21.8. Schematic depicting the
distribution of several
jejunal and ileal arteries.

The caudal mesenteric artery (1, Fig. 21.9) arises
from the abdominal aorta (2) near the level of
the 5th lumbar intervertebral disc.

The two primary branches of the caudal
mesenteric artery are the left colic (3) and cranial
rectal (4) arteries.

The **LEFT COLIC ARTERY** courses cranially in
the mesenteric attachment (dorsal surface) of the
descending colon (5); the terminal branches of
the left colic artery anastomose with those of the
middle colic artery (6). The **CRANIAL RECTAL**
(pl. recti; straight) **ARTERY** passes along the
mesenteric attachment of the rectum (7),
supplying blood to the cranial portion of the
rectum (see pp. 318 for middle and caudal rectal
arteries).

The **HEPATIC PORTAL VEIN** drains blood to the liver from much of the abdominal viscera. Upon entering the porta (entrance) of the liver, the hepatic portal vein divides into a smaller right and larger left branch. The sinusoidal capillaries of the liver receive blood from terminal branches of the hepatic portal vein.

The hepatic portal vein is formed by the **GASTRODUODENAL VEIN** (1, Fig. 21.10), which collects blood from the **RIGHT GASTRIC, RIGHT GASTROOMENTAL**, and **CRANIAL PANCREATICODUODENAL VEINS**; the **SPLENIC VEIN** (2), which collects blood from **PANCREATIC, LEFT GASTRIC, SHORT GASTRIC**, and **LEFT GASTROOMENTAL VEINS**; the **CRANIAL MESENTERIC VEIN** (3), which drains the **CAUDAL PANCREATICODUODENAL, JENUNAL, ILEAL**, and **COMMON COLIC VEINS**; and the **CAUDAL MESENTERIC VEIN** (4), which is formed by **LEFT COLIC** and **CRANIAL RECTAL VEINS**.

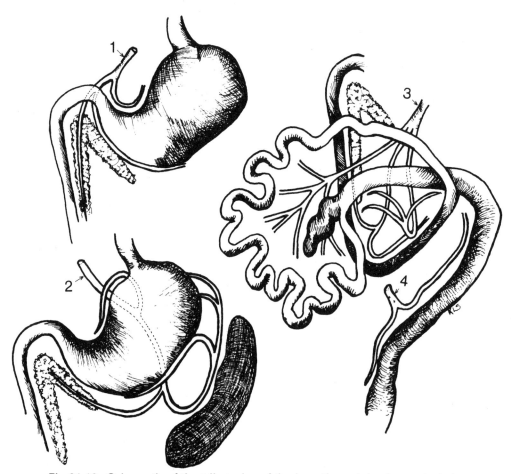

Fig.21.10. Schematic of the tributaries of the hepatic portal vein, ventral view.

Unit VIII

Lymphoreticular System

The one chapter on the lymphatic system will introduce the reader to the various lymph vessels, lymph nodes, lymph nodules, and tonsils in the body, which protect the animal against infectious agents.

Contents:

351

Chapter 22

LYMPHORETICULAR— LYMPHATIC SYSTEM

Objectives: To be able to identify the major lymphatic vessels and organs in the body and be able to predict routes by which infection might spread along the lymphatic pathway.

Superficial Cervical Lymphocenter: Superficial Cervical Lymph Nodes

Axillary Lymphocenter: Accessory Axillary and Axillary Lymph Nodes

Popliteal Lymphocenter: Popliteal Lymph Node

Inguinofemoral Lymphocenter: Superficial Inguinal Lymph Nodes (Mammary and Scrotal)

Iliosacral Lymphocenter: Medial Iliac, Hypogastric, and Sacral Lymph Nodes

Iliofemoral Lymphocenter: Iliofemoral Lymph Nodes

Celiac Lymphocenter: Hepatic, Splenic, Gastric, and Pancreaticoduodenal Lymph Nodes

Cranial Mesenteric Lymphocenter: Jejunal Lymph Nodes; Right and Middle Colic Lymph Nodes

Caudal Mesenteric Lymphocenter: Caudal Mesenteric Lymph Nodes

Lumbar Lymphocenter: Aortic and Renal Lymph Nodes

Ventral Thoracic Lymphocenter: Sternal Lymph Nodes

Mediastinal Lymphocenter: Cranial Mediastinal Lymph Nodes

Bronchial Lymphocenter: Left, Right, and Middle Tracheobronchial Lymph Nodes

Parotid Lymphocenter: Parotid Lymph Nodes

Mandibular Lymphocenter: Mandibular Lymph Nodes

Retropharyngeal Lymphocenter: Medial Retropharyngeal Lymph Node

Deep Cervical Lymphocenter: Cranial, Middle, and Caudal Deep Cervical Lymph Nodes

Right and Left Tracheal Trunks, Right Lymphatic Duct, Thoracic Duct, Cisterna Chyli, Palatine Tonsils, Pharyngeal Tonsils,

Approximately 15% of the body weight is composed of interstitial fluid; this water, which is bound to the colloidal matrix between cells, is primarily derived from the blood vascular system. Approximately 40 ml/hr of this interstitial fluid is returned to the venous system in a 20 lb dog.

The lymphatic system is a part of the circulatory system that functions to recirculate the interstitial fluid back into the bloodstream. Structures of the lymphatic system are generally present in all regions of the body except the central nervous system, bulb of the eye, bone marrow, and within skeletal muscle; however, lymphatic vessels are abundant in the fascial clefts between muscles.

The lymphatic system of the dog (Fig. 22.1) consists of **LYMPH VESSELS, LYMPH NODES,** and **LYMPH NODULES.** Lymph vessels are present as **AFFERENT VESSELS** (1), which drain extracellular tissue fluid toward lymph nodes (2), and **EFFERENT VESSELS** (3), which drain fluid from the lymph nodes and lymph nodules toward the venous system.

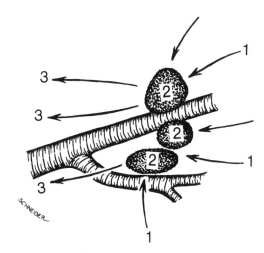

Fig. 22.1. Afferent lymph flow to and efferent lymph flow away from lymph nodes.

When lymph nodes are interconnected in series, an efferent lymph vessel of one node is an afferent vessel for the next lymph node of the series (Fig. 22.2).

Lymph nodes and vessels are quite variable in both location and number; those groups of lymph nodes that occur constantly in the same region of all species and drain similar body regions via afferent lymph vessels are termed **LYMPHOCENTERS.** Lymph nodes filter out

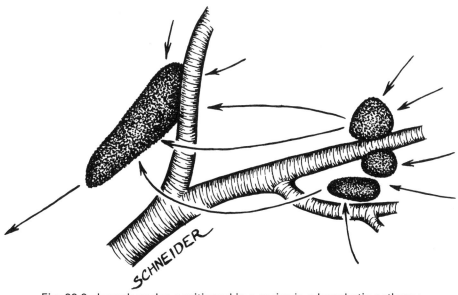

Fig. 22.2. Lymph nodes positioned in a series in a lymphatic pathway.

foreign substances from the lymph and produce lymphocytes and plasma cells (which function in the immune response of the body).

The lymphatic vessels that drain interstitial fluid from the intestines function also to carry long-chain fats (stearic and palmitic acids) from the viscera to the bloodstream.

All efferent lymphatic vessels eventually drain into veins at the cranial thoracic aperture (Fig. 22.3). Efferent vessels in the region of the cranial thoracic aperture include **RIGHT** (1) and **LEFT** (2) **TRACHEAL TRUNKS**, the **THORACIC DUCT** (3), and the **RIGHT LYMPHATIC DUCT** (4).

These lymph vessels drain into an external jugular vein (5), a subclavian vein (6), a brachiocephalic vein (7), or a combination of these structures.

When describing the distribution of this highly variable system in subsequent paragraphs, the term "cranial thoracic aperture" is used as a generality.

The smallest lymphatic vessels are termed **LYMPHATIC CAPILLARIES** and the largest are named **LYMPHATIC TRUNKS**, or **PLEXI** (plek' see, sing. plexus; braid or network) if they occur as branching networks.

The terminal ends of lymph capillaries are closed, i.e., the capillary lumen is capped and not structurally open to the interstitial "space" (Fig.22.4). Valves that prevent backflow of lymph are more numerous and effective in lymph vessels than they are in veins.

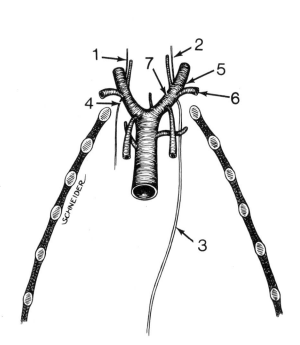

Fig. 22.3. Schematic of the lymphatic drainage into veins at the cranial thoracic aperture, ventral view.

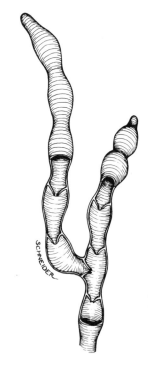

Fig. 22.4. Schematic of the terminal portions of lymph capillaries.

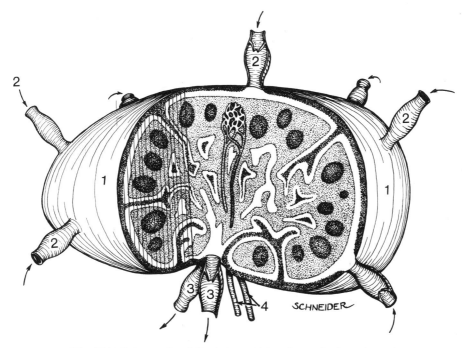

Fig.22.5. Schematic of the internal structure of a lymph node.

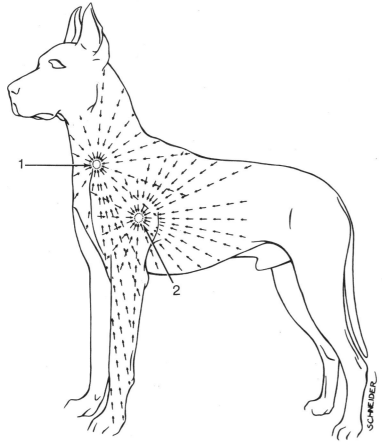

Fig. 22.6. Schematic of the left superficial cervical and axillary
lymphocenters, lateral view.

Lymph nodes (1, Fig. 22.5) are supplied by a number of afferent lymph vessels (2), which enter the node in the dog through the convex surface. One to several efferent lymph vessels (3) drain fluid from the concave surface or hilus of the lymph node. Blood vessels (4) also enter and leave the hilus of a lymph node; the walls of the smallest blood vessels (capillaries) within the lymph node are thickened, thus ensuring a greater degree of separation between blood and lymph.

The thoracic limb and superficial structures of the cranial portion of the trunk are drained by lymph vessels (Fig. 22.6) carrying lymph to either the superficial cervical lymphocenter (1) or the axillary lymphocenter (2).

357

The **SUPERFICIAL CERVICAL LYMPHOCENTER** (Fig. 22.7) usually consists of two **SUPERFICIAL CERVICAL LYMPH NODES** (1), which are located deep to the omotransversarius muscle and cranial to the supraspinatus muscle.

The superficial cervical lymph nodes drain the caudal surface of the head, lateral surface of the neck, ventral surface of the cranial thoracic region, and most of the thoracic limb. Efferent vessels drain deeply into the venous system at the cranial thoracic aperture.

The **AXILLARY LYMPHOCENTER** (Fig. 22.8) consists of **PROPER** (1) and **ACCESSORY** (2) **AXILLARY LYMPH NODES** situated in the axillary space superficial to the first to second and third intercostal spaces, respectively. Usually the accessory axillary and proper axillary lymph nodes are present as one node each (if the accessory axillary lymph node is present at all). The axillary lymphocenter drains fluid from the surface of the thorax and cranial portion of the abdomen and from much of the thoracic limb. The efferent vessels of the axillary lymphocenter course cranially around the 1st rib to enter the venous system in the region of the cranial thoracic aperture.

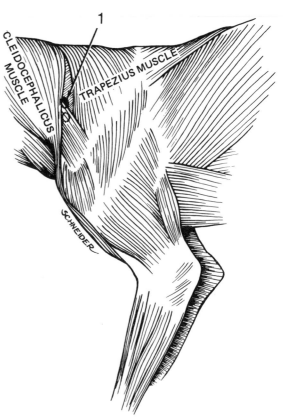

Fig.22.7. Left superficial cervical lymph nodes, lateral view.

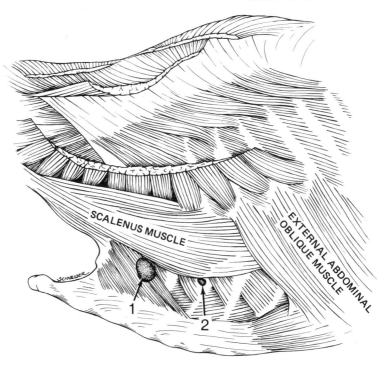

Fig.22.8. Left axillary lymph nodes, lateral view with the left thoracic limb removed.

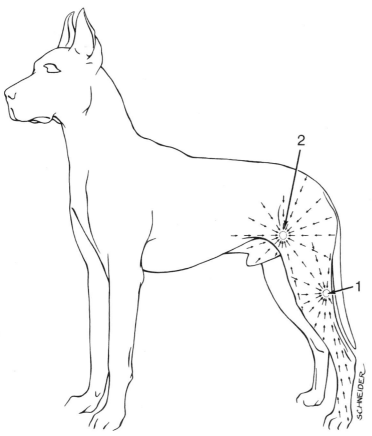

Fig.22.9. Schematic of the left popliteal and inguinofemoral lymphocenters, lateral view.

The pelvic limb and superficial structures of the caudal portion of the trunk are drained by lymph vessels (Fig. 22.9) carrying lymph to either the popliteal (1) or inguinofemoral (2) lymphocenters.

The **POPLITEAL LYMPHOCENTER** (Fig. 22.10), which consists of one **POPLITEAL LYMPH NODE** (1), is situated deep to the biceps femoris muscle in the popliteal space. Afferent vessels of the popliteal lymph node drain the entire crus and pes as well as much of the lateral and caudal femoral regions. Efferent vessels from the popliteal lymphocenter pass either along with the ischiatic nerve or with the femoral blood vessels to drain into large lymph nodes (medial iliac lymph nodes) located near the origin of the external iliac vessels.

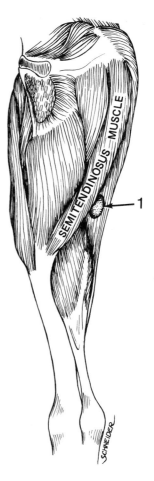

Fig.22.10. Right popliteal lymph node, caudomedial view.

The **INGUINOFEMORAL LYMPHOCENTER** (Fig. 22.11) is usually composed of two **SUPERFICIAL INGUINAL LYMPH NODES** (1) situated in the superficial fascia, ventral to the cranial border of the pubic symphysis.

In the bitch the superficial inguinal lymph nodes are termed **MAMMARY LYMPH NODES** since they receive afferent vessels from the caudal mammary glands; the superficial inguinal lymph nodes of the dog are called **SCROTAL LYMPH NODES**, even though they are located dorsal to the body of the penis and drain fluid from both the scrotum and prepuce.

The superficial inguinal lymph nodes collect fluid via afferent lymph vessels from the caudoventral half of the trunk, from the ventral pelvic region (including the vulva or prepuce and scrotum), from the medial femoral and crural regions, and from the lateral femoral and gluteal regions. Lymph nodules are present in the surface layer of the prepuce. The efferent vessels of the superficial inguinal lymph nodes also convey their contents to the medial iliac lymph node.

The **ILIOSACRAL LYMPHOCENTER** (Fig. 22.12) in the dog is composed of three groups of lymph nodes within the abdominal and pelvic cavities (medial iliac, hypogastric, and sacral); these three groups of lymph nodes are situated adjacent to the external iliac, internal iliac, and median sacral arteries.

The **MEDIAL ILIAC LYMPH NODES** (1) are large nodes, one on each side of the abdominal aorta, between the origins of the deep circumflex iliac and external iliac arteries. Afferents carry

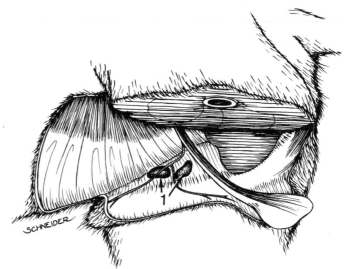

Fig.22.11. Left superficial inguinal lymph nodes, left pelvic limb transected and removed.

lymph to the medial iliac lymph nodes from the inguinofemoral and popliteal lymphocenters, the hypogastric and sacral lymph nodes, and lymph nodes associated with the caudal mesenteric artery (caudal mesenteric lymphocenter).

HYPOGASTRIC LYMPH NODES (2) are situated along the medial surface of the internal iliac artery near the origin of the median sacral artery; the hypogastric lymph nodes are easily confused with **SACRAL LYMPH NODES** (3), which are positioned next to the median sacral artery.

The sacral lymph nodes are considered to be a subgroup of the medial iliac lymph nodes. Afferent lymphatic vessels of the hypogastric nodes drain the structures supplied by vascular branches of the internal iliac artery—in particular, the rectum, anus, external genitalia, urinary bladder, urethra, uterus, prostate, and ductus deferens.

The sacral lymph nodes are small nodes that filter lymph collected from the tail; they drain via efferent vessels into the medial iliac lymph nodes. Efferent vessels from the iliosacral lymphocenter drain cranially into small lymph nodes scattered along the abdominal aorta or into relatively large interconnecting vessels surrounding the aorta (**LUMBAR TRUNK**).

The **ILIOFEMORAL LYMPHOCENTER** in the dog usually consists of the **ILIOFEMORAL LYMPH NODE** (4, Fig. 22.12), which when present is positioned between the internal and external iliac veins as they converge to form the common iliac vein.

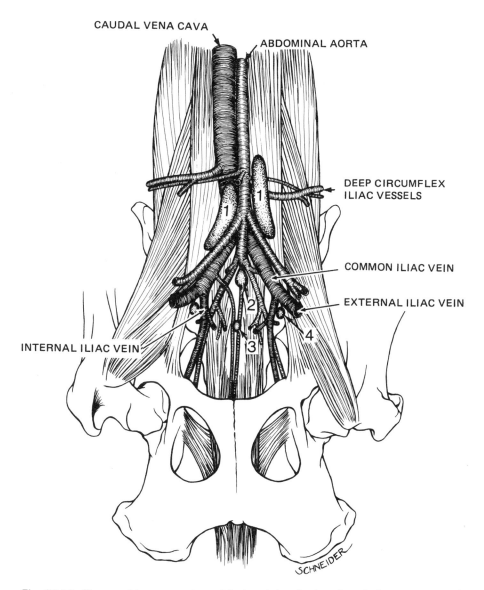

Fig. 22.12. Iliosacral lympocenter, with the abdominal wall and viscera removed, ventral view.

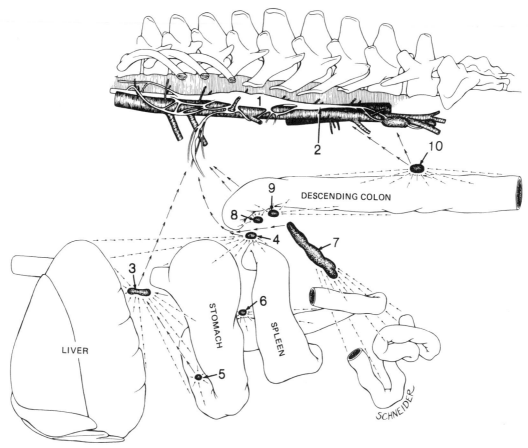

Fig. 22.13. Schematic of the celiac, cranial mesenteric and caudal mesenteric lymphocenters, left lateral view.

The abdominal viscera is protected by three lymphocenters (celiac, cranial mesenteric, and caudal mesenteric) that filter fluid collected from the viscera (Fig. 22.13).

Efferent vessels of the cranial mesenteric and celiac lymphocenters drain into the **CISTERNA CHYLI** (kie' lie; juice) (1), a dilated cranial continuation of the lumbar trunks dorsolateral to the abdominal aorta at a level between the 1st and 4th lumbar vertebrae.

The caudal mesenteric lymphocenter drains via efferents into the lumbar trunk (2), the medial iliac lymph nodes, or into small scattered lumbar aortic lymph nodes.

The **CELIAC LYMPHOCENTER** consists of two **HEPATIC LYMPH NODES** (3), one on each side of the hepatic portal vein; **SPLENIC LYMPH NODES** (4), along the splenic vessels; **GASTRIC LYMPH NODES** (5), near the right gastric artery when present; and **PANCREATICODUODENAL LYMPH NODES** (6), in mesentery supporting the pancreas and duodenum.

The **CRANIAL MESENTERIC LYMPHOCENTER** consists of large **JEJUNAL LYMPH NODES** (7) and **RIGHT** (8) and **MIDDLE** (9) **COLIC LYMPH NODES.**

The jejunal lymph nodes are present usually as two elongated nodes that receive afferent vessels from the jejunum and ileum.

362

The right and middle colic lymph nodes are positioned along the correspondingly named vessels. Circular lymph nodules, approximately 3 mm in diameter, in the walls of the cecum and colon are quite visible in the gas-distended large intestine. The efferent vessels of these nodules drain into the colic lymph nodes.

The **CAUDAL MESENTERIC LYMPHOCENTER** is represented by several **CAUDAL MESENTERIC LYMPH NODES** (10) that receive afferent lymphatic flow from that portion of the intestine served by the left colic and cranial rectal vessels.

Afferent vessels from lymph nodules in the wall of the descending colon and cranial portion of the rectum carry lymph to the caudal mesenteric lymphocenter.

The small lumbar aortic lymph and renal nodes (some 17 or more) form the **LUMBAR LYMPHOCENTER**. These lymph nodes filter lymph carried through afferent vessels from the parietal peritoneum, kidney, adrenal glands, ovaries and testes, and epaxial structures and the efferent flow from the medial iliac lymph nodes via the lumbar trunk.

Efferents of the lumbar lymphocenter drain into either the lumbar trunk or into the cisterna chyli.

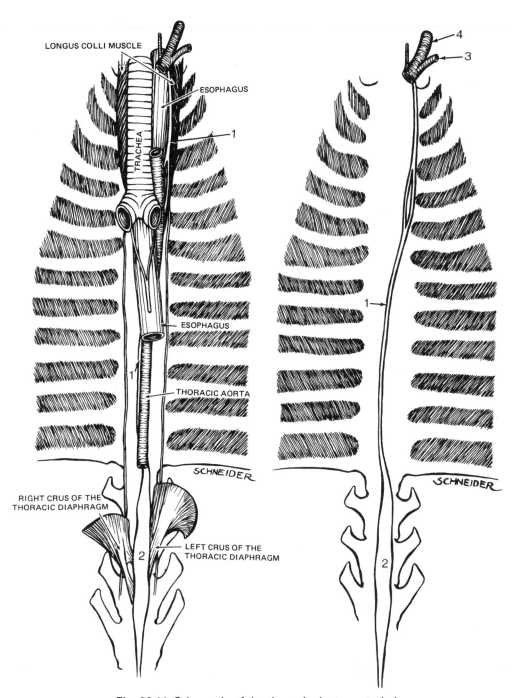

LONGUS COLLI MUSCLE

ESOPHAGUS

TRACHEA

1

ESOPHAGUS

1

THORACIC AORTA

SCHNEIDER

RIGHT CRUS OF THE
THORACIC DIAPHRAGM

2

LEFT CRUS OF THE
THORACIC DIAPHRAGM

4

3

1

SCHNEIDER

2

Fig. 22.14. Schematic of the thoracic duct, ventral view.

The **THORACIC DUCT** (1, Fig. 22.14) is the thoracic portion of the large lymphatic vessel that carries lymph along the dorsal wall of the abdominal cavity, i.e., it extends from the cisterna chyli (2) to the cranial thoracic aperture, where it joins a vein. The thoracic duct arises from the cisterna chyli between the right and left diaphragmatic crura and courses cranially along the right dorsal surface of the thoracic aorta (here it may be a plexus rather than a trunk). At approximately the level of the 6th thoracic vertebra it passes craniolaterally to the left across the dorsal surface of the aorta.

As observed from the left, the thoracic duct cranial to the heart courses cranioventrally in the groove between the esophagus and left longus colli muscle to the area where the left subclavian (3) and external jugular (4) veins join.

The thoracic duct terminates as a single or branched vessel, and it may discharge into any of the veins near the cranial thoracic aperture; however, it most likely will discharge its contents into the venous system near the junction of left subclavian and left external jugular veins.

Within the thoracic cavity are four lymphocenters (dorsal thoracic, ventral thoracic, mediastinal, and bronchial). The **DORSAL THORACIC LYMPHOCENTER**, if present in the dog, is represented by **INTERCOSTAL LYMPH NODES** in the 5th to 7th intercostal spaces, near the intervertebral disc. Afferent drainage is from the parietal pleura, epaxial structures, and thoracic wall; efferent flow is to the cranial mediastinal lymph nodes of the mediastinal lymphocenter.

The **VENTRAL THORACIC LYMPHOCENTER** (Fig. 22.15) is represented by **STERNAL LYMPH NODES** (1), one on each side, that are positioned along the cranioventral surface of the internal thoracic artery (2). The sternal lymph nodes receive afferent flow from the parietal pleura, mediastinum, thymus, ventral thoracic wall, and thoracic diaphragm. Peritoneal fluid absorbed into afferent lymph vessels on the caudal surface of the thoracic diaphragm is conducted to the sternal nodes.

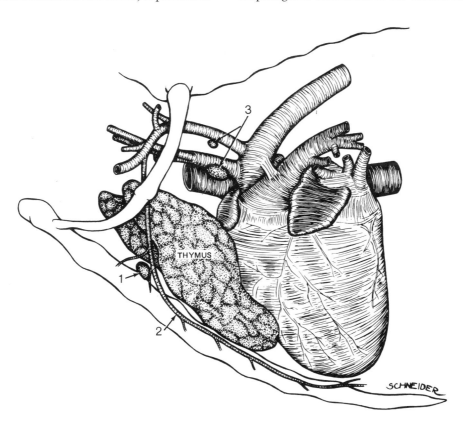

Fig.22.15. Sternal and cranial mediastinal lymph nodes, left lateral view.

The **MEDIASTINAL LYMPHOCENTER** in the dog is represented by lymph nodes present only in that portion of the mediastinum cranial to the heart, termed **CRANIAL MEDIASTINAL LYMPH NODES** (3). These lymph nodes are scattered along the major vessels cranial to the heart (cranial vena cava, costocervical trunk, subclavian) and filter lymph received from the thymus, trachea, esophagus, and heart and the drainage area supplied by the costocervical trunk plus the efferent drainage of the dorsal thoracic and bronchial lymphocenters.

Efferent vessels from the cranial mediastinal lymphocenter drain into the venous system at the cranial thoracic aperture.

The **BRONCHIAL LYMPHOCENTER** (Fig. 22.16) is composed of **RIGHT TRACHEOBRONCHIAL LYMPH NODE** (1), **LEFT TRACHEOBRONCHIAL LYMPH NODE** (2), **MIDDLE TRACHEOBRONCHIAL LYMPH NODE** (3), and **PULMONARY LYMPH NODES.**

The small pulmonary lymph nodes are located near the terminal end of the primary bronchi, often within the angle of bifurcation of primary into secondary bronchi. The pulmonary lymph nodes receive afferent vessels from the smaller airways and lung tissue; efferent vessels carry fluid from the pulmonary lymph nodes to the tracheobronchial lymph nodes. The three tracheobronchial lymph nodes are situated at the tracheal bifurcation into primary bronchi: a node adjacent to the right azygous vein at the right craniolateral surface of the tracheal bifurcation, a node on the left craniolateral surface of the tracheal bifurcation, and a V-shaped node between the primary bronchi near their origin from the trachea.

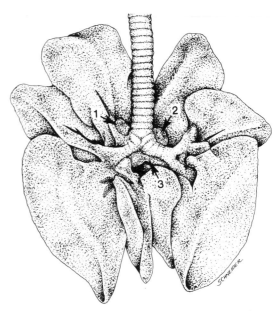

Fig.22.16. Tracheobronchial lymph nodes, ventral view.

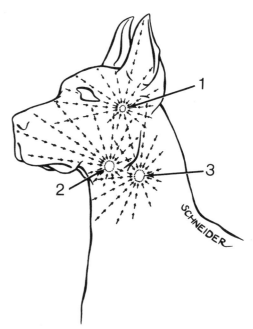

Fig.22.17. Schematic of the left parotid, mandibular, and retropharyngeal lymphocenters, lateral view.

366

Efferent vessels from the bronchial lymphocenter drain into the cranial mediastinal lymph nodes.

The lymph nodes of the head (Fig. 22.17) belong to one of three centers: parotid (1), mandibular (2), or retropharyngeal (3).

The **PAROTID LYMPHOCENTER** (Fig. 22.18) in the dog usually consists of a single **PAROTID LYMPH NODE** (1) situated near and partly under the rostral border of the parotid salivary gland (2). The parotid lymph node filters lymph received from the surface structures of the nasal, frontal, orbital (including eyelids), and auricular regions; and from the temporomandibular joint, parotid salivary gland, and lacrimal gland. Efferents carry lymph to the retropharyngeal lymphocenter. Lymph nodules are present on the deep surface of the semilunar conjunctival fold (see p.16).

(DIFFERENCES TO BE NOTED IN THE CAT: Two parotid nodes are the SUPERFICIAL and DEEP PAROTID NODES. The larger superficial parotid lymph node is on the caudal surface of the parotid salivary gland. The smaller deep parotid lymph node is deep to the rostral portion of the parotid salivary gland.)

The **MANDIBULAR LYMPHOCENTER** consists usually of two to three **MANDIBULAR LYMPH NODES** (3) situated on the surface of the head caudoventral to the masseter muscle and craniolateral to the basihyoid; these nodes are situated both within and dorsal to the angle formed by the bifurcation of the linguofacial vein (4) into lingual and facial veins.

The mandibular lymph nodes receive lymph from the nasal, superior labial, inferior labial, mental, orbital (including palpebrae), zygomatic, temporal, masseteric, buccal, and intermandibular regions as well as from the tongue and temporomandibular joint. Efferent vessels pass from the mandibular lymph node to the retropharyngeal lymphocenter.

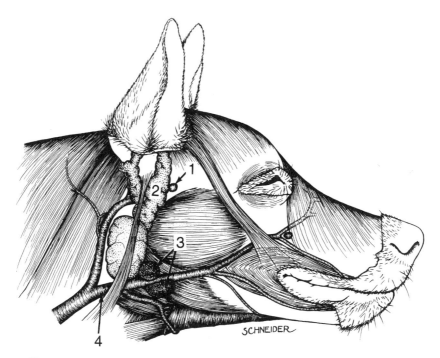

Fig. 22.18. Right parotid and mandibular lymph nodes, lateral view.

The **RETROPHARYNGEAL LYMPHOCENTER** (Fig. 22.19) of the dog is formed by the large **MEDIAL RETROPHARYNGEAL LYMPH NODE** (1) situated ventral to the transverse process of the atlas (2).

Afferent lymph vessels carry lymph from the deep portions of the head and neck, deep portion of the external ear, salivary glands, larynx, cranial portions of the trachea and esophagus, and thyroid glands. Lymph nodules of the nasal and oral passages and **PALATINE** and **PHARYNGEAL TONSILS** of the pharynx drain into the retropharyngeal lymphocenter.

The efferent vessels of the parotid and mandibular lymphocenters are also afferent vessels of the medial retropharyngeal lymph node. On each side, efferents of the medial retropharyngeal lymph node form a **TRACHEAL TRUNK**, which courses along the carotid sheath to the cranial thoracic aperture.

Three groups of lymph nodes situated along the trachea form the **DEEP CERVICAL LYMPHOCENTER**. When present, these small lymph nodes are observed as single nodes on each side of the trachea near the level of the thyroid gland (**CRANIAL DEEP CERVICAL LYMPH NODES**), middle third of the trachea (**MIDDLE DEEP CERVICAL LYMPH NODES**), and caudal third of the trachea (**CAUDAL DEEP CERVICAL LYMPH NODES**). Afferent vessels from the thyroid gland, larynx, trachea, and esophagus enter the deep cervical lymphocenter; efferent vessels from the deep cervical lymphocenter enter the tracheal trunks, thoracic duct, right lymphatic duct, or a major vein at the level of the 1st rib.

The **RIGHT LYMPHATIC DUCT**, when present, is a combination of the efferents of the superficial cervical lymph nodes and the right tracheal trunk.

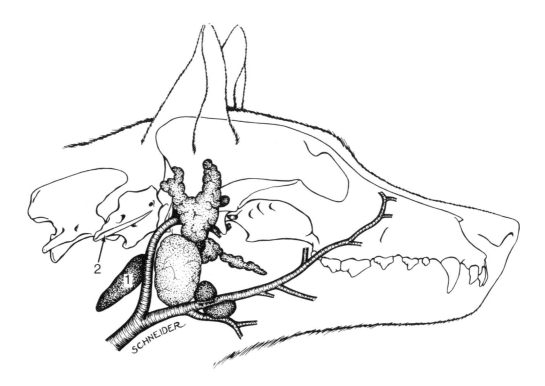

Fig.22.19. Schematic of the right medial retropharyngeal, parotid, and mandibular lymph nodes, lateral view.

Unit IX

Peripheral Nervous System

The following six chapters will introduce the reader to the grossly identifiable structures of the nervous system, excluding those of the brain and spinal cord.

Contents:

Chapter 23

PERIPHERAL NERVOUS SYSTEM— INTRODUCTION

Objectives: To introduce some basic concepts of the nervous system.

Major divisions: Central and Peripheral Nervous Systems; Autonomic Nervous System composed of Sympathetic and Parasympathetic systems

Cells: Neurons and Glial Cells

Neuron: Dendrites, Neuron Body, and Axon

Nuclei and Ganglia

Synapses, Myoneural Junctions, Motor Endplates

Meninges (Dura Mater, Arachnoid Membrane, and Pia Mater) and Epineurium

Afferent and Efferent Impules and Fibers

Exteroception, Interoception, and Proprioception

Reflex and Reflex Arc

Myelinated and Nonmyelinated Fibers; Neurolemma, Endoneurium, Perineurium, and Nerve Fascicles

Spinal Nerves: Dorsal and Ventral Roots; Spinal Ganglia; Dorsal, Ventral, and Communicating Rami

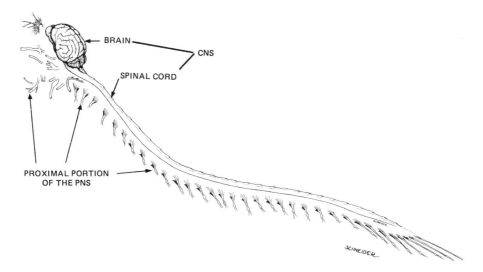

Fig.23.1. Central and peripheral portions of the nervous system.

Although the nervous system is one unit both functionally and structurally, it is arbitrarily divided into two major divisions (Fig. 23.1): the **CENTRAL NERVOUS SYSTEM (CNS)** and the **PERIPHERAL NERVOUS SYSTEM (PNS)**. The CNS consists of the **BRAIN** and **SPINAL CORD**.

The **PNS** consists of **CRANIAL NERVES** and **SPINAL NERVES**.

The nervous system is composed of cells specialized for receiving stimuli and conducting waves of excitation (nerve impulses). These nerve cells (**NEURONS**) are present in living tissues throughout the body. Neurons are not the only cell type present in the nervous system. **GLIAL** (neuroglial) **CELLS** are various cell types (present throughout the nervous system) that support the functions of neurons but do not have specialized powers of irritability and conductivity.

Each neuron (Fig. 23.2) is composed of a **NEURON BODY** (1) and various processes. **DENDRITES** (2) are processes that transmit impulses to nerve cell bodies; **AXONS** (3) are processes that transmit impulses away from the nerve cell body.

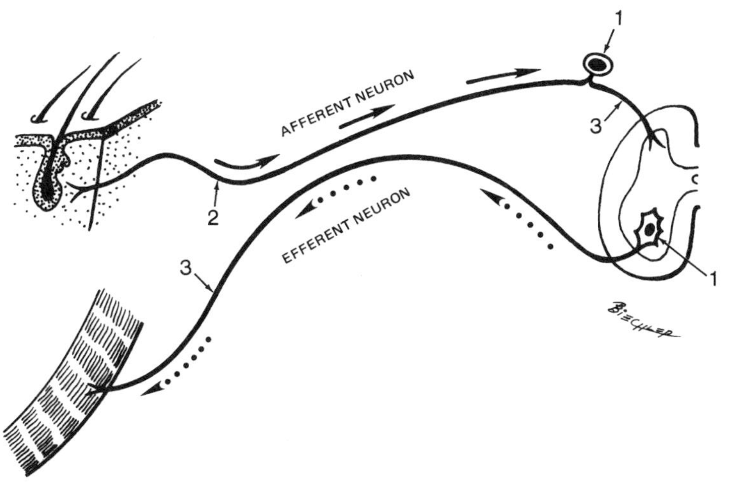

A transverse section of an axon or a dendrite is microscopic in size; however, many neuronal processes are quite long, e.g., those processes that span the distance between the distal portions of the manus or pes and the spinal cord.

Fig.23.2. Portions of neurons of the peripheral nervous system.

373

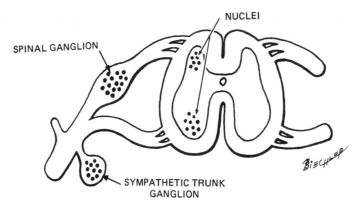

Fig.23.3. Concentrations of neuron bodies in the
CNS and PNS.

Localized concentrations of nerve cell bodies
within the brain and spinal cord are termed
NUCLEI (sing. nucleus) (Fig.23.3).Those nerve
cell bodies that are situated peripheral to the
CNS are usually located in specific places with
numerous other cell bodies of other neurons;
these accumulations of nerve cell bodies in the
PNS are called **GANGLIA** (sing. ganglion).

Three general types of cells stimulated by
impulses carried by a neuron are other neurons,
muscle cells (skeletal, cardiac, and smooth), and
gland cells.

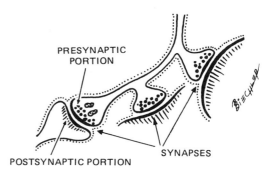

Fig.23.4. Diagram of three synapses.

Neurons that excite or inhibit other neurons do
so at cellular junctions named synapses. The
most common type of mammalian **SYNAPSE**
(Fig. 23.4) is an area where a very fine cleft
separates two neurons and chemical transmitters
produced by the one diffuse across to and
activate the other.

Neurons that excite skeletal muscle cells do so at
MOTOR ENDPLATES, or **MYONEURAL
JUNCTIONS** (Fig. 23.5); during stimulation,
chemical transmitters pass from the neuron to
the muscle cell across a narrow cleft at the motor
endplate.

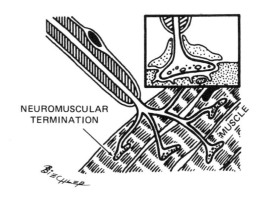

Fig.23.5. Diagram of a myoneural
junction.

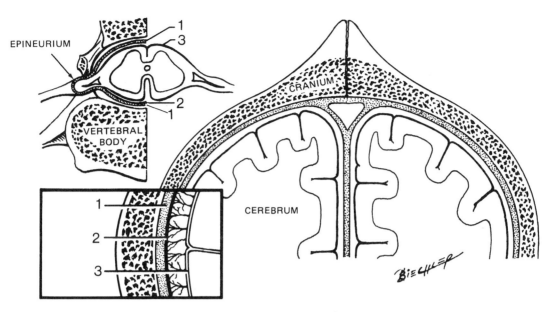

Fig.23.6. Diagram of the meninges and epineurium.

Both divisions of the nervous system, central and peripheral, are encased in a protective tissue layer. The layer around the CNS is in the form of three membranes, collectively termed the **MENINGES** (Fig. 23.6). The outermost meningeal layer of the CNS, the **DURA MATER** (1), is continuous with the **EPINEURIUM**, or outermost covering of nerves belonging to the PNS.

The other two layers are the delicate **ARACHNOID MATER** (2) and the **PIA MATER** (3).

The dog has 12 pairs of cranial nerves and approximately 36 pairs of spinal nerves (the caudal nerves are variable in number). It is through these neural pathways that information from the body parts reaches the CNS (afferent or sensory pathway) and by which impulses from the CNS reach their target or effector site (efferent or motor pathway).

AFFERENT NERVE FIBERS conduct impulses from receptors to the CNS; **EFFERENT NERVE FIBERS** conduct impulses away from the CNS to their terminations on muscle, gland, or other nerve cells.

Each sensory neuron of a peripheral nerve may have a hundred or more peripheral branches, some of which terminate in the skin and others that terminate on blood vessels, glands, muscles, and joints deep to the skin. Sensations received from the body by the CNS include exteroceptive, interoceptive, and proprioceptive sensations. Touch, pressure, temperature, and noxious sensations from the skin are **EXTERO-CEPTIVE SENSATIONS**. Perceptions of pain, burning, and pressure from visceral organs of the thorax and abdomen are **INTEROCEPTIVE SENSATIONS**. **PROPRIOCEPTIVE SENSATIONS** are those resulting from muscle tension and alterations in angulation of joints.

Generally, the fewer muscle fibers innervated by a single motor neuron the finer and more precise is the movement produced. The eyeball is an example of a structure that can be moved by very precise and coordinated muscular contractions.

375

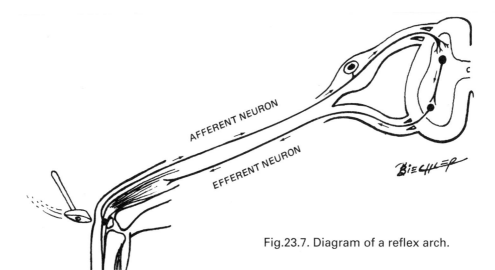

Fig.23.7. Diagram of a reflex arch.

Stimuli, either external to or within the body, elicit neurally controlled activity called **REFLEXES**. A reflex, or involuntary response, involves transmission of impulses over a **REFLEX ARC** usually consisting of a peripheral receptor or dendritic ending and its afferent neuron, one or more synapses in the **CNS**, and an efferent neuron (Fig. 23.7).

Most actions of the dog involve reflexes, some of which include the patellar tendon-stretch reflex, pupillary-light reflex, corneal-touch reflex, and carotid sinus reflex. Reflex activity frequently is modified by impulses originating from other centers in the **CNS**.

The epineurium is the superficial layer of connective tissue that forms a sheath or casing around a peripheral nerve (Fig. 23.8). A number of bundles (**FASCICLES**) of axons, each contained within its own connective tissue sheath or **PERINEURIUM**, are situated deep to the epineurium. Each axon is in turn ensheathed in a layer of cells, collectively named the **NEUROLEMMA**.

Larger axons are insulated by a **MYELIN LAYER**, which is formed by spirals of the external cell membrane of the neurolemmal cells and is situated between the axon and the remainder of the neurolemma.

Myelin is a white, glistening, fatty material that imparts to the nerve its white appearance. Neurons with little myelin are described as being **NONMYELINATED**.

MYELINATED NERVE FIBERS transmit nerve impulses more rapidly than nonmyelinated fibers. Each axon and its neurilemma cells are supported by a thin connective tissue sheath called the **ENDONEURIUM**.

Of the 36 pairs of spinal nerves in the dog, 8 are cervical (one more than the number of corresponding vertebrae), 13 are thoracic, 7 are lumbar, 3 are sacral, and 4–7 are caudal. The spinal nerves or their branches exit from the vertebral column bilaterally through intervertebral foramina; three exceptions to the preceding occur: the first cervical and first two sacral spinal nerves exit from the vertebral canal through foramina surrounded by bone.

Each spinal nerve (1, Fig. 23.9) is attached to the spinal cord by two roots, a **DORSAL** (2) and a **VENTRAL** (3) **ROOT**. Each root, in turn, is composed of a number of rootlets. Afferent impulses enter the spinal cord through the

376

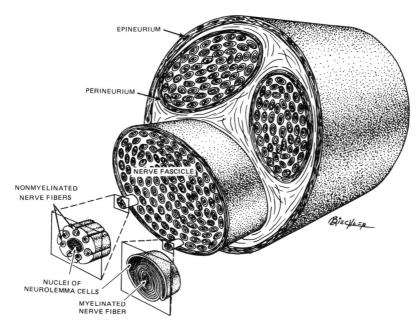

Fig.23.8. Composition of a peripheral nerve.

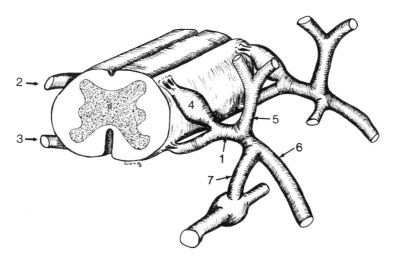

Fig.23.9. Schematic of a segment of the spinal cord and the roots
and proximal branches of spinal nerves.

The nerve cell bodies of motor neurons are situated in the spinal cord. Distal to the junction of dorsal and ventral roots, the spinal nerve contains both sensory and motor nerve fibers.

A typical spinal nerve branches into two primary rami (dorsal and ventral) near the level of the intervertebral foramen; each of these primary rami conducts both afferent and efferent impulses. The **DORSAL RAMUS** (ramus, pl. rami; branch) (5), typically as in the thoracic region, divides into a **MEDIAL BRANCH**, which innervates the spinal meninges and epaxial muscles, and a **LATERAL BRANCH**, which innervates primarily the skin. The

rootlets of the dorsal root of each spinal nerve. In each dorsal root an enlargement, the **SPINAL GANGLION** (4), is the result of an assemblage of nerve cell bodies of the sensory neurons contained in each spinal nerve. Efferent impulses leave the spinal cord through the rootlets of the ventral root of each spinal nerve.

VENTRAL RAMUS (6), supplies hypaxial structures.

Most spinal nerves have a **COMMUNICATING RAMUS** (7) with the sympathetic portion of the autonomic nervous system; these junctions of spinal nerves with communicating branches occur near the intervertebral foramina.

Neurons are classified functionally (Table 23.1) according to the nature of the impulse (sensory or motor) and type of structure innervated (somatic or visceral).

Motor innervation of skeletal muscle (**GSE**) takes place through a one-neuron span from the **CNS** to the motor endplate (Fig. 23.10). Sensory innervation from the skin, skeletal muscle, and joints (**GSA**) and from the viscera and visceral pleura and peritoneum (**GVA**) also occurs in a one neuron system spanning the distance from the receptor to the spinal cord.

Motor innervation of smooth muscle, cardiac muscle, and glands (**GVE**) occurs through a two-neuron span from the spinal cord to the effector site.

Another commonly used term for the **GVE** system is the **AUTONOMIC NERVOUS SYSTEM** (**ANS**); impulses of this important efferent system arise and exit from the **CNS** through four cranial nerves (III, VII, IX, and X), all the thoracic spinal nerves, the first five or six lumbar spinal nerves, and the sacral spinal nerves.

Efferent fibers to visceral structures, arising from the brain through cranial nerves III, VII, IX, and X and from the sacral segment of the spinal

Table 23.1. Functional classification of neurons in spinal nerves.

	Direction of Impulse	Functional Class
Sensation		
Pain, temperature, touch	To CNS	General somatic afferent (GSA)
Fullness from distention of the alimentary canal, Pain from lack of blood in the viscera	To CNS	General visceral afferent (GVA)
Changes in chemical content	To CNS	General visceral afferent (GVA)
Joint or muscle movement	To CNS	General proprioceptive (GP)
Action		
Fiber contraction in most skeletal muscles	From CNS	General somatic efferent (GSE)
Fiber contraction in skeletal muscle derived from mesoderm of the brachial arch	From CNS	Special visceral efferent (SVE)
Fiber contraction in smooth and cardiac muscle	From CNS	General visceral efferent (GVE)
Secretion by glands	From CNS	General visceral efferent (GVE)

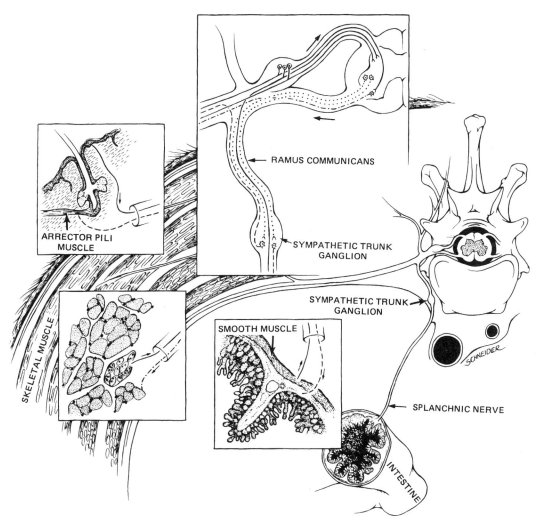

Fig.23.10. Schematic of the pathway of sensory fibers from and motor fibers to the skin, skeletal muscles, and digestive tract.

cord, form the **PARASYMPATHETIC PORTION OF THE ANS,** which is concerned with vegetative functions such as digestion and absorption. Although the parasymphathetic nerve fibers arise from the craniosacral region of the body, some of them are distributed throughout the thoracic and abdominal cavities.

Efferent fibers to visceral structures that arise from the thoracolumbar portion of the spinal cord form the **SYMPATHETIC PORTION OF THE ANS.** Although the sympathetic fibers arise from the thoracic and lumbar portions of the CNS, they are distributed with peripheral nerves and blood vessels to all parts of the body. The sympathetic nervous system is concerned with the "flight or fight" state of the body.

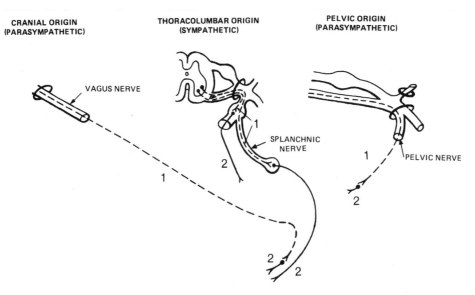

Fig.23.11. Pathway of autonomic fibers.

Nerves observed within the thoracic, abdominal, and pelvic cavities are, with few exceptions, autonomic and contain **GVE** fibers; however, **GVA** fibers are also present in these nerves to the viscera.

The **GVE** nerves in the major cavities of the body may be parasympathetic, sympathetic, or both; the individual fibers may be **PREGANGLIONIC** (1) or **POSTGANGLIONIC** (2, Fig. 23.11). Each of the divisions of efferent systems consists of two neurons connecting the **CNS** with the structure innervated.

The nerve cell body of the proximal or preganglionic neuron is situated in either the thoracolumbar portion of the spinal cord (sympathetic), sacral portion of the spinal cord (parasympathetic), or brain (parasympathetic); the nerve cell body of the distal or postganglionic neuron is generally in a ganglion situated proximal to the structure innervated (sympathetic neuron) or in the structure innervated (parasympathetic neuron).

Anastomoses between blood vessels that course along in the connective tissue of peripheral nerves are so plentiful that a nerve may be freed from its attachments for a considerable distance (15 cm in some cases) during surgery without appreciable damage being done.

Nerve fibers are organized in a "wavy" or undulating pattern in peripheral nerves. This undulating pattern permits the stretching of nerves without harm to individual nerve fibers; the perineurium is a tough layer of connective tissue that takes up most of the tension produced during stretching.

Nerves may be paralyzed in various degrees of severity by pressure. The more mild paralysis results from anoxia due to interference with blood flow. More severe paralysis may be due to destruction of axons and their connective tissue sheaths. Neural processes within peripheral nerves are capable of regeneration; this regenerative process is dependent to a large extent upon the integrity of the connective tissue sheaths surrounding the axons and nerve fascicles.

Chapter 24

PERIPHERAL NERVOUS SYSTEM— THORACIC LIMB

Objectives: To identify the major nerves to muscle and skin of the thoracic limb and to understand the effects of specific nerve damage at various levels, proximo-distally, in the thoracic limb.

Cervical Intumescence and Brachial Plexus

Nerves from the Brachial Plexus to extrinsic muscles: Brachiocephalic Nerve; Cranial Pectoral Nerves; Long, Lateral and Dorsal Thoracic Nerves; Caudal Pectoral Nerves

Nerves from the Brachial Plexus to intrinsic muscles: Suprascapular Nerve, Musculocutaneous Nerve, Axillary Nerve, Radial Nerve, Median Nerve, Ulnar Nerve

Branches of the Radial Nerve: Superficial Branch of the Radial nerve and its Medial and Lateral Branches; Deep Branch of the Radial Nerve

Cutaneous Branches: Cranial, Lateral, Caudal, and Medial Cutaneous Antebrachial Nerves

Nerves of the Manus: Dorsal Common Digital Nerves, Palmar Common Digital Nerves, Palmar Metacarpal Nerves

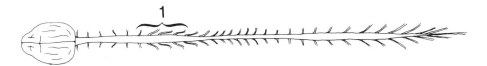

Fig.24.1. Cervical intumescence, dorsal view.

The nerves that innervate the muscles, skin, and joints of the thoracic limb arise from or reach the spinal cord at the level of the 5th cervical through 1st thoracic vertebrae. Due to the many afferent and efferent neurons that pass between structures of the limb and spinal cord, this region is enlarged, nearly filling the vertebral canal. This localized enlargement of the spinal cord is termed the **CERVICAL INTUMESCENCE** (in " tu-mes' ens; swelling) (1, Fig. 24. 1).

The ventral rami of a number of spinal nerves, usually C6, C7, C8, and T1, interconnect distal to the vertebral column, forming a tangle or network of nerve trunks. This tangle, called the **BRACHIAL PLEXUS** (1, Fig. 24.2), supplies nerves to the thoracic limb.

A couple of nerves to the thoracic limb are direct continuations of the ventral rami and are not formed by the plexus, i.e., the intercostobrachial nerves are lateral branches of intercostal nerves (see p. 438).

Distal to the brachial plexus, individual nerves supplying extrinsic and intrinsic structures of the thoracic limb may be identified; many of these nerves are formed by fibers from more than one level of the spinal cord.

The spinal nerves that supply ventral rami to the brachial plexus exit from the vertebral canal between vertebrae as follows:

C6 between the 5th and 6th cervical vertebrae; C7 between the 6th and 7th cervical vertebrae; C5 between the 7th cervical and the 1st thoracic vertebrae; and T1 between the 1st and 2nd thoracic vertebrae (Fig. 24.2).

The brachial plexus is situated within the axillary space at a level cranial to the 1st rib, ventral to the scalenus muscle, and dorsal to the pectoralis muscles. Those spinal nerves that innervate extrinsic structures of the thoracic limb include the brachiocephalic, cranial pectoral, long thoracic, thoracodorsal, lateral thoracic, and caudal pectoral nerves.

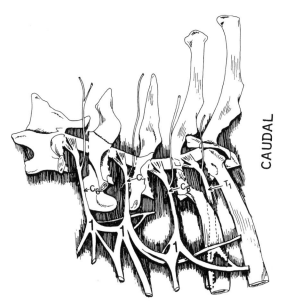

Fig.24.2. Left brachial plexus, lateral view.

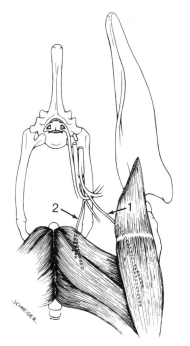

Fig.24.3. Brachiocephalic nerve, cranial view.

A muscular branch of the **BRACHIOCEPHALIC NERVE** (1, Fig. 24.3) enters the brachiocephalicus muscle near the clavicular intersection, cranial to the humeral articulation. A cutaneous branch of the brachiocephalic nerve innervates the skin of the cranial humeral region.

The **CRANIAL PECTORAL NERVES** (2) are usually present as two nerves that pass ventrally to supply the superficial pectoral muscle.

The **LONG THORACIC NERVE** (1, Fig. 24.4) courses caudally on the superficial surface of the serratus ventralis muscle, which it innervates.

The **THORACODORSAL NERVE** (2) courses caudally on the deep surface of the latissimus dorsi muscle, which it innervates.

A superficial nerve, which may be confused with the more deeply and more dorsally situated thoracodorsal, is the **LATERAL THORACIC**

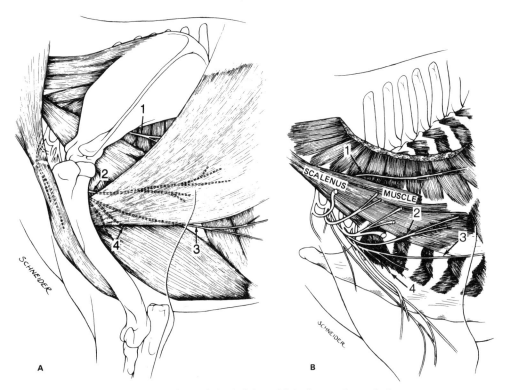

Fig.24.4. Branches of the left brachial plexus, lateral view.

NERVE (3). It courses caudally near the ventral margin of the latissimus dorsi and dorsolateral border of the deep pectoral muscles and innervates the cutaneous trunci muscle. Cutaneous branches, which pass from the lateral thoracic nerves to the skin, are fibers that reach the lateral thoracic from lateral cutaneous branches of intercostal nerves (**INTERCOSTOBRACHIAL NERVES**, see p. 438).

Three or four nerve branches innervate the deep pectoral muscle; these **CAUDAL PECTORAL NERVES** (4) usually arise from the brachial plexus in common with the lateral thoracic nerve.

Other nerves to extrinsic muscles of the thoracic limb, some of which are described on page 436 include the accessory nerve (to the trapezius, omotransversarius, and cleidocephalicus muscles) and ventral branches of cervical and thoracic spinal nerves (to the cleidocephalicus, rhomboideus, and omotransversarius muscles).

Nerves to the intrinsic structures of the thoracic limb (Figs. 24.5, 24.6) are the suprascapular (1), subscapular (2), musculocutaneous (3), axillary (4), radial (5), median (6), and ulnar (7) nerves.

Since these nerves may be involved in injuries of the thoracic limb or may evidence, through their loss of function, damage to the spinal cord, they are of considerable importance to the veterinarian.

Nerves that distribute fibers to the antebrachial region and/or manus are the musculocutaneus, axillary, radial, median, and ulnar nerves.

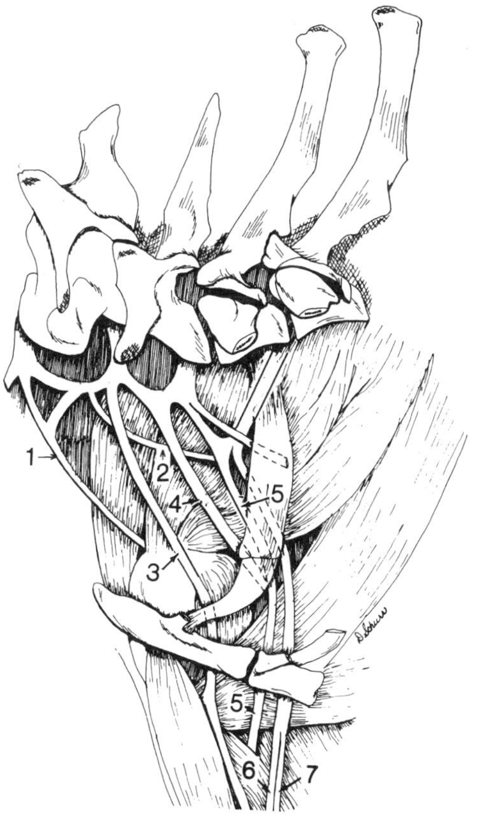

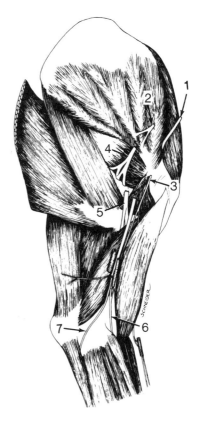

Fig.24.5. Branches of the right brachial plexus, medial view.

Fig.24.6. Nerves to the left thoracic limb, medial view.

The **SUPRASCAPULAR NERVE** (1, Fig. 24.6; 1, Fig. 24.7) courses around the cranial border of the scapula to supply the supraspinatus and infraspinatus muscles. Note that this nerve passes between the supraspinatus and subscapularis muscles to reach the scapular notch, through which it attains the lateral surface of the scapula. The suprascapular nerve is susceptible to damage from pressure applied to the craniodistal border of the scapula; a severely damaged suprascapular nerve will result in atrophy of the supraspinatus and infraspinatus muscles.

The **SUBSCAPULAR NERVES** (2, Fig. 24.6) innervate the subscapularis muscle. Branches of these nerves will not be observed on the lateral or superficial surface of the scapula since they enter the deep surface of the subscapularis.

The **MUSCULOCUTANEOUS NERVE** (3, Fig. 24.6; 1, Fig. 24.8) courses down the medial surface of the brachium in contact with the biceps brachii muscle and in close assocation with the cranial border of the major artery of the arm (brachial artery). A small branch (2) of the musculocutaneous nerve separates off from the parent trunk, proximal and deep to the humeral articulation, and innervates the coracobrachialis muscle. On the proximal medial surface of the brachium a proximal muscular branch (3) of the musculocutaneus supplies the biceps brachii muscle. On the distal third of the medial surface of the brachium the musculocutaneous nerve splits into two branches; fibers of one branch (4) join with the median nerve (5) and are distributed distally with the various branches of the median nerve to carpal and digital flexor muscles.

The other branch (6), a continuation of the musculocutaneous nerve, crosses the deep (lateral) surface of the distal portion of the biceps brachii, innervates the brachialis muscle at the level of the cubital articulation, and continues as a small cutaneous nerve. This **MEDIAL CUTANEOUS ANTEBRACHIAL NERVE** (7) supplies the skin on the craniomedial portion of the antebrachium.

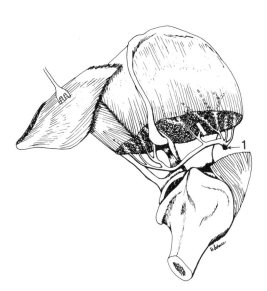

Fig.24.7. Right shoulder dissected to demonstrate the suprascapular nerve, lateral view.

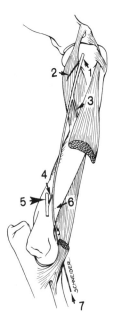

Fig.24.8. Musculocutaneous nerve and deep structures of the left thoracic limb, medial view.

The **AXILLARY NERVE** (1, Fig. 24.9) is a large nerve bundle that spans the axillary space to reach the caudomedial surface of the shoulder. It passes between the subscapular and teres major muscles at the level of the neck of the scapula, supplying muscular branches to the teres major, teres minor, deltoideus, and the caudal part of the subscapularis muscles. A fracture through the neck of the scapula may involve the axillary nerve.

A portion of the axillary nerve, the **CRANIAL LATERAL CUTANEOUS BRACHIAL NERVE**, observed superficially between the deltoideus and lateral head of the triceps brachii muscles, provides innervation to the skin of the craniolateral surface of the brachium. Fibers of the cranial lateral cutaneous brachial nerve continue into the antebrachium as the **CRANIAL CUTANEOUS ANTEBRACHIAL NERVE** and provide innervation to the cranial surface of the antebrachium.

The **RADIAL NERVE** (2) is the largest and most important (in terms of locomotion) nerve of the brachial plexus. Within the axillary space, the radial nerve is parallel and adjacent to the common trunk (3) of the median and ulnar nerves. The radial nerve crosses the axilla to the caudal surface of the brachium where it enters the tricipital muscle mass, passing distally between the long and medial heads of the triceps brachii muscle.

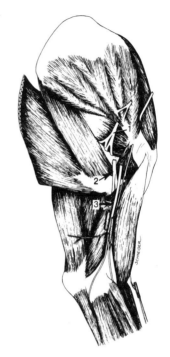

Fig.24.9. Nerves to the left thoracic limb, medial surface.

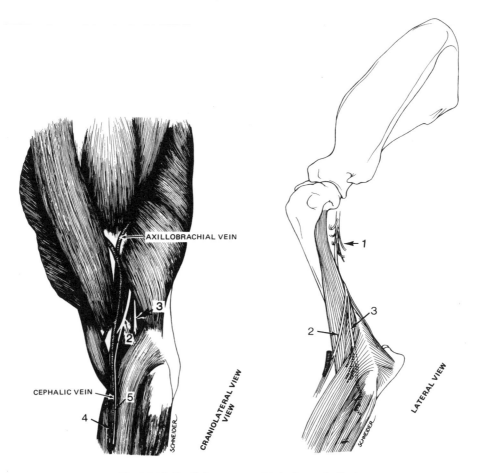

Fig.24.10. Radial nerve and left thoracic limb.

Near the level at which the radial nerve enters the tricipital muscle, some muscular branches (1, Fig. 24.10) supply the long head, accessory head, and medial head of the triceps brachii muscle.

The main continuation of the radial nerve courses distally between the triceps brachii and the brachialis muscles. The radial nerve and brachialis muscle are positioned in a spiralling pattern from the caudal border of the humerus (proximally) to the craniolateral border of the humerus (distally).

The radial nerve provides muscular branches to the lateral head of the triceps brachii muscle and the anconeus muscle near the distal portion of the brachium.

Deep to the lateral head of the triceps brachii muscle, the radial nerve divides into superficial (2) and deep (3) branches.

The **SUPERFICIAL BRANCH OF THE RADIAL NERVE** may be located in the fascia beneath the skin on the distal lateral surface of the brachialis muscle. It divides into **MEDIAL** (4) and **LATERAL** (5) **BRANCHES**. The smaller (medial) branch, which may be joined by fibers of the cranial cutaneous antebrachial nerve (of the axillary), is situated on the medial surface of the cephalic vein and craniolateral to the medial cutaneous antebrachial nerve (of the musculocutaneous).

The medial branch of the superficial branch of the radial nerve (1, Fig. 24.11) in the metacarpal region is named the **DORSAL COMMON DIGITAL NERVE I** (2). (The designation of I, II, III, or IV is made according to whether the common digital nerve is situated superficial to the 1st, 2nd, 3rd, or 4th intermetacarpal space.)

The dorsal common digital nerve supplies the dorsal axial surface of digit I and the dorsal abaxial surface of digit II as the **DORSAL PROPER DIGITAL NERVES.**

The lateral branch (3) of the superficial branch of the radial nerve courses along the lateral surface of the cephalic vein. Near the level of the cubital articulation the **LATERAL CUTANEOUS ANTEBRACHIAL NERVE** (4) arises from the lateral branch of the superficial radial to supply the skin of the craniolateral portion of the antebrachium.

The lateral branch of the superficial branch of the radial nerve divides over the dorsal surface of the metacarpus into **DORSAL COMMON DIGITAL NERVES II, III,** and **IV** (5–7, respectively). Each of the dorsal common digital nerves divides, forming two dorsal proper digital nerves (e.g., dorsal common digital nerve II divides into two dorsal proper digital nerves: one supplying the dorsal axial surface of digit II and the other supplying the dorsal abaxial surface of digit III).

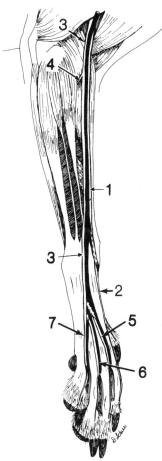

Fig.24.11. Medial and lateral branches of the superficial branch of the radial nerve in the right thoracic limb, craniolateral view.

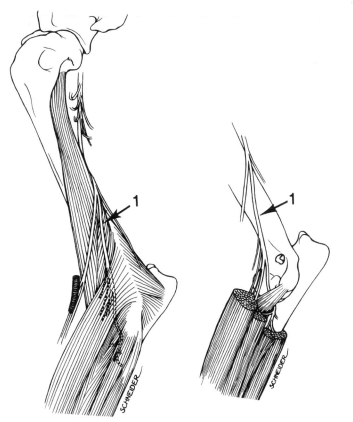

Fig.24.12. Deep branch of the radial nerve and deep structures of the left thoracic limb, lateral view.

At the transverse level of the cubital articulation, the median nerve, brachial artery, and ulnar nerve are quite superficially situated near the medial epicondyle (3) of the humerus; therefore, they are vulnerable to injury at this level.

On the distal medial surface of the brachium the **COMMUNICATING BRANCH (4) OF THE MUSCULOCUTANEOUS NERVE** joins the median nerve.

The median nerve passes deep to the pronator teres muscle (5), where it provides nerve branches to a number of muscles of the caudomedial (flexor) muscle group. It continues distally along the antebrachium between the flexor carpi radialis (6) and deep digital flexor (7) muscles to reach the carpus.

(*DIFFERENCE TO BE NOTED IN THE CAT: The median nerve passes through the supracondylar foramen.*)

The **DEEP BRANCH OF THE RADIAL NERVE** (1, Fig. 24.12) enters the antebrachium deep to the extensor carpi radialis muscle and divides into a number of branches that supply the craniolateral (extensor) group of muscles of the antebrachium.

The **MEDIAN NERVE** (1, Fig. 24.13) is usually bound to the ulnar nerve (2) by connective tissue in the axilla and proximal brachial regions. The median nerve is positioned on the medial surface of the brachium, deep to the skin and superficial pectoral muscle, caudal to the brachial artery, and cranial to the ulnar nerve.

The **ULNAR NERVE** (2, Fig. 24.13) is situated along the caudal surface of the median nerve (1) in the brachium.

The **CAUDAL CUTANEOUS ANTEBRACHIAL NERVE** (8) branches caudally away from the ulnar nerve in the distal half of the brachium; it courses superficial to the olecranon and the flexor carpi ulnaris muscle to reach a caudolateral position on the antebrachium.

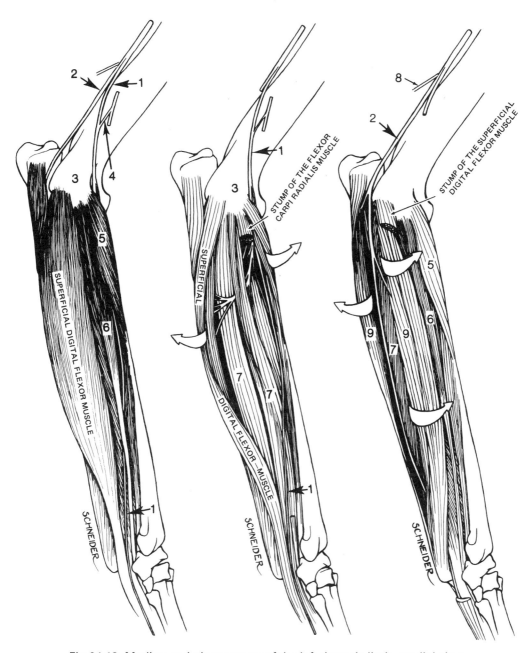

Fig.24.13. Median and ulnar nerves of the left thoracic limb, medial view.

The main continuation of the ulnar nerve passes distally over the caudal surface of the medial humeral epicondyle to reach the flexor muscles of the antebrachium.

Muscular branches of the ulnar nerve supply many of the caudomedial antebrachial muscles. In the proximal portion of the antebrachium the ulnar nerve is situated between the deep digital flexor (7) and flexor carpi ulnaris (9) muscles.

391

The median nerve (Fig. 24.14) branches in the metacarpal region to form the **PALMAR ABAXIAL DIGITAL NERVE I** and the **PALMAR COMMON DIGITAL NERVES I, II,** and **III** (1, 2, and 3, respectively), each of which divides into two **PALMAR PROPER DIGITAL NERVES.**

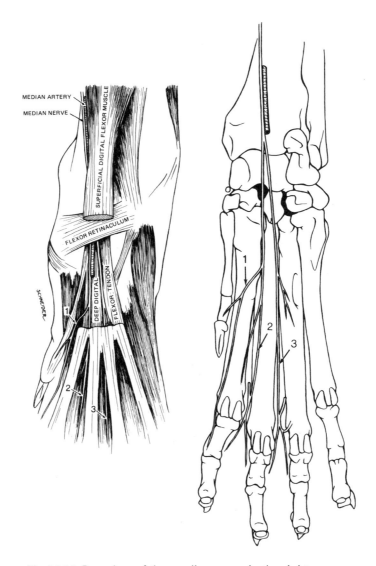

Fig.24.14. Branches of the median nerve in the right manus, palmar view.

The ulnar nerve divides into two branches, a smaller **DORSAL BRANCH** (1, Fig. 24.15) and the larger **PALMAR BRANCH** (2).

The dorsal branch of the ulnar nerve passes between the flexor carpi ulnaris and extensor carpi ulnaris muscles to reach the lateral surface of the distal antebrachium. The **DORSAL ABAXIAL DIGITAL NERVE V** (3) is the continuation of the dorsal branch.

The palmar branch of the ulnar nerve passes through the carpal canal, where it divides into

SUPERFICIAL and **DEEP BRANCHES**.

The superficial branch of the ulnar nerve subdivides into the **PALMAR COMMON DIGITAL NERVE IV** (4) and the **PALMAR ABAXIAL DIGITAL NERVE V** (5).

The deep branch of the ulnar subdivides into **PALMAR METACARPAL NERVES I, II, III,** and **IV**, each of which combines with a palmar common digital nerve before contributing to the formation of two palmar proper digital nerves.

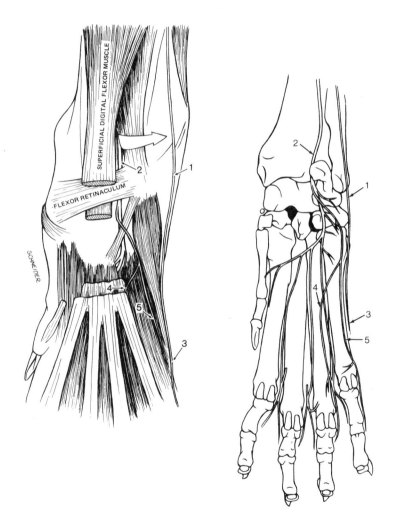

Fig.24.15. Branches of the ulnar nerve in the right manus, palmar view.

393

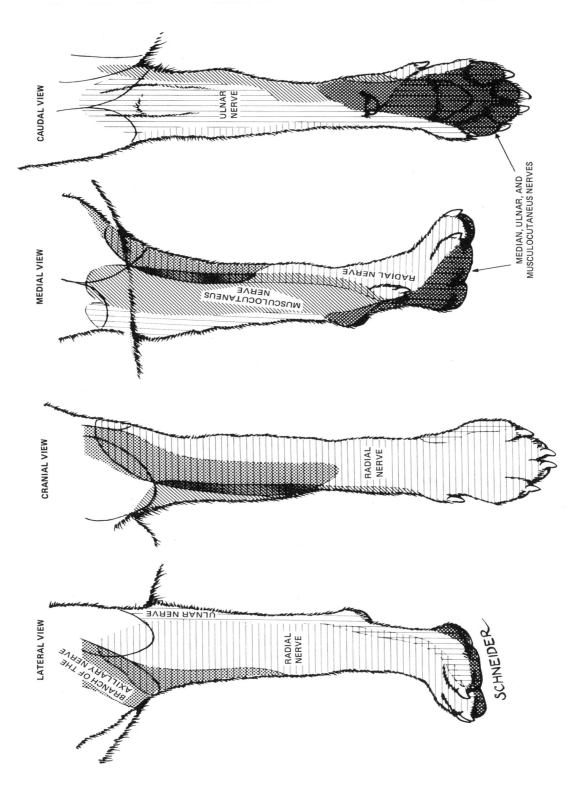

Fig.24.16. Sensory branches of individual nerves to the skin of the left thoracic limb (modified from Kitchell et al. 1983. *Am. J. Vet. Res.* 41: 61–76).

The nerves that conduct innervation from the skin of the thoracic limb (Fig. 24.16) include the axillary, intercostobrachial, radial, musculocutaneous, utnar, and median nerves. A summary of muscle and cutaneous innervation is given in Table 24.1.

Although a cutaneous nerve provides innervation to an area of skin, portions of the same area may also be supplied by several other nerves (zones of overlap). A more limited portion of this cutaneous area, innervated by a single cutaneous nerve, is termed the autonomous zone for that nerve.

Table 24.1. Innervation of the thoracic limb.

Muscle	Nerve
Supraspinatus, Infraspinatus	Suprascapular
Deltoideus, Teres major, Teres minor	Axillary
Biceps brachii, Brachialis	Musculocutaneus
Triceps brachii, Anconeus	Radial
Craniolateral muscles of antebrachium (extensors of carpus and digits)	Radial
Caudaomedial muscles of antebrachium (flexors of carpus and digits)	Ulnar, Median, Musculocutaneus
Sensory Region	**Cutaneous Branches***
Craniolateral brachium	Axillary
Caudal brachium	Intercostobrachial
Caudolateral brachium	Radial
Cranial antebrachium	Axillary, Radial
Lateral antebrachium	Radial
Caudal antebrachium	Ulnar
Medial antebrachium	Musculocutaneus
Palmar manus	Median, Ulnar
Lateral manus	Ulnar
Dorsal manus	Radial

*The suprascapular, subscapular, lateral thoracic, thoracodorsal, and cranial and caudal pectoral nerves in the dog lack cutaneous afferent fibers.

Chapter 25

PERIPHERAL NERVOUS SYSTEM— PELVIC LIMB

Objectives: To identify the major nerves to muscle and skin of the pelvic limb and to understand the effects of specific nerve damage at various levels, proximodistally, in the thoracic limb.

Lumbar Intumescence, Lumboscaral Plexus and Lumbosacral Trunk

Nerves of the Pelvic Limb: Lateral Cutaneous Femoral Nerve, Femoral Nerve, Saphenous Nerve, Obturator Nerve, Cranial and Caudal Gluteal Nerves, Ischiatic Nerve

Branches of the Ischiatic Nerve: Muscular Branches, Common Fibular and Tibial Nerves

Branches of the Common Fibular Nerve: Lateral Cutaneous Sural, Superficial and Deep Fibular Nerves

Branches of the Tibial Nerve: Caudal Cutaneous Sural, Lateral and Medial Plantar Nerves

Nerves in the Pes: Dorsal Common Digital and Dorsal Metatarsal Nerves; Plantar Common Digital and Plantar Metatarsal Nerves

The nerves supplying the pelvic limb are derived variably from the ventral branches of the last five lumbar and all three sacral spinal nerves. Because of the great number of neurons carrying information to and from the pelvic limb, there is also an enlargement in the spinal cord between the levels of the 4th lumbar and 2nd sacral spinal nerve-spinal cord junctions (3rd to 5th lumbar vertebral levels).

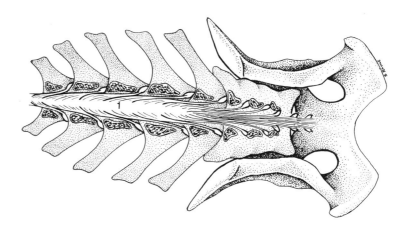

Fig.25.1. Caudal portion of the spinal cord, dorsal view with dorsum of the lumbar and sacral vertebrae removed.

Since the spinal cord extends caudally only as far as the 6th to 7th lumbar vertebrae in the dog, the second pair of sacral spinal nerves arises from the spinal cord at the level of the 5th lumbar vertebra (Fig. 25.1). This enlargement of the caudal portion of the spinal cord is termed the **LUMBAR INTUMESCENCE** (1). The ventral rami of lumbar and spinal nerves form a network of interconnecting fibers known as the **LUMBOSACRAL PLEXUS**.

(DIFFERENCE TO BE NOTED IN THE CAT: The spinal cord extends caudally, variably, to the level of the 6th lumbar to 3rd sacral vertebrae.)

The nerves, formed at the lumbosacral plexus that innervate structures of the pelvic limb (Fig. 25.2) include the lateral cutaneous femoral (1), femoral (2), obturator (3), lumbosacral trunk (4), and caudal cutaneous femoral (5) nerves.

The **LATERAL CUTANEOUS FEMORAL NERVE** (1) passes through the psoas minor muscle and exits through the abdominal wall with the deep circumflex iliac vessel, reaching the superficial fascia near the ventral surface of the tuber coxae. Superficial branches of the lateral cutaneous femoral nerve supply the skin of the cranial gluteal, cranial femoral, and lateral genual regions.

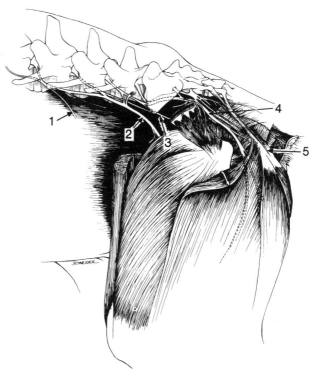

Fig.25.2. Nerves formed at the left lumbosacral plexus, with the ilium excised and the gluteal muscles removed, lateral view.

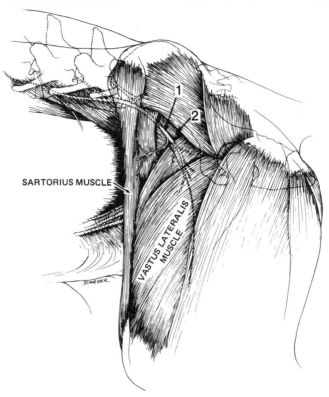

SARTORIUS MUSCLE

VASTUS LATERALIS MUSCLE

Fig.25.3. Left femoral nerve and pelvic limb, with the tensor
fasciae latae removed, lateral view.

The fibers of the **FEMORAL NERVE** (1, Fig. 25.3) originate primarily from the 5th lumbar segment of the spinal cord. The femoral nerve is formed from the lumbosacral plexus within the iliopsoas muscle (2) and accompanies the iliopsoas muscle through the muscular lacuna to reach the pelvic limb.

The major part of the femoral nerve is not observed superficially since it divides into a number of branches that enter the proximal portion of the quadriceps femoris muscle.

The femoral nerve innervates the iliopsoas (the sartorius in some dogs) and extensor muscles of the stifle (cranial thigh muscles).

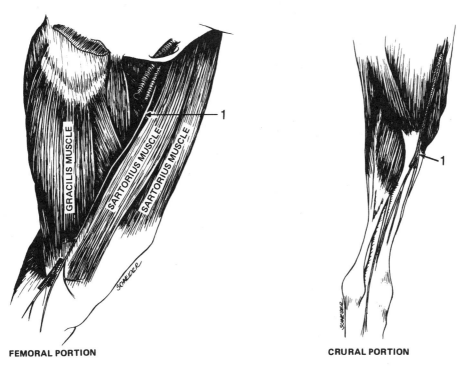

Fig.25.4. Left saphenous nerve, medial view of the pelvic limb.

The **SAPHENOUS NERVE** (1, Fig. 25.4) is a branch of the femoral nerve, from which it separates within the iliopsoas muscle. In some dogs a proximal branch of the saphenous nerve supplies the sartorius muscle.

The saphenous nerve is superficially positioned as it courses distally with the femoral vessels through the femoral triangle, across the superficial surface of the vastus medialis muscle, and on down the medial surface of the crus in close association with branches of saphenous blood vessels.

Cutaneous branches of the saphenous nerve supply the skin of the medial femoral, medial crural, and dorsomedial tarsal regions. Digits I (when present) and II receive cutaneous innervation via the terminal branches of the saphenous nerve.

The **OBTURATOR NERVE** (1, Figs. 25.5, 25.6) is also formed from the lumbosacral plexus within the iliopsoas muscle. This nerve courses

caudomedially to lie within the cranial pelvic aperture (pelvic inlet), deep to the ilium. It reaches the adductor muscles superficial to the

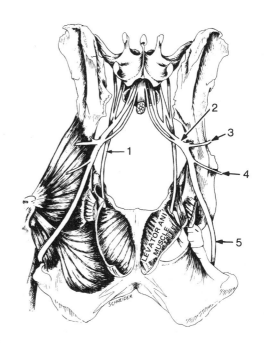

Fig.25.5. Pelvic girdle and caudal portion of the lumbosacral plexus, caudodorsal view.

401

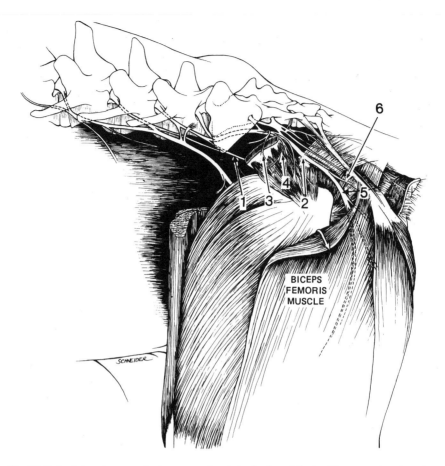

Fig.25.6. Left lumbosacral plexus and pelvic limb, with the ilium excised and the gluteal muscles removed, lateral view.

os coxae by passing along the obturator groove and out through the obturator foramen.

During parturition (particularly in large domestic animals or in certain breeds of dog such as the Boston terrier) the obturator nerves are susceptible to pressure as they are pressed by the fetus against the pelvic girdle. The obturator nerve innervates the external obturator, pectineus, gracilis, and adductor muscles.

The major nerve to the pelvic limb is the **LUMBOSACRAL TRUNK** (2, Figs. 25.5, 25.6), which arises primarily (via the lumbosacral plexus) from the ventral rami of the last two lumbar and first sacral spinal nerves (L6, L7, and Sl). The lumbosacral trunk near its origin is situated in the dorsal portion of the pelvic cavity

between the parietal peritoneum and the ventromedial surface of the ilium.

In its caudolateral course to the major ischiatic notch the lumbosacral trunk branches, forming the **CRANIAL GLUTEAL** (3) and **CAUDAL GLUTEAL** (4) **NERVES**. The main extrapelvic continuation of the lumbosacral trunk, distal to the major ischiatic notch, is the ischiatic nerve (5).

The cranial gluteal nerve arises from the lumbosacral trunk, crosses the dorsal surface of the ilium near the cranial margin of the major ischiatic notch with the cranial gluteal vessels, and innervates the middle gluteus, deep gluteus, and tensor fasciae latae muscles.

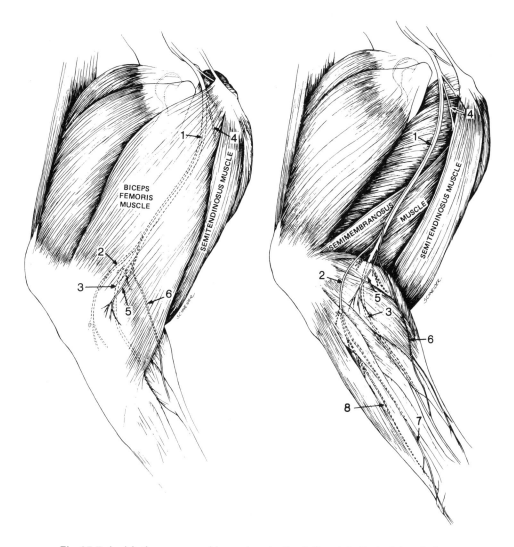

Fig.25.7. Ischiatic nerve and branches in the left pelvic limb, lateral view.

The caudal gluteal nerve usually branches away from the lumbosacral trunk near the dorsal margin of the major ischiatic notch and supplies the superficial gluteal muscle. A muscular branch (6) from the lumbosacral trunk (or, more distally, from the ischiatic nerve) supplies the internal obturator, gemellus, and quadratus femoris muscles.

The **ISCHIATIC NERVE** (1, Fig. 25.7), a continuation of the lumbosacral trunk distal to the major ischiatic notch, consists of two large nerves bound together by connective tissue. These two nerves, the common fibular

(peroneal) (2) and tibial (3) nerves, supply most of the intrinsic structures of the pelvic limb (those not supplied by the lateral cutaneous femoral, femoral, obturator, gluteal, and caudal cutaneous femoral nerves).

The ischiatic nerve courses distally between the superficial and deep gluteal muscles, then between the biceps femoris (superficially) and gemellus, internal obturator, quadratus femoris, and adductor muscles (deeply). The ischiatic nerve is vulnerable in this location to careless injections made into the caudal thigh muscles.

403

One or more large **MUSCULAR BRANCHES** (4) from the caudal surface of the proximal portion of the ischiatic nerve supply the biceps femoris, caudal crural abductor, semitendinosus, and semimembranosus muscles.

A small proximal cutaneous branch of the tibial nerve passes distally with the caudal crural abductor muscle and provides sensory innervation to the skin in the popliteal region.

A cutaneous branch of the common fibular nerve, either proximal or distal to the level at which the common fibular and tibial portions of the ischiatic nerve separate from each other, enters and passes through the biceps femoris muscle. This **LATERAL CUTANEOUS SURAL** (su'ral; calf of the leg) **NERVE** (5) passes through connective tissue between two portions of the biceps femoris muscle and supplies the skin of the lateral crural region.

Another cutaneous nerve, the **CAUDAL CUTANEOUS SURAL NERVE** (6), arises from the tibial nerve a short distance distal to the origin of the lateral cutaneous sural from the common peroneal nerve. The caudal cutaneous sural nerve, located caudal to the tibial nerve, courses distally to the popliteal region, where the cutaneous nerve is associated with the caudal surface of the gastrocnemius muscle.

The caudal cutaneous sural nerve divides into a number of small branches supplying the skin of the caudal tarsal region. One terminal branch passes craniomedially between the superficial and deep digital flexor tendons, joins the tibial nerve, and in some dogs provides innervation to the skin of the plantar metatarsal region.

The **COMMON FIBULAR NERVE**, located superficial to the lateral head of the gastrocnemius muscle and deep to the distal portion of the biceps femoris muscle, supplies the fibularis longus muscle with innervation and divides into two branches: the superficial (7) and deep (8) fibular nerves, both of which course distally through the crus parallel to each other, one more superficially and the other more deeply situated.

The **SUPERFICIAL FIBULAR NERVE** (7), near its origin from the common fibular nerve, is adjacent to the caudal border of the fibularis longus muscle and superficial to the lateral head of the deep digital flexor muscle; it courses craniodistally deep to the fibularis longus tendon to lie superficial to the long digital extensor tendon and proximal extensor retinaculum.

A small branch (1, Fig. 25.8) separates from the superficial fibular nerve (2), near the tarsocrural articulation to course along the dorsolateral surface of the tarsus and metatarsus. This small lateral branch is the **DORSAL ABAXIAL DIGITAL NERVE V.**

The superficial fibular nerve branches over the dorsal surface of the tarsal bones and proximal metatarsus to supply the superficial part of the innervation to the digits. (The superficial nerves of the metatarsal region are designated **COMMON DIGITAL NERVES**; the deep nerves of the metatarsal region are designated **METATARSAL NERVES**.)

The dorsal nerves to the digits that receive innervation via the superficial peroneal nerve are the **DORSAL COMMON DIGITAL NERVES II, III,** and **IV** (3–5), which are located in the second, third, and fourth intermetatarsal spaces, respectively, and the **DORSAL ABAXIAL DIGITAL NERVE II** (6). If a dew claw is present, the last named nerve would be the **DORSAL COMMON DIGITAL NERVE I.**

Each of the dorsal common digital nerves divide into two **DORSAL PROPER DIGITAL NERVES,** an **AXIAL** and an **ABAXIAL NERVE.**

The **DEEP FIBULAR NERVE** (7) also passes into the fascial cleft separating the deep digital flexor muscle (caudally) and the fibularis longus muscle (cranially).

Branches of the deep fibular nerve supply the fibularis longus, long digital extensor, and cranial tibial muscles. The deep fibular nerve courses distally with a major artery of the crus, the cranial tibial artery (8), to the tarsocrural articulation where it is situated deep and medial to the superficial fibular nerve.

The deep fibular nerve and cranial tibial artery pass distally deep to the proximal extensor retinaculum. The deep fibular nerve divides in the tarsal region to become **DORSAL METATARSAL NERVES II, III,** and **IV** (9–11, respectively), each of which combines with a dorsal common digital nerve (II, III, or IV) to supply nerve fibers to the digits.

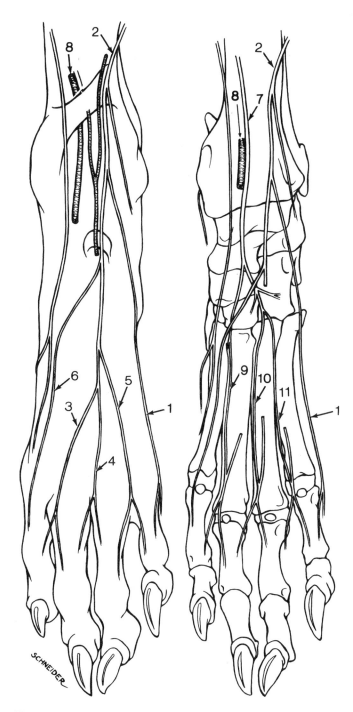

Fig.25.8. Branches of the superficial and deep fibular nerves in the left pes, dorsal view.

The **TIBIAL NERVE** (Fig. 25.9) courses distally through the popliteal region and enters the crus between the lateral and medial heads of the gastrocnemius muscle.

Muscular branches of the tibial nerve supply the gastrocnemius, superficial digital flexor, popliteus, and deep digital flexor muscles.

In the crural region the tibial nerve (1) is situated between the superficial digital flexor and deep digital flexor muscles. Proximal to the tarsal articulation, a terminal branch (2) of the laterally situated caudal cutaneous sural nerve joins the tibial nerve.

The tibial nerve separates into two nerves near the tarsocrural articulation: a smaller, more superficial medial plantar nerve (3) and a larger, deeper lateral plantar nerve (4), both of which

pass distally across the medial surface of the calcaneus tarsal bone into the pes.

The **MEDIAL PLANTAR NERVE** (3) courses through the tarsal region along the medial surface of the superficial digital flexor tendon.

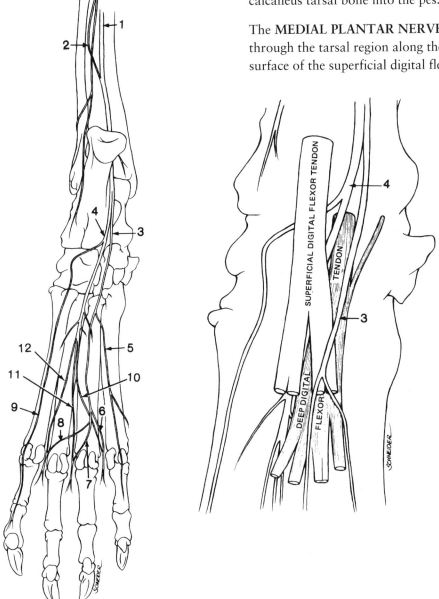

Fig.25.9. Distribution of the tibial nerve in the left pes, plantar view.

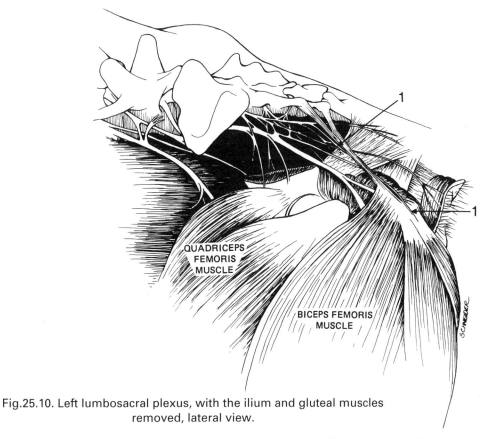

Fig.25.10. Left lumbosacral plexus, with the ilium and gluteal muscles removed, lateral view.

In the proximal metatarsal region the medial plantar nerve branches into the **PLANTAR ABAXIAL DIGITAL NERVE II** (5) and the parent trunk of the superficial plantar nerves of the distal metatarsus: **PLANTAR COMMON DIGITAL NERVES II, III,** and **IV** (6–8, respectively).

The **LATERAL PLANTAR NERVE** (4) passes distally into the fascia between the tendons of the superficial digital flexor and deep digital flexor muscles.

It then branches to form the **PLANTAR ABAXIAL DIGITAL NERVE V** (9) and the deep plantar nerves of the metatarsus, **PLANTAR METATARSAL NERVES II, III,** and **IV** (10–12, respectively). The plantar metatarsal nerves combine with the plantar common digital nerves near the distal metatarsal region. The combined nerve trunks thus formed divide into **PLANTAR AXIAL** and **ABAXIAL PROPER DIGITAL NERVES.**

The **CAUDAL CUTANEOUS FEMORAL NERVE** (1, Fig. 25.10) courses caudolaterally, deep to the sacrotuberous ligament, in the ischiorectal fossa to appear superficially on the semitendinosus muscle at the ischiatic tuberosity.

The terminal branches of the caudal cutaneus femoral nerve, the **CAUDAL CLUNIAL** (kloo' ne-al; buttocks) **NERVES,** supply fibers to the skin of the caudal and lateral femoral regions.

Nerves that conduct sensory innervation from the skin of the pelvic limb (Fig. 25.11) include the lateral cutaneous femoral; saphenous; and

407

branches of the tibial, common fibular, and
caudal cutaneous femoral nerves. A summary of
muscle and cutaneous innervation is given in
Table 25.1.

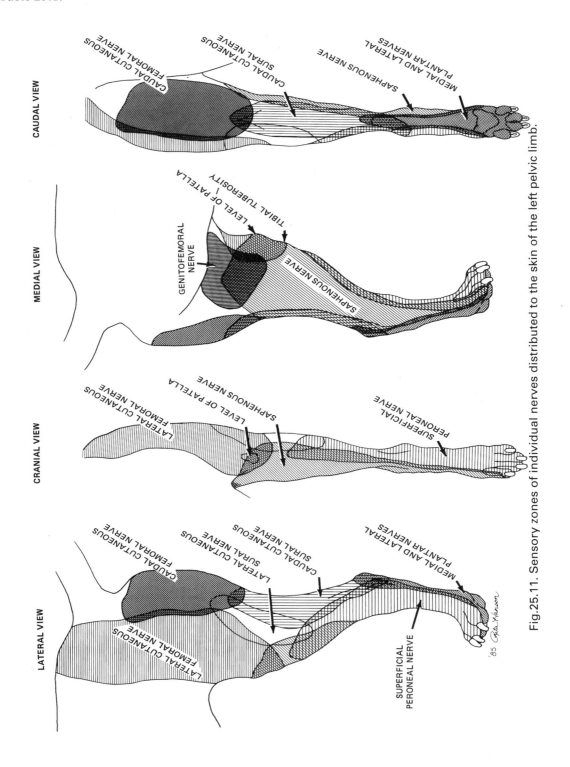

Fig.25.11. Sensory zones of individual nerves distributed to the skin of the left pelvic limb.

Table 25.1. Innervation of the pelvic limb.

Muscle	Nerve
Middle gluteus, deep gluteus, tensor fasciae latae	Cranial gluteal
Superficial gluteus	Caudal gluteal
Quadriceps femoris, iliopsoas, sartorius	Femoral
Biceps fenoris, caudal crural abductor, semitendinosus, semimembranosus	Muscular branches of the ischiatic
External obturator, pectineus, gracilis, adductor	Obturator
Internal obturator, gemellus, quadratus femoris	Muscular branch of the lumbosacral trunk
Craniolateral muscles of the crus (flexors of the tarsus, extensors of the digits)	Deep fibular
Caudal muscles of the crus (extensors of the tarsus, flexors of the digits, popliteus)	Tibial
Region	**Cutaneous Branches**
Cranial gluteal, craniolateral femoral	Lateral cutaneous femoral
Medial femoral and crural, dorsomedial tarsal	Saphenous
Caudal femoral	Caudal cutaneous femoral
Lateral crural	Lateral cutaneous sural
Caudal crural	Caudal cutaneous sural
Dorsal pes	Superficial and deep fibular
Plantar pes	Lateral and medial plantar

Chapter 26

PERIPHERAL NERVOUS SYSTEM—HEAD

Objectives: To identify the major cranial nerves and study the distribution of their fibers. Also, Identify ganglia associated with nerve cell bodies of sensory and autonomic nerves. Provide an understanding of extrinsic eye musculature such that innervation of oculomotor, trochlear, and abducens cranial nerves may be studied.

Olfactory, Optic, Oculomotor, Trochlear, Trigeminal, Abducens, Facial, Vestibulocochlear, Glossopharyngeal, Vagus, Accessory, and Hypoglossal

Branches of the Trigeminal Nerve: Mandibular, Maxillary, and Ophthalmic Nerves

Branches of the Mandibular Nerve: Auriculotemporal, Mylohyoid, Inferior Alveolar, Lingual, Buccalis, and Masticatory Nerves

Branches of the Maxillary Nerve: Infraorbital Nerves, Superior Alveolar Nerves, Pterygopalatine Nerve, and Zygomatic Nerve

Branches of the Pterygopalatine Nerve: Minor Palatine, Major Palatine, and Caudal Nasal Nerves

Branches of the Zygomatic Nerve: Zygomaticofacial and Zygomaticotemporal Nerves

Branches of the Facial Nerve: Caudal Auricular, Ventral Buccal, Dorsal Buccal, and Auriculopalpebral Nerves

Branches of the Glossopharyngeal Nerve: Carotid Sinus, Tonsilar, and Lingual Branches

Portions and Branches of the Right and Left Vagus Nerves: Distal Ganglion of the Vagus and Cranial Laryngeal Nerve

Parasympathetic Ganglia: Ciliary, Pterygopalatine, and Otic Ganglia

Sympathetic Ganglion: Cranial Cervical Ganglion

Periorbita, Chorda Tympani

Extrinsic Muscles of the Eye: Dorsal, Medial, Ventral and Lateral Recti muscles; Dorsal and Ventral Oblique Muscles, Levator Palpebrae Superioris, Retractor Bulbi

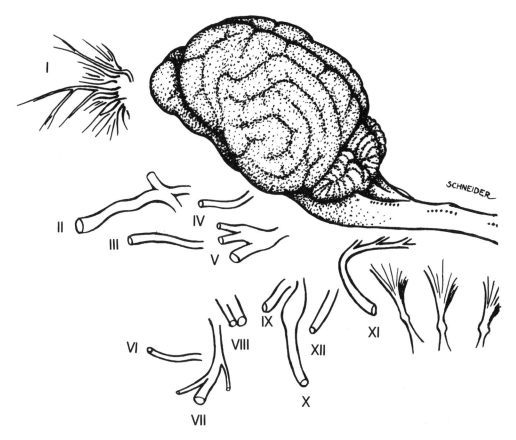

Fig.26.1. Left cranial nerves I–XII, lateral view.

The **CRANIAL NERVES I** through XII (Figs. 26.1; 26.2), numbered relative to their origin from the brain (rostral to caudal), are as follows:
I = olfactory, II = optic,
III = oculomotor,
IV = trochlear,
V = trigeminal,
VI = abducens,
VII = facial,
VIII = vestibulocochlear,
IX = glossopharyngeal,
X = vagus,
XI = accessory,
XII = hypoglossal.

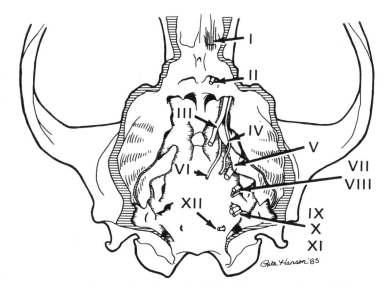

Fig.26.2. Ventral internal surface of skull, with stumps of cranial nerves I–XII exiting from the cranial cavity through foramina, dorsal view.

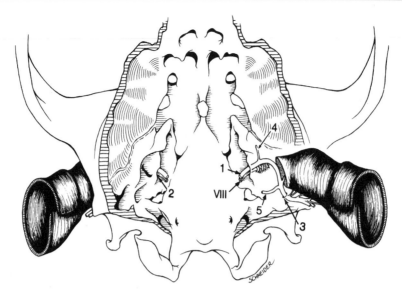

Fig.26.3. Schematic of the ventral surface of the cranial cavity,
illustrating the course of the facial and vestibulocochlear nerves in the petrous temporal bone.

A number of superficial nerve branches may be observed on the surface of the head deep to the skin, superficial fascia, and platysma muscle. Nearly all of these superficial nerves contain both efferent and afferent fibers; the majority of the superficial fibers to muscle are of the cranial nerve VII (facial), and most of the cutaneous fibers belong to branches of cranial nerve V (trigeminal).

The **FACIAL NERVE** (1, Fig. 26.3) emerges from the cranial cavity by passing into the internal acoustic meatus (2) of the petrous temporal bone and exiting from the skull through the stylomastoid foramen (3). During its course through the temporal bone of the skull, small parasympathetic preganglionic fibers (4) branch away from the facial nerve. An auricular branch (5) of the vagus nerve joins with the facial nerve in the petrous temporal bone (see pp. 116, 411).

As the facial nerve emerges from the stylomastoid foramen, caudoventral to the ear, it branches deep to or within the

parotid salivary gland into four or more large branches: the caudal auricular (1), ventral buccal (2), dorsal buccal (3), and auriculopalpebral (4) subdivisions (Fig. 26.4). The **CAUDAL AURICULAR NERVES** (1) arise from the facial nerve before or as the parent nerve emerges through the stylomastoid foramen, pass deep to the proximal lateral border of the auricular cartilage, and supply the caudal and dorsal auricular muscles.

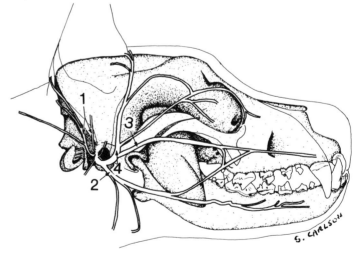

Fig.26.4. Schematic of the branches of the right facial nerve,
lateral view.

414

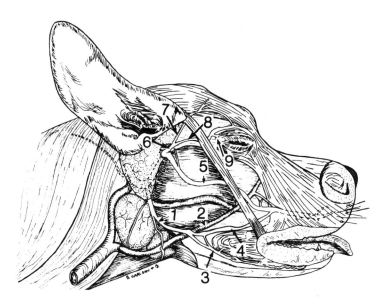

Fig.26.5. Branches of the right facial nerve, lateral view.

The **VENTRAL BUCCAL BRANCH OF THE FACIAL NERVE** (1, Fig. 26.5) appears superficially between the rostroventral surface of the parotid salivary gland and the masseter muscle; it courses rostrally across the masseter muscle, superficial to the facial vein (2), and divides into two major components.

One terminal portion of the ventral buccal branch (3) innervates the buccinator and orbicularis oris muscles of the lower jaw; the other terminal portion (4) passes rostrodorsally to combine with the **DORSAL BUCCAL BRANCH OF THE FACIAL NERVE** (5). The dorsal buccal branch courses rostrodorsally past the rostral margin of the parotid salivary gland and then superficially across the dorsal portion

of the masseter muscle. Branches of the dorsal buccal branch innervate the buccinator and orbicularis oris muscles of the upper jaw.

The **AURICULOPALPEBRAL NERVE** (6), deep to the parotid salivary gland, courses rostrodorsally, dividing into **ROSTRAL AURICULAR** (7) and **ZYGOMATIC** (8) branches. The zygomatic branch passes rostrodorsally over the zygomatic arch and temporalis muscle. Palpebral branches (9) of the zygomatic portion of the auriculopalpebral supply the orbicularis oculi muscle; the zygomatic branch also supplies the levator nasolabialis muscle with innervation.

415

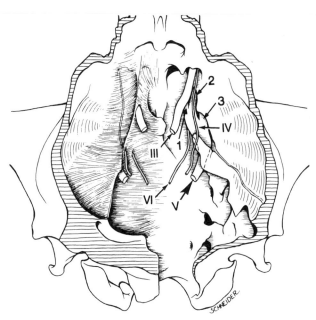

Fig.26.6. Ventral surface of cranial cavity, illustrating ophthalmic, maxillary, and mandibular divisions of right trigeminal nerve.

The rostral auricular branch passes dorsally near the rostral edge of the base of the ear, sending branches to the rostral auricular muscles. Near the stylomastoid foramen a branch nerve courses ventrally from the facial nerve to innervate the caudal portion of the digastricus muscle.

Cranial nerve V, the **TRIGEMINAL NERVE** (Fig. 26.6), divides into three large branches prior to exiting from the skull: the ophthalmic (1), maxillary (2), and mandibular (3) divisions.

Subsequent to exiting from the cranial cavity via the oval foramen, the **MANDIBULAR NERVE** (Figs. 26.7, 26.8) branches into a dorsal and ventral trunk. The dorsal trunk of the mandibular nerve, containing fibers of the buccalis, masticatory, and pterygoid nerves, crosses the superficial surface of the lateral pterygoid muscle.

The **INFERIOR ALVEOLAR NERVE** (5) enters the mandibular canal through the mandibular foramen. Small branches leave the inferior alveolar nerve within the mandibular canal to supply the roots of all the mandibular teeth.

Several **MENTAL NERVES** branch from the inferior alveolar nerve, exit from the rostral portion of the mandible through the mental foramina, and supply the lips and skin of the chin. The **LINGUAL NERVE** (6) courses rostrally into the tongue.

The **LINGUAL NERVE** (1, Fig. 26.9), a branch of the mandibular nerve, passes rostroventrally medial to the mandible and lateral to the styloglossus muscle. It supplies fibers to the mucosa of a portion of the pharynx, the rostral two-thirds of the tongue, and the floor of the mouth.

416

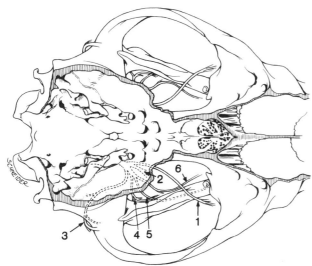

Fig.26.7. Schematic of the branches of the mandibular
nerve, dorsal view.

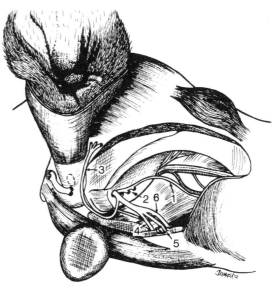

Fig.26.8. Branches of the right mandibular nerve with the caudal
portion of the mandible removed, lateral view.

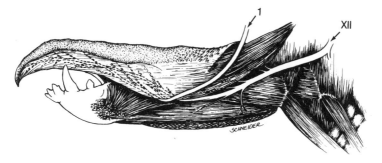

Fig.26.9. Tongue and associated structures, with the left mandible
removed, left lateral view.

417

The **MAXILLARY NERVE** (1, Figs. 26.10, 26.11) reaches the pterygopalatine fossa from the cranial cavity by passing into the alar canal through the round foramen and then rostrally out the rostral alar foramen.

Within the pterygopalatine fossa the maxillary nerve is usually present as several nerves, two or three side by side and one deep.

The superficial branches of the maxillary nerve are called **INFRAORBITAL NERVES** (2, Figs. 26.10, 26.11). Both the terminal maxillary and the infraorbital portions of this nerve supply sensory branches to the roots of the teeth.

These sensory branches are the **SUPERIOR ALVEOLAR NERVES** (3, Figs. 26.10, 26.11). Branches of the infraorbital nerves exit from the infraorbital canal through the infraorbital foramen to innervate the skin of the upper lip and muzzle.

The deep branch of the maxillary nerve, the **PTERYGOPALATINE NERVE** (4, Fig. 26.11) courses rostrally and divides into the minor palatine, major palatine, and caudal nasal nerves. The **MINOR PALATINE NERVE** (5, Fig. 26.11) is a small branch that courses ventrally over the superficial surface of the medial pterygoid muscle to reach the soft palate, which it innervates.

The **MAJOR PALATINE NERVE** (6, Figs. 26.10, 26.11) enters the caudal palatine foramen, travels through the palatine canal, and exits through the major and minor palatine foramina to innervate the soft structures of the

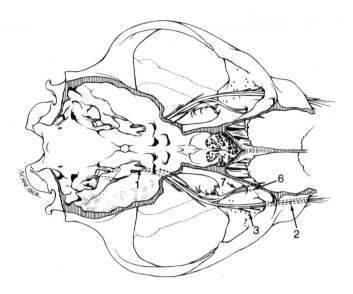

Fig.26.10. Schematic of the maxillary nerve and its branches, dorsal view.

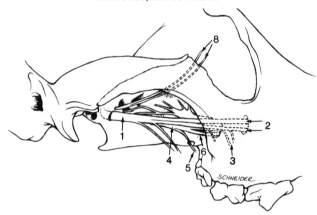

Fig.26.11. Schematic of the maxillary nerve and its branches, lateral view.

hard palate. The **CAUDAL NASAL NERVE** (7, Fig. 26.10) enters the sphenopalatine foramen and supplies innervation to the soft structures of the nasal septum, ventral concha, and maxillary recess.

The **ZYGOMATIC NERVE** (8, Fig. 26.11) is a proximal branch of the maxillary nerve that often leaves the alar canal through a separate foramen (small alar foramen) dorsal to the

418

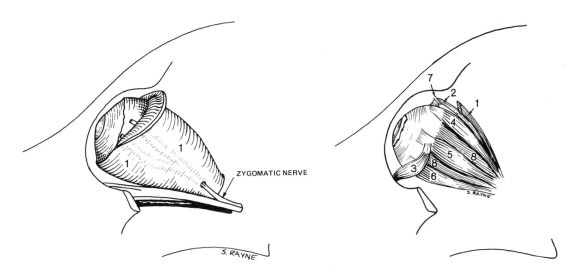

Fig.26.12. Periorbita, lateral view.

Fig.26.13. Extrinsic musles of the eye, lateral view.

rostral alar foramen. The zygomatic nerve passes into the apex of the cone-shaped muscular fascia, where it may be observed as two nerves (the **ZYGOMATICOTEMPORAL** and **ZYGOMATICOFACIAL BRANCHES**) on the lateral surface of the orbital muscles and fat. The zygomatic nerve supplies fibers to the lacrimal gland and to the lateral portion of the superior and inferior palpebrae.

The extrinsic eye muscles; oculomotor, trochlear, abducens, optic, zygomatic, and ophthalmic nerves; and blood vessels of the eye are all enclosed by a cone-shaped muscular fascia, the **PERIORBITA** (1, Fig. 26.12).

The superficial set of muscles of the eye (Fig. 26.13), observed when the muscular fascia is removed, are the levator of the superior palpebra (1), the dorsal (2) and ventral (3) obliques, and four straight muscles. The **LEVATOR PALPEBRAE SUPERIORIS** arises from the skull near the optic canal and inserts as a flat tendon in the superior palpebra.

The straight muscles are named according to their position relative to the optic nerve: **DORSAL RECTUS** (4), **LATERAL RECTUS** (5), **VENTRAL RECTUS** (6), and **MEDIAL RECTUS**. The four recti muscles arise from the skull near the optic canal and insert on the four surfaces of the eyeball (dorsal, lateral, ventral, and medial).

The **DORSAL OBLIQUE MUSCLE** (2) arises from the skull near the optic canal, passes rostrally superficial and dorsomedial to the cone formed by the recti muscles, and inserts by a long tendon on the outer fibrous layer of the eyeball. Its tendon of insertion is anchored to the orbital surface of the frontal bone by a cartilaginous pulley or **TROCHLEA** (7); from the trochlea the tendon passes laterally to insert on the dorsal surface of the eyeball.

The **VENTRAL OBLIQUE MUSCLE** (3) arises from the rostral portion of the orbital surface of the palatine bone and courses laterally around the ventral surface of the eyeball to insert on the lateral surface of the eyeball.

419

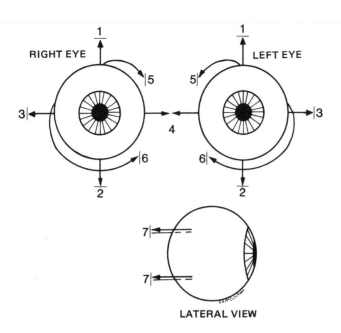

Fig.26.14. Schematic illustrating the points of insertion by extrinsic eye muscles on the bulb of the eye.

A cone of four muscle fascicles are positioned around the optic nerve deep to the four recti muscles. These fascicles are the **RETRACTOR BULBI MUSCLES** (8). They arise from the skull near the orbital fissure and insert on the eyeball posterior to the insertion of the recti muscles.

The extrinsic muscles, described briefly above, function as follows with respect to the anterior surface of the bulb of the eye (Fig. 26.14): 1) dorsal rectus levates it, 2) ventral rectus depresses it, 3) lateral rectus pulls it laterally, 4) medial rectus pulls it medially, 5) dorsal oblique rotates or swivels the dorsal surface ventromedially, 6) ventral oblique rotates or swivels the ventral surface dorsomedially, and 7) the retractor bulbi pulls it posteriorly.

When contracting simultaneously, the two oblique muscles pull the anterior portion of the eyeball medially.

The **OPHTHALMIC NERVE** (Figs. 26.15, 26.16) emerges from the orbital fissure and supplies afferent fibers to many structures of the orbital, nasal, and frontal regions via the **FRONTAL** (1), **LACRIMAL** (2), and **NASOCILIARY** (3) **NERVES**.

The frontal nerve is sensory to the middle of the superior palpebra. Branches of the nasociliary are sensory to the medial commissure, cornea, bulbar conjunctiva, iris, and ciliary body; one branch, the **INFRATROCHLEAR NERVE** (4), is visible near the medial commissure, ventral to the trochlea.

In addition to the ophthalmic nerve, three other cranial nerves (oculomotor, trochlear, and abducens) provide innervation to periorbital structures.

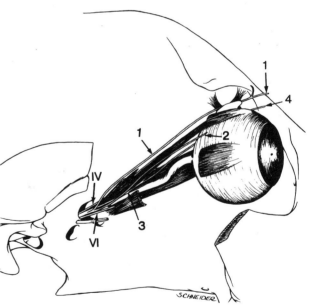

Fig.26.15. Nerves: trochlear, abducens, and branches of the ophthalmic, with several extrinsic muscles of the right eye removed, lateral view.

420

The oculomotor, trochlear, and abducens all emerge from the cranial cavity through the orbital fissure. These three cranial nerves (III, IV, and VI) innervate the seven extrinsic muscles of the eyeball and one of the superior palpebra.

Cranial nerve III, the **OCULOMOTOR NERVE** (1, Figs. 26.17, 26.18), enters the muscular fascia from the orbital fissure and courses along the ventrolateral surface of the optic nerve and ophthalmic blood vessels to innervate the levator palpebrae superioris; ventral oblique; and dorsal, medial, and ventral recti muscles.

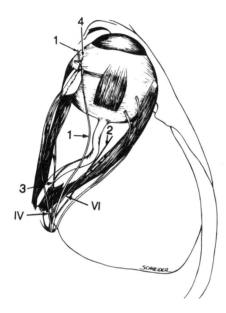

Fig.26.16. Nerves: trochlear, abducens, and branches of the ophthalmic, dorsal view of the right eye.

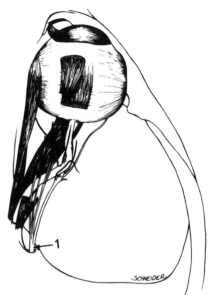

Fig.26.17. Right oculomotor nerve and branches, with several extrinsic eye muscles removed, dorsal view.

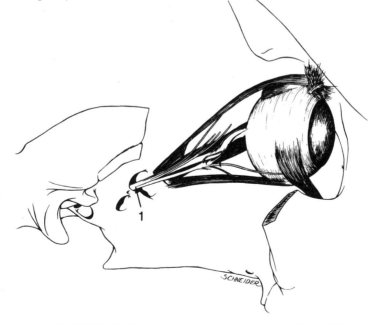

Fig.26.18. Right oculomotor nerve and branches, with several extrinsic eye muscles removed, lateral view.

421

Cranial nerve IV, the **TROCHLEAR NERVE** (1, Fig. 26.19), upon entering the periorbita from the orbital fissure, innervates the dorsal oblique muscle.

Cranial nerve VI, the **ABDUCENS** (ab-du' senz; to abduct) **NERVE** (2), after exiting from the cranial cavity through the orbital fissure, enters the periorbita and innervates the retractor bulbi and lateral rectus muscles. Retraction of the eyeball indirectly puts pressure on the base of the semilunar conjunctival fold, resulting in protrusion of the fold.

The numerous afferent **OLFACTORY** (cranial I) **NERVES** pass directly from the olfactory mucosa of the nasal cavity through foramina of the cribriform lamina of the ethmoid bone to the olfactory bulbs of the brain.

Cranial nerve II, the **OPTIC NERVE** (1, Fig. 26.20), containing afferent fibers arising in the retina, passes through the optic canal to reach the brain. The optic nerve is deep to extrinsic muscles of the bulb of the eye.

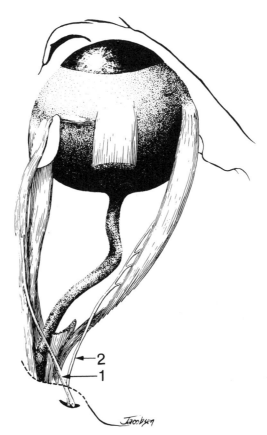

Fig.26.19. Right trochlear and abducens nerves with several extrinsic eye muscles removed, dorsal view.

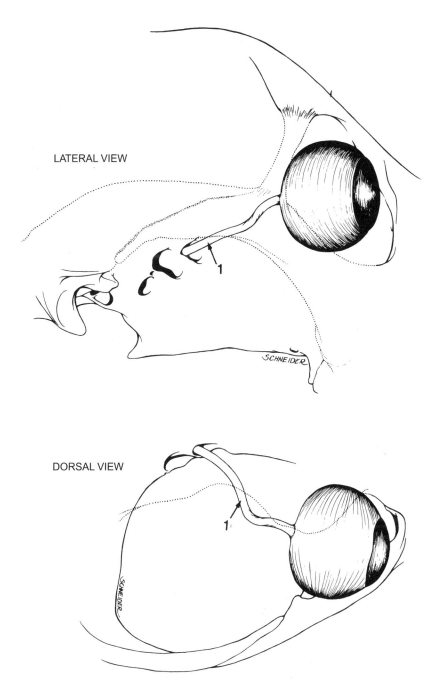

LATERAL VIEW

DORSAL VIEW

Fig.26.20. Bulb of the eye and extracranial portion of the optic nerve.

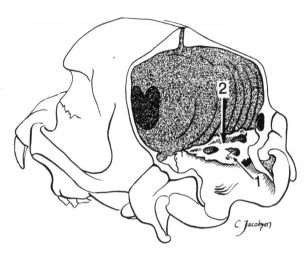

Fig.26.21. Right vestibulocochlear nerve, entering the right petrous temporal bone.

Cranial nerve VIII, the **VESTIBULOCO-CHLEAR NERVE** (1, Fig. 26.21), enters the internal acoustic meatus from the cranial cavity along with the facial nerve (see p. 414). The vestibular portion is concerned with balance and the cochlear portion with hearing. Neither the vestibular nor the cochlear portion of cranial nerve VIII may be seen on the superficial surface of the skull since both innervate structures of the inner ear, which is contained within the petrous temporal bone (2).

Cranial nerve XII, the **HYPOGLOSSAL NERVE** (1, Figs. 26.22, 26.23), exits from the skull through the hypoglossal canal. This nerve, medial to the accessory nerve and lateral to the vagus nerve at the canal, crosses the lateral surface of the external carotid artery and hyoglossal muscle to enter the tongue.

The hypoglossal nerve supplies innervation to the extrinsic muscles of the tongue (genioglossus, hyoglossus, and styloglossus) as well as to the intrinsic tongue musculature.

A small branch of the hypoglossal nerve (2, Fig. 26.22) forms a loop with a branch of the 1st cervical spinal nerve (3, Fig. 22.22). This loop is termed the **ANSA** (an " sah; handle) **CERVICALIS** (see p. 435).

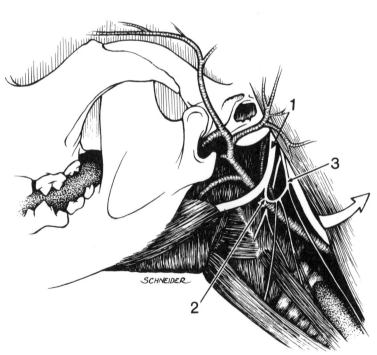

Fig.26.22. Position of the left hypoglossal nerve relative to the carotid arteries, vagosympathetic trunk, and digastricus musle, lateral view.

424

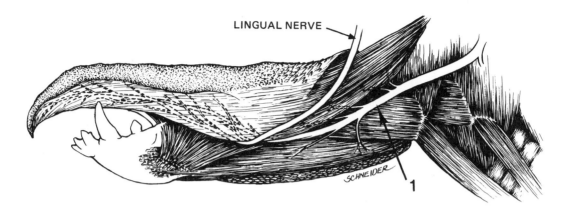

Fig.26.23. Distribution of the left hypoglossal nerve in the tongue, with the left mandible removed, lateral view.

Cranial nerve X, the vagus nerve, extends caudally into the neck, thorax, and abdomen; the vagus and its branches are closely associated with sympathetic fibers arising from the spinal cord in thoracolumbar segments. The **VAGUS NERVE** (1, Fig. 26.24) emerges from the tympanooccipital fissure in common with the glossopharyngeal (2) and accessory (3a, 3b) nerves.

Nerve cell bodies of sensory fibers carried within the vagus are present in one of two ganglia; one ganglion is located proximal and the other distal to the tympanooccipital fissure.

These two ganglia are called the **PROXIMAL** (4) and **DISTAL** (5) **GANGLIA OF THE VAGUS.**

The distal ganglion of the vagus is closely united by connective tissue with an accumulation of sympathetic postganglionic nerve cell bodies, the **CRANIAL CERVICAL GANGLION** (6).

Extracranial branches of the vagus to the head and neck regions include the **COMMUNICATING RAMUS** with the **GLOSSO-PHARYNGEAL NERVE** (7), **PHARYNGEAL BRANCHES** (8), and the **CRANIAL LARYNGEAL NERVE** (9). The cranial laryngeal nerve branches from the vagus at the level of the distal ganglion.

Within the skull an **AURICULAR BRANCH OF**

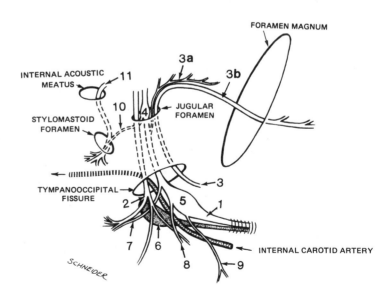

Fig.26.24. Schematic of the positions of the facial, glossopharyngeal, vagus, and accessory nerves relative to each other, and to the cranial cervical ganglion and interanal carotid artery.

425

THE VAGUS (10, Fig. 26.24; 1, Fig. 26.25) passes through a portion of the petrous temporal bone to join the facial nerve (11, Fig. 26.24; 2, Fig. 26.25). Sensory fibers of the auricular branch of the vagus reach the luminal surface of the external acoustic meatus with internal auricular branches of cranial nerve VII (3, Fig. 26.25). Irritation of the acoustic meatus by ear mites in young dogs may result in vomiting; the sensory inputs from the ear and the alimentary canal through the vagus apparently are not differentiated by the brain in the young dog.

Cranial nerve XI, the **ACCESSORY NERVE**, which has its origin both from the cervical portion of the spinal cord and the medulla oblongata, exits from the cranial cavity through the jugular foramen. Prior to emerging from the tympanooccipital fissure, the portion of the accessory nerve that originates from the medulla oblongata, the **INTERNAL BRANCH** (3a, Fig. 26.24), separates off and exits through the tympanooccipital fissure with the vagus nerve.

The **EXTERNAL BRANCH OF THE ACCESSORY NERVE** (3b) passes into and through the sternomastoideus and cleidomastoideus muscles caudoventral to the mandibular salivary gland and dorsolateral to the medial retropharyngeal lymph node. The accessory nerve, which innervates the cleidomastoideus, sternomastoideus, sternohyoideus, omotransversarius, and trapezius muscles, is described with the trunk innervation (see p. 436).

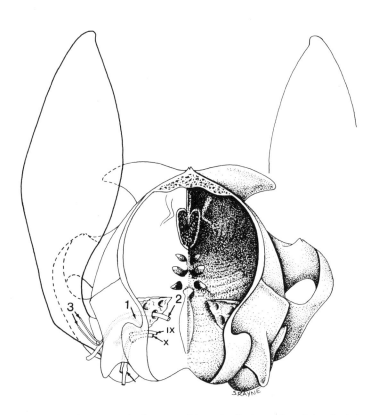

Fig.26.25. Schematic of the positional relationship of the facial and vagus nerves, caudal view.

The **GLOSSOPHARYNGEAL NERVE** (1, Fig. 26.26) enters the jugular foramen and exits from the skull through the tympanooccipital fissure. Two ganglia, **PROXIMAL** and **DISTAL**, of cranial nerve IX are present within the skull. The glossopharyngeal nerve divides to form several branches (pharyngeal, lingual, tonsillar, and carotid sinus).

The **PHARYNGEAL BRANCH** (2) courses rostrally, medial to the stylohyoid, and with fibers from the vagus and sympathetic trunk forms the **PHARYNGEAL PLEXUS**. The pharyngeal plexus supplies the mucous membrane of the dorsal wall of the pharynx with fibers.

The **CAROTID SINUS BRANCH** (3) courses caudoventrally to the bulbous origin of the internal carotid from the common carotid artery. The **LINGUAL BRANCHES** (4) supply the caudal one-third of the tongue with nerve fibers. The **TONSILAR BRANCHES** supply fibers to the lateral pharyngeal wall, including the palatine tonsil.

Parasympathetic fibers originating from nerve cell bodies in nuclei of the CNS are carried from the brain by four cranial nerves: oculomotor, facial, glossopharyngeal, and vagus. These parasympathetic fibers branch away from the four above-mentioned cranial nerves and join other nerves during their course to various glands and smooth muscle fibers.

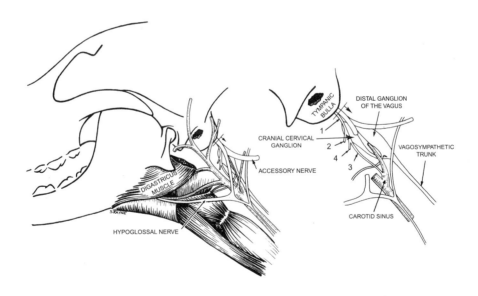

Fig.26.26. Left cranial nerves IX–XII, cranial sympathetic ganglion, and internal carotid artery adjacent to the occipitotympanic fissure, lateral view.

Preganglionic parasympathetic fibers carried from the brain in the oculomotor nerve (1, Fig. 26.27) branch away from the oculomotor to reach the **CILIARY GANGLION** (2).

The cell bodies of postganglionic parasympathetic neurons are present in the ciliary ganglion; parasympathetic axons (3) are distributed from the ciliary ganglion to the internal structures of the eyeball, where innervation results in constriction of the pupil and an alteration in the curvature of the eyeball, allowing the lens to become thicker.

Parasympathetic fibers carried from the brain in the facial and glossopharyngeal nerves leave these nerves, exit from the skull, and join branches of the trigeminal nerve to reach the various salivary glands and glands of the nasal and oral mucosa.

Parasympathetic preganglionic fibers carried from the brain by the facial nerve exit from the skull through the minute pterygoid foramen as the **NERVE OF THE PTERYGOID CANAL** (1, Fig. 26.28).

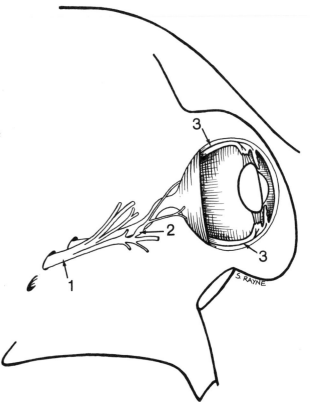

Fig.26.27. Schematic of the distribution of the parasympathetic fibers to the iris and ciliary body, lateral view.

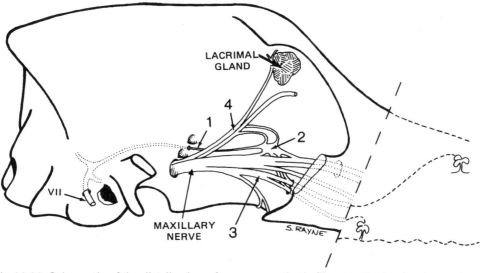

Fig.26.28. Schematic of the distribution of parasympathetic fibers to the lacrimal, nasal, and palatine glands, lateral view.

These preganglionic fibers synapse with postganglionic fibers in the **PTERYGOPALATINE GANGLION** (2), which is situated on the lateral surface of the medial pterygoid muscle, dorsal to the pterygopalatine nerve (3).

Postganglionic parasympathetic fibers span the gap between the thin, flat pterygopalatine ganglion and the pterygopalatine nerve; postganglionic parasympathetic fibers may course in a retrograde direction to reach the lacrimal gland via the zygomatic nerve (4), or they may supply numerous nasal and palatine glands via branches of the pterygopalatine nerve.

The **CHORDA** (kor' dah; cord) **TYMPANI** (drum) (1, Fig. 26.29) is a small nerve that separates from the facial nerve (2), exits from the skull, and joins with the lingual nerve (3).

The chorda tympani passes rostroventrally deep to the mylohyoid and inferior alveolar nerves to join the lingual nerve near the inferior alveolar-lingual bifurcation.

The chorda tympani contains preganglionic parasympathetic fibers destined for the mandibular and sublingual salivary glands, preganglionic parasympathetic fibers to glands of the rostral two-thirds of the tongue and floor of the mouth, and afferent fibers from taste receptors in the rostral two-thirds of the tongue.

Preganglionic parasympathetic fibers reach the mandibular and sublingual salivary glands by passing from the chorda tympani to the lingual nerve and then branching caudally, at the level of the styloglossus muscle, to enter ganglia near the glands.

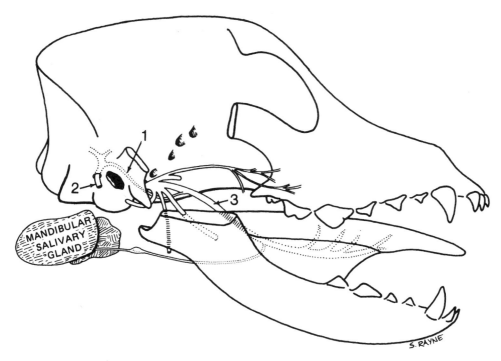

Fig.26.29. Schematic of the distribution of parasympathetic fibers to the mandibular and sublingual salivary glands, glands of the rostral portion of the tongue, and glands of the oral mucosa, lateral view.

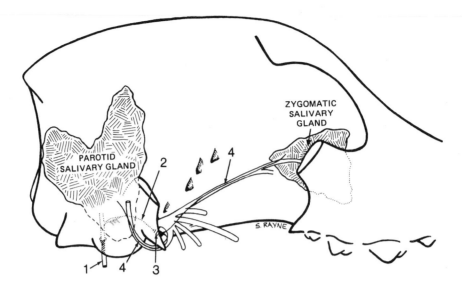

Fig.26.30. Schematic of the distribution of parasympathetic fibers to the parotid and zygomatic salivary glands.

Preganglionic parasympathetic fibers (Fig. 26.30) also branch from the glossopharyngeal nerve (1) within the skull and pass out of the skull as the **MINOR PETROSAL NERVE** (2) to the **OTIC GANGLION** (3) near the oval foramen. Postganglionic parasympathetic fibers (4) join the auriculotemporal and buccalis nerves to reach the parotid and zygomatic salivary glands.

Nerve fibers within the vagus include preganglionic parasympathetic (GVE) and GVA, SVE, SVA, and GSA.

(DIFFERENCES TO BE NOTED IN THE CAT: Striated muscle fibers of the lateral rectus and levator palpebrae superioris muscles insert on the third eyelid. Thus the third eyelid— semilunar conjunctival fold—may be drawn over the cornea of the cat independent of retraction of the eyeball.)

Some clinically useful reflexes are given in Table 26.1; a summary of the innervation of the head is listed in Table 26.2.

Table 26.1. Clinically useful reflexes in the head.

Structure Stimulated	Stimulus	Sensory Pathway	Motor Pathway	Action
Cornea	Air	Opthalmic of trigeminal	Auriculopalpebral of facial	Close palpebral fissure
Palpebrae				
Superior palpebra, medial commissure	Touch	Opthalmic	Auriculopalpebral	Close palpebral fissure
Lateral commissure, inferior palpebra	Touch	Zygomatic of the maxillary division of the trigeminal	Auriculopalpebral	Close palpebral fissure
Retina	Movement toward the eye	Optic nerve	Auriculopalpebral	Close palpebral fissure
Retina	Light	Optic nerve	Oculomotor (para-sympathetic fibers)	Constriction of pupil

Table 26.2. Summary of the innervation of the head.

Muscle	Cranial Nerve	Primary Branch	Secondary Branch
Facial expression:			
Platysma, levator nasolabialis, orbicularis oris orbicularis oculi, zygomaticus, buccinator, auricular	Facial		
Mastication:			
Close jaws temporalis, masseter, medial and lateral pterygoideus	Trigeminal	Mandibular	
Open jaws—digastricus	Trigeminal Facial	Mandibular	Mylohyoid
Tongue:			
Genioglossus, hyoglossus, styloglossus, intrinsic	Hypoglossal		
Extrinsic eye:			
Dorsal rectus, medial rectus, ventral rectus, ventral oblique, levator plapebrae superioris	Oculomotor		
Dorsal oblique	Trochlear		
Lateral rectus, retractor bulbi	Abducens		
Extrinsic pharyngeal:			
Hyopharyngeus, thyropharyngeus, cricopharyngeus	Glossopharyngeal		
Extrinsic laryngeal:			
Cricothyroideus	Vagus	Cranial laryngeal	
Cricoarytenoideus dorsalis, cricoarytenoideus lateralis, thyroarytenoideus	Vagus	Recurrent laryngeal	Caudal laryngeal

Cutaneous or Mucosal Region	Secondary Branch	Primary Branch	Nerve
Dorsal and lateral nasal, superior labial	Infraorbital	Maxillary	Trigeminal
Inferior labial, mental	Inferior alveolar	Mandibular	Trigeminal
Cheek	Buccal	Mandibular	Trigeminal
Eyelids and cornea:			
Superior palpebrae, medial commissure	Frontal Infratrochlear	Opthalmic	Trigeminal
Inferior palpebrae, lateral commissure	Zygomatic	Maxillary	Trigeminal
Ear:			
Tragic margin	Auriculotemporal	Mandibular Major occipital	Trigeminal Second cervical
Concave surface		Internal auricular	Facial
Antitragic margin		Internal auricular Major auricular	Facial Second cervical
Convex surface		Major occipital Major auricular	Second cervical

Chapter 27

PERIPHERAL NERVOUS SYSTEM—TRUNK

Objectives: To identify the major nerves to muscle and skin of the neck, rib cage, and abdominal wall.

Cervical Spinal Nerves: Major Occipital Nerve, Major Auricular Nerve, Transverse Nerve of the Neck, Phrenic Nerve

Thoracic Spinal Nerves: Dorsal Rami with Lateral and Medial Branches; Ventral Rami (Right and Left Intercostal Nerves and Right and Left Costoabdominal Nerve) with Lateral Cutaneous, Ventral Cutaneous, and Muscular Branches

Lumbar Spinal Nerves: Dorsal Rami with Lateral and Medial Branches; Ventral Rami (Right and Left Cranial and Caudal Iliohypogastric Nerves; Right and Left Ilioinguinal, Lateral Cutaneous Femoral, and Genitofemoral Nerves). Other branches studied in Chapter 25, "Pelvic Limb."

Sacral Spinal Nerves: Dorsal Rami with Lateral and Medial Branches; Ventral Rami forming the Right and Left Sacral Plexuses from which the Right and Left Pudendal Nerves are formed

Branches of each Pudendal Nerve: Superficial and Deep Perineal Nerves; Caudal Rectal Nerve; Dorsal Nerve of Clitoris/Penis

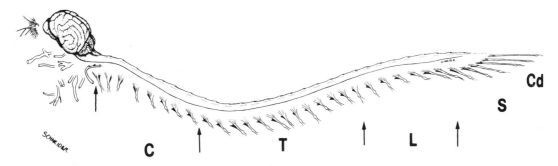

Fig.27.1. Spinal nerves, lateral view.

The trunk is innervated by 8 pairs of **CERVICAL**, 13 pairs of **THORACIC**, 7 pairs of **LUMBAR**, and 3 pairs of **SACRAL SPINAL NERVES** (Fig. 27.1). Seven of the eight pairs of cervical spinal nerves exit from the vertebral canal through intervertebral foramina (the 1st cervical spinal nerve emerges from the 1st cervical vertebra through the lateral vertebral foramen). Thus the cervical spinal nerves emerge from the vertebral column at intervals equal to the length of one vertebra.

The 1st (most cranial) cervical spinal nerve divides near the lateral vertebral foramen into a dorsal and ventral ramus. The dorsal and ventral rami of C1 usually do not reach the surface of the neck.

The **DORSAL RAMUS** supplies epaxial neck musculature (including the capital obliques, dorsal recti muscles, the semispinalis capitis, and splenius).

The **VENTRAL RAMUS** (1, Fig. 27.2) courses caudoventrally, initially deep to the medial retropharyngeal lymph node and distally next to the vagosympathetic trunk (2). The ventral ramus of C1 often forms a junction with a branch of the hypoglossal nerve, forming the **ANSA CERVICALIS,** or cervical loop (3).

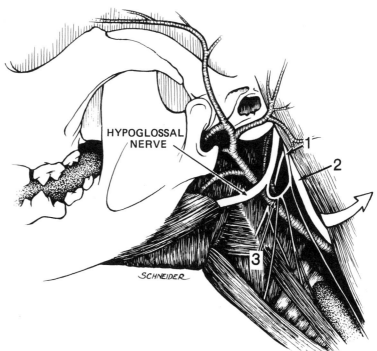

Fig.27.2. Topographical relationship of the ansa cervicalis with the vagosympathetic trunk and carotid arteries, left lateral view.

435

The ventral ramus of C1 innervates the sternothyroideus and sternohyoideus muscles.

The part of the **ACCESSORY** (cranial XI) **NERVE** (1, Fig. 27.3) that arises from the cervical portion of the spinal cord is termed the **EXTERNAL BRANCH** (see p. 426). It courses caudally from the tympanooccipital fissure, through the sterno- and cleidomastoideus muscles, which it innervates, and on caudally deep to the cleidocervicalis and omotransversarius muscles.

Branches of the ventral rami of a number of cervical spinal nerves (C2, C3, and C4) join the accessory nerve as the cranial nerve courses past them. The accessory nerve is the sole innervator of the trapezius muscle.

The roots of the 2nd cervical spinal nerve exit from the intervertebral foramen between the atlas and axis. The **SPINAL GANGLION** and the junction of dorsal and ventral roots are peripheral to the vertebral column.

The dorsal ramus of C2 (the **MAJOR OCCIPITAL NERVE**) innervates the semispinalis capitis and splenius muscles, then supplies fibers to the skin of the caudal auricular and parietal regions.

The ventral ramus of C2 courses caudoventrally between the sternooccipitalis and cleidomastoideus muscles. Superficially positioned adjacent to the transverse process of the atlas, the ventral ramus of C2 divides into a major auricular nerve and a transverse nerve of the neck. The **MAJOR AURICLAR NERVE** (2) courses craniodorsally to innervate the skin of

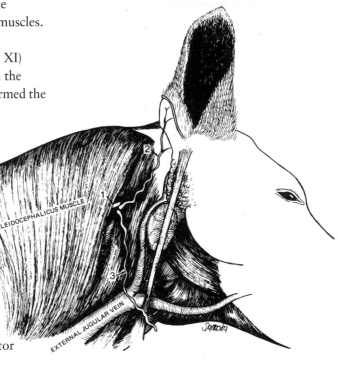

Fig.27.3. Surface of the head and neck depicting the positions of the right accessory nerve and branches of the ventral ramus of the 2nd cervical spinal nerve.

the convex surface of the ear.

The **TRANSVERSE NERVE OF THE NECK** (3) courses rostrally, superficial to the large veins of the head, supplying fibers to the platysma and the skin of the laryngeal and intermandibular regions.

Cervical spinal nerves 2–8 are characterized by relatively small dorsal rami, with medial subbranches supplying the skin of the dorsal cervical region and lateral subbranches supplying the epaxial muscles. Ventral rami of C3–C5 may be located deep to the omotransversarius muscle, through which they traverse. These ventral rami supply hypaxial muscles and the skin of the ventral and lateral cervical regions.

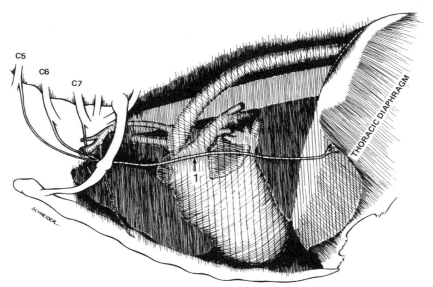

Fig.27.4. Left phrenic nerve, lateral view.

Caudal branches of the ventral rami of C5–C7 unite to form the **PHRENIC NERVE** (1, Fig. 27.4), which passes caudally deep to the 1st rib to innervate the thoracic diaphragm. The phrenic nerve of each side is situated within the lamina of connective tissue (mediastinum) separating right and left portions of the thoracic cavity, medial to the lungs and lateral to the base of the heart. On the surface of the diaphragm the phrenic nerve divides into ventral, lateral, and dorsal branches.

Each of the 13 **THORACIC SPINAL NERVES** (Fig. 27.5) exits from the vertebral canal through an intervertebral foramen immediately caudal to the corresponding vertebra (e.g., the 6th thoracic spinal nerve emerges from the vertebral canal through the foramen formed by the caudal vertebral notch of the 6th thoracic vertebra and the cranial vertebral notch of the 7th thoracic vertebra). Each thoracic spinal nerve divides into a dorsal (1) and a ventral (2) ramus.

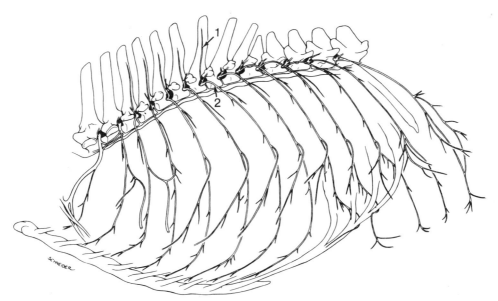

Fig.27.5. Portions of the rib cage and left thoracic spinal nerves, lateral view.

437

The **DORSAL RAMUS** (1, Fig. 27.6) of a thoracic spinal nerve bifurcates into medial and lateral branches. The **MEDIAL BRANCH** (2) of the dorsal ramus supplies the epaxial muscles and the meninges of the spinal cord; the **LATERAL BRANCH** (3) courses dorsolaterally between the longissimus and iliocostalis muscles and divides into a **MEDIAL CUTANEOUS** (4) and a **LATERAL CUTANEOUS** (5) **BRANCH.** Branches of the **VENTRAL RAMI** (6) of thoracic spinal nerves are **MUSCULAR** (7), **LATERAL CUTANEOUS** (8), and **VENTRAL CUTANEOUS** (9) **BRANCHES.**

The lateral cutaneous branches course laterally and may be observed superficially on the lateral surface of the external abdominal oblique muscle near the ventral border of the latissimus dorsi muscle.

The lateral cutaneous branches of T2 and T3 intercostal nerves are relatively large nerves that innervate the skin of the tricipital and olecranon regions; these nerves are named the **INTERCOSTOBRACHIAL NERVES.** A number of the lateral cutaneous branches supply fibers to the thoracic mammary glands; these fibers are named the **LATERAL MAMMARY BRANCHES.**

The ventral cutaneous branches of the ventral rami of the thoracic spinal nerves enter the skin in the sternal region. Nerve fibers that arise from the ventral cutaneous branches and innervate the thoracic mammary glands are termed the **MEDIAL MAMMARY BRANCHES.** Each of the ventral portions of the last thoracic ventral rami are situated abdominally as the costal arch curves cranioventrally.

Each of the ventral rami (1, Fig. 27.7) of the thoracic spinal nerves courses through the thoracic wall in contact with blood vessels next

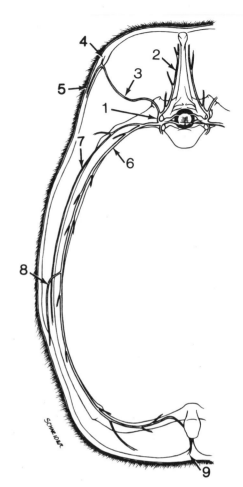

Fig.27.6. Branches of a thoracic spinal nerve, caudal view.

to the caudal border of the correspondingly numbered rib (the ventral ramus of the 1st thoracic spinal nerve is an exception since most of the nerve joins the brachial plexus).

Since each ventral ramus of each thoracic spinal nerve is situated in an interval between two adjacent ribs, they are named **INTERCOSTAL NERVES.** The one exception to the intercostal location occurs caudally where the ventral ramus of the 13th spinal nerve is situated near the caudal surface of the last rib; the ventral ramus of T13 is named the **COSTOABDOMINAL NERVE** (2).

438

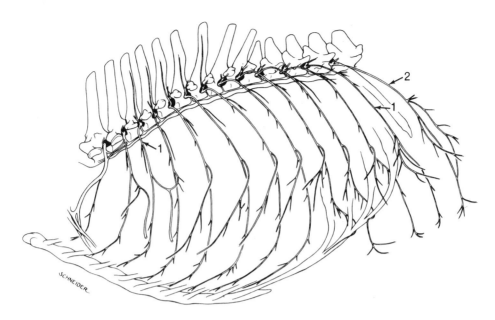

Fig.27.7. Left intercostal nerves and the costoabdominal nerve, lateral view.

The seven **LUMBAR SPINAL NERVES** (Fig. 27.8) also divide into **DORSAL** (1) and **VENTRAL** (2) **RAMI.** The dorsal rami supply medial branches to the epaxial musculature and lateral branches to the skin of the dorsolateral lumbar and sacral regions.

The lateral cutaneous branches of the caudal several lumbar spinal nerves are also known as the **CRANIAL CLUNIAL NERVES.**

The ventral rami of the first several lumbar spinal nerves, oriented in series parallel with the ventral rami of the caudal thoracic spinal nerves, are named the cranial iliohypogastric (3), caudal iliohypogastric (4), ilioinguinal (5), lateral cutaneous femoral (6), and genitofemoral nerves. The ventral ramus of the 1st lumbar spinal nerve, named the **CRANIAL ILIOHYPOGASTRIC NERVE** (3), emerges deep to the abdominal wall

from the quadratus lumborum. It innervates some of the parietal peritoneum and a segment of the quadratus lumborum, passes ventrolaterally through the dorsal aponeurosis of the transversus abdominis muscle, and divides into a lateral and a medial branch. The lateral

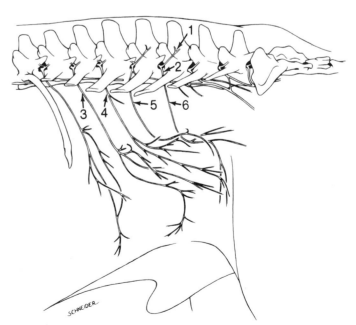

Fig.27.8. Left costoabdominal and lumbar spinal nerves, lateral view.

439

branch passes through the internal abdominal oblique muscle to course ventrally between the two abdominal oblique muscles.

This lateral branch innervates both oblique muscles, then passes through the external abdominal oblique as the **LATERAL CUTANEOUS BRANCH,** which innervates a vertical band of skin in the ventrolateral abdominal region.

The medial branch courses ventrally on the superficial surface of the transversus abdominis muscles, which it innervates in part. A ventral portion of the medial branch innervates the rectus abdominis muscle in part and passes out to the skin as the **VENTRAL CUTANEOUS BRANCH.**

The ventral ramus of the 2nd lumbar spinal nerve, the **CAUDAL ILIOHYPOGASTRIC NERVE** (4), is similar in pattern and innervation to the cranial iliohypogastric nerve. It innervates the skin of the cranial femoral region.

The ventral ramus of the 3rd lumbar spinal nerve is named the **ILIOINGUINAL NERVE** (5); the ilioinguinal nerve, which also receives fibers from the 4th lumbar nerve, supplies cutaneous fibers via the lateral cutaneous branch to the skin of the craniolateral femoral region.

The **LATERAL CUTANEOUS FEMORAL NERVE** (6), formed primarily by the ventral ramus of the 4th lumbar nerve, courses laterally with the deep circumflex iliac vessels and supplies the lateral surface of the femoral and genual regions.

The **GENITOFEMORAL NERVE** (1, Fig. 27.9) contains fibers that arise from ventral rami of both the 3rd and 4th lumbar spinal nerves; the proximal portion of this nerve, deep to the abdominal wall, courses caudoventrally on the surface of the external iliac artery.

The genitofemoral nerve exits from the abdominal cavity through the inguinal canal to supply the cremaster muscle and the skin of the inguinal, medial femoral, and preputial regions in the dog, or the caudal abdominal mammary gland in the bitch.

The dorsal rami of the three **SACRAL SPINAL NERVES** exit from the vertebral canal through the dorsal sacral foramina. Each of these dorsal rami divides into a medial branch (supplying the dorsal muscles of the tail) and a lateral cutaneous branch.

The three lateral cutaneous branches of the dorsal sacral rami, named the **MIDDLE CLUNIAL NERVES,** innervate the skin of the superficial gluteal and proximal caudolateral femoral regions.

The **SACRAL PLEXUS** is formed by ventral rami of the three sacral spinal nerves and by a contribution of fibers from the ventral rami of the 6th and 7th lumbar spinal nerves.

The bilaterally paired **PUDENDAL NERVE** of the bitch (1, Fig. 27.10) arises from the sacral plexus and crosses the dorsolateral surface of the coccygeus muscle in association with the internal pudendal artery.

The **SUPERFICIAL PERINEAL NERVE** (2), a branch of the pudendal nerve, courses laterally across the external anal sphincter and innervates the skin of the perineum and the dorsal vulvar region via **DORSAL LABIAL NERVES.**

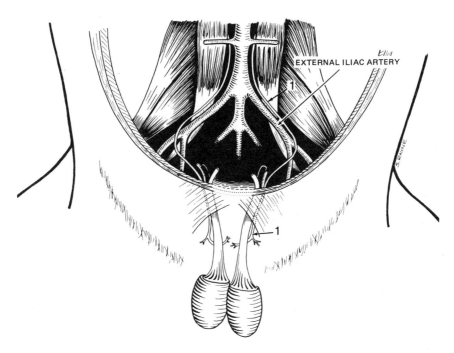

Fig.27.9. Genitofemoral nerve and distribution, ventral view.

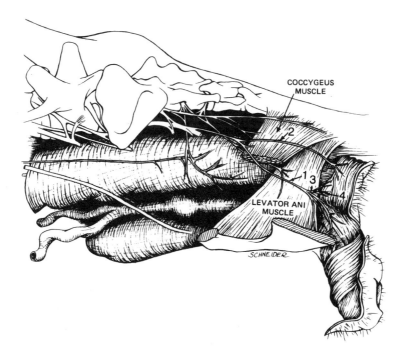

Fig.27.10. Left pudendal nerve and its branches in the bitch, lateral view with left limb removed.

The **DEEP PERINEAL NERVES** (3) branch caudally off the pudendal nerve and innervate the urethralis, ischiourethralis, ischiocavernosus, constrictor vestibuli, and constrictor vulvae muscles.

The **CAUDAL RECTAL NERVE** (4), usually a branch of a deep perineal nerve, innervates the external anal sphincters. The **DORSAL NERVE OF THE CLITORIS** is a branch of the pudendal nerve that innervates the body and glans of the clitoris.

The pudendal nerve of the dog (1, Fig. 27.11) courses caudally in association with the internal pudendal artery across the dorsolateral surface of the coccygeus.

The superficial perineal nerve (2) and its terminal branch, the **DORSAL SCROTAL NERVE** (3), have a distribution similar to that in the bitch. The deep perineal nerves (4) innervate the retractor penis, urethralis, ischiourethralis, bulbospongiosus, and ischiocavernosus muscles.

The caudal rectal nerve (5) innervates the external anal sphincter.

The **DORSAL NERVE OF THE PENIS** (6) is the distal continuation of the pudendal nerve along the dorsum of the root and body and into the glans of the penis.

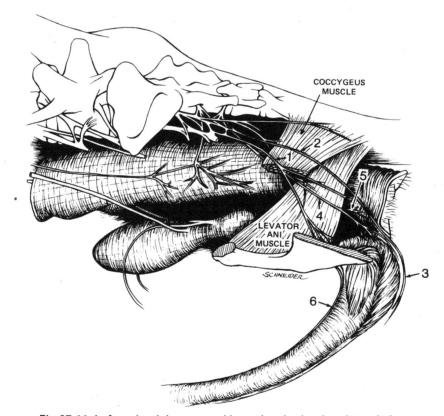

Fig.27.11. Left pudendal nerve and branches in the dog, lateral view.

Chapter 28

PERIPHERAL NERVOUS SYSTEM—VISCERA

Objectives: To identify the major nerves to the smooth muscle and glands of the digestive, respiratory, urinary, reproductive, and cardiovascular systems, as well as to the cardiac muscle of the heart. To provide a basis for understanding the function of the autonomic nervous system.

Autonomic Nervous System (General Visceral Efferent or GVE pathway): Sympathetic and Parasympathetic Nervous Systems

Vagosympathetic Trunk: Sympathetic pathway to head and Parasympathetic pathway to visceral structures in neck, thorax, and cranial abdomen

Cranial nerves carrying parasympathetic fibers from the brain: Oculomotor, Facial, Glossopharyngeal, and Vagus

Branches of the Right and Left Vagus Nerve: Cranial Laryngeal Nerve, Recurrent Laryngeal Nerve, Dorsal and Ventral Branches (which unite dorsally and ventrally with that of the other side to/from the Dorsal and Ventral Vagal Trunks)

Pelvic Nerve and Pelvic Plexus

Sympathetic pathways: Right and Left Communicating Rami between Spinal Nerves T1–L3 and the Right and Left Sympathetic Trunks, Sympathetic Trunk Ganglia, Cervicothoracic Ganglia, Ansa Subclavia, Middle Cervical Ganglia, Cervical Sympathetic Trunks, Cranial Cervical Ganglia; Right and Left Major Splanchnic, Lessor Splanchnic, and Lumbar Splanchnic Nerves; Celiac, Cranial Mesenteric, and Caudal Mesenteric Ganglia; Right and Left Hypogastric Nerves

Nerves to the viscera contain both sensory and motor fibers. Sensory fibers from viscera are termed general visceral afferent (**GVA**); GVA fibers carry impulses from baro- and chemoreceptors in blood vessels of the neck and thorax and from pain receptors in the thoracic, abdominal, and pelvic cavities. Impulses resulting from noxious stimuli may be carried from pleura and peritoneum through both visceral or parietal pathways (Fig. 28.1). The nerve cell bodies of afferent fibers belonging to both visceral and parietal pathways are situated in spinal ganglia of the various spinal nerves.

The parietal pleura and peritoneum are associated with sensory endings that respond to tactile, thermal, and chemical stimuli; impulses generated in the afferent fibers are carried through the same nerve trunks as are impulses from muscle and skin. In contrast to the parietal lining, touching or incising visceral structures is not perceived by the brain; pain in visceral structures is the result of a diffuse stimulation, as from distention of the gut or lack of blood (ischemia) in an area. The pain of a heart attack is largely due to ischemic cardiac tissue.

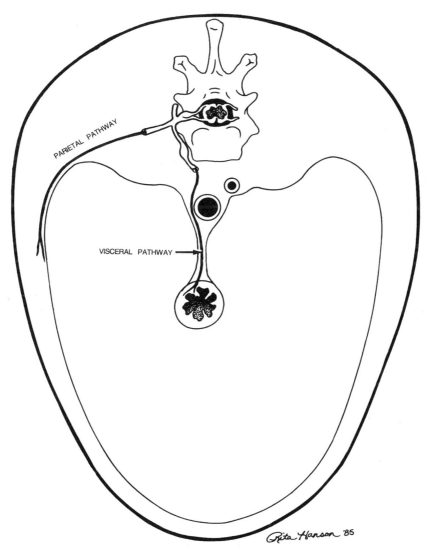

Fig.28.1. Schematic of the pathways by which fibers reach the viscera and serous membranes from the spinal cord.

A sensation of pain in the viscera is often felt on the surface of the body (referred pain). Referred pain probably results when GVA fibers share a common termination in the CNS with general somatic afferent (GSA) fibers.

The brain associates impulses over the GSA pathway with external events and may not distinguish the GVA as a separate input. The surface area to which visceral pain is referred often has a common embryological origin with the visceral structure from which the pain impulse arises. Subsequent to the change in positions of many organs during development, visceral pain in the postnatal animal may be interpreted as coming from an area of the body some distance away from the irritated organ.

The **AUTONOMIC NERVOUS SYSTEM** (ANS) is generally defined as the system of GVE fibers. The term **GENERAL VISCERAL EFFERENT** (GVE) describes motor innervation to visceral structures. **VISCUS** refers to an organ in one of the three large cavities of the body; however, in addition to viscera, the ANS supplies innervation to smooth muscle of blood vessels, smooth muscles of the eye, and many glands that are not restricted to the body cavities.

Anatomically and pharmacologically the ANS is divided into two units (Table 28.1): **SYMPATHETIC** and **PARASYMPATHETIC**. These two divisions are antagonistic in function, with the sympathetic portion of the **ANS** preparing the body for greater skeletomuscular activity and the parasympathetic portion preparing the body for quiet digestive-type activity.

In general, each structure innervated by the sympathetic portion of the ANS is also innervated by the parasympathetic portion, and vice versa. Some exceptions to this dual innervation are sweat glands, arrector pili muscles, adrenal glands, testes, kidney, and smooth muscle of blood vessels, all of which receive little parasympathetic innervation.

Continuous stimulation at a low level by both parasympathetic and sympathetic portions of the ANS produces a maintained state of partial contraction (tone) in visceral structures. Each portion can exert both positive and negative effects by either increasing or decreasing the number of impulses above or below the normal level.

Table 28.1. A comparison of the two portions of the autonomic nervous system.

Characteristic	Parasympathetic Portion	Sympathetic Portion
Number of neurons in series from CNS to effector organ	1 preganglionic 1 postganglionic	1 preganglionic 1 postganglionic
Location of preganglionic nerve cell bodies	Nuclei in the brain and sacral portion of the spinal cord	Nuclei in the thoracolumbar portion of the spinal cord
Location of postganglionic nerve cell bodies	In ciliary, pterygopalatine, otic, mandibular, and sublingual ganglia of head or near structures innervated in thoracic and abdominal cavities	In sympathetic trunk, cranial cervical, middle cervical, cervicothoracic, celiac, cranial mesenteric, and caudal mesenteric ganglia
Function	For quiet, vegetative functions	For active, stressful situations

The sympathetic nerve fibers extend from the thoracic and lumbar segments of the spinal cord to all regions of the body. The parasympathetic fibers extend from the brain and sacral segment of the spinal cord to visceral structures.

Each **VAGUS** (cranial X) **NERVE** (1, Fig. 28.2) extends caudally through the neck in association with fibers of the **SYMPATHETIC TRUNK** (2), which carry efferent impulses toward the head. The vagus and sympathetic trunk, bound together by connective tissue, are collectively named the **VAGOSYMPATHETIC TRUNK** (3).

The sympathetic trunk is composed predominantly of preganglionic sympathetic fibers. The **CRANIAL CERVICAL GANGLION** (4) is an aggregation of nerve cell bodies, which are part of postganglionic sympathetic nerve fibers that are distributed with blood vessels and cranial nerves to nearly all parts of the head.

Right and left vagus nerves separate from right and left sympathetic trunks near the level of the 1st ribs; a sympathetic ganglion, the **MIDDLE CERVICAL GANGLION** (5), may be observed near the level at which each vagus and sympathetic trunk separate.

The **RIGHT VAGUS NERVE** (1, Fig. 28.3) courses caudally ventral to the right subclavian artery and vein, the main vessels of the thoracic limb, giving off a number of branches as it passes caudally dorsal to the base of the heart.

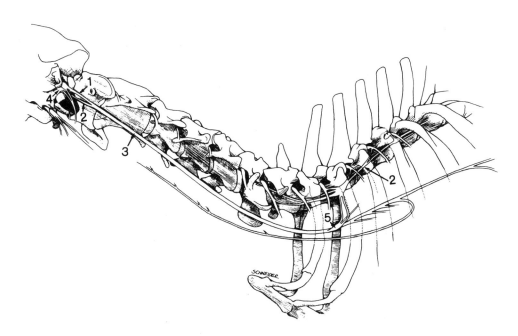

Fig.28.2. Cervical and cranial thoracic portions of the left vagus nerve, ventrolateral view.

One relatively large branch, the **RIGHT RECURRENT LARYNGEAL NERVE (2)**, curves craniodorsally around the right subclavian artery, then courses cranially toward the larynx in contact with the trachea and next to the right longus capitis muscle. The right recurrent laryngeal nerve innervates the esophagus and trachea.

The **RIGHT CAUDAL LARYNGEAL NERVE**, a terminal branch of the right recurrent laryngeal, innervates all of the intrinsic laryngeal muscles on the right side except for the cricothyroideus. A number of nerve fibers branch from the vagus or recurrent laryngeal nerve near the base of the heart; some of these fibers are cardiac branches and some are bronchial branches.

The **LEFT VAGUS NERVE** (3) separates from the sympathetic trunk near the left middle cervical ganglion and continues caudally past the base of the heart.

The **LEFT RECURRENT LARYNGEAL NERVE** (4) curves dorsomedially around the aorta and then passes cranially toward the larynx between the trachea and esophagus.

The branches of the left recurrent laryngeal nerve are the same as those of the right side.

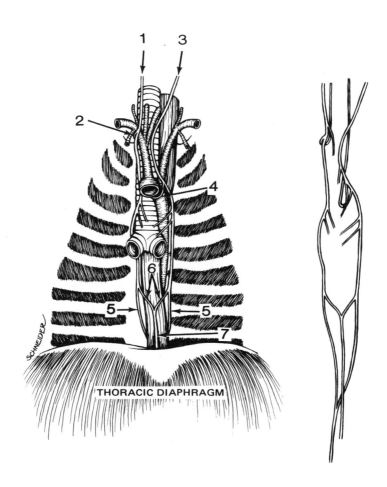

Fig. 28.3. Thoracic portion of the right and left vagus nerves, ventral view.

Bronchial and cardiac branches arise from the vagus near the base of the heart. Both right and left vagi divide into dorsal (5) and ventral (6) branches dorsal to the caudal portion of the base of the heart.

The right and left ventral vagal branches unite on the ventral surface of the esophagus to form the **VENTRAL VAGAL TRUNK** (7), which supplies fibers to the esophagus and then passes caudally through the esophageal hiatus of the diaphragm. Right and left dorsal vagal branches course along the right and left dorsolateral aspects of the esophagus, respectively, and fuse with each other near the thoracic diaphragm. The **DORSAL VAGAL TRUNK** supplies fibers to the esophagus and continues caudally through the esophageal hiatus with the esophagus and ventral vagal trunk.

In the abdominal cavity, the dorsal (1, Fig. 28.4) and ventral (2) vagal trunks may be located along the lesser curvature of the stomach. The ventral vagal trunk supplies fibers to the liver, gall bladder, bile duct, pancreas, and parietal surface and pylorus of the stomach. The dorsal vagal trunk innervates the cardiac and visceral regions of the stomach as well as the pylorus. A **CELIAC BRANCH** (3) of the dorsal vagal trunk passes caudodorsally to a plexus around the origin of two malor unpaired arteries that supply the viscera. Nerve fibers pass along these arteries and their branches to much of the abdominal viscera.

The **PELVIC NERVE** (4) carries parasympathetic fibers to the caudal abdominal and pelvic viscera; it also is a carrier of GVA fibers. The pelvic nerve arises as branches of the ventral rami of sacral spinal nerves. Right and

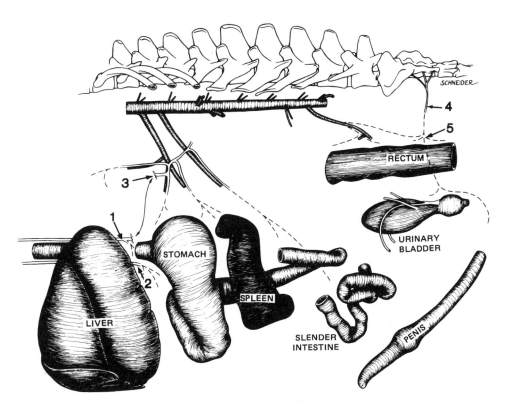

Fig.28.4. Schematic of the distribution of parasympathetic fibers in the abdominal and pelvic cavities, lateral view.

left pelvic nerves each form a **PELVIC PLEXUS** (5) on the lateral surface of the caudal portion of the rectum within the pelvic cavity. Preganglionic parasympathetic fibers extend from the spinal cord through this plexus to reach the rectum, urinary bladder, uterus, descending colon, etc.

Preganglionic sympathetic neurons arise from the spinal cord and enter the sympathetic trunk ganglia between the 1st thoracic and 4th to 5th lumbar spinal cord segments. Although sympathetic fibers seldom arise from the spinal cord cranial to TI or caudal to L5, they gain access to all areas of the body by leaving the sympathetic trunk to be distributed with cranial nerves, spinal nerves, and blood vessels.

Preganglionic neurons (1, Fig. 28.5) pass to **SYMPATHETIC TRUNK GANGLIA** (2) through **COMMUNICATING RAMI** (3); some of the preganglionic neurons synapse in the first ganglion entered, or in a sympathetic trunk ganglion located either more cranially or more caudally, while others synapse in a ganglion (4) located within the abdominal cavity. Postganglionic sympathetic neurons (5) pass through a communicating ramus to a spinal nerve and thus innervate glands of the skin or blood vessels of the body wall; pass to various parts of the body wall with blood vessels; or pass out to the viscera with blood vessels or nerves of the thoracic, abdominal, and pelvic cavities.

In the region of the thoracic inlet, medial to the 1st rib, each middle cervical ganglion, right and left (1, Fig. 28.6), is connected to a cranial cervical ganglion by the cervical portion of the sympathetic trunk (2) and to the **CERVICOTHORACIC GANGLION** (3) by means of the **ANSA SUBGLAVIA** (4). The ansa (or "loop") is a nerve that passes caudodorsally,

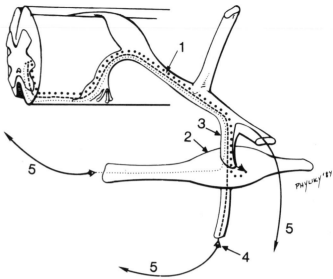

Fig.28.5. Some possible sympathetic pathways through which impulses may pass in going from the spinal cord to the effector site.

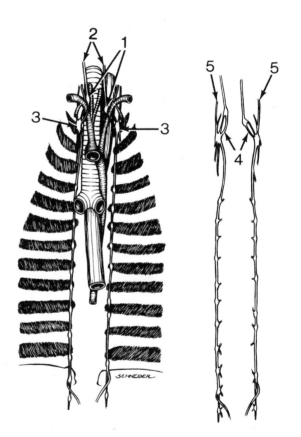

Fig.28.6. Thoracic portion of the sympathetic nervous system, ventral view.

around the ventral surface of the subclavian artery, from the middle cervical ganglion to the cervicothoracic ganglion.

In general, preganglionic sympathetic fibers emerging from the spinal cord through thoracic spinal nerves cranial to T5 pass cranially in the sympathetic trunk, while those arising caudal to T5 pass caudally in the sympathetic trunk.

Some of the preganglionic neurons pass cranially to synapse in the cranial cervical ganglion, while others synapse in either the middle cervical or the cervicothoracic ganglion.

Postganglionic sympathetic fibers separate from the cervicothoracic ganglion, ansa subclavia, and middle cervical ganglion and pass to structures of the thoracic cavity or course along with blood vessels to the body wall.

The **VERTEBRAL NERVE** (5) is a sympathetic postganglionic pathway or plexus that passes craniodorsally with the vertebral artery through the transverse foramina of cervical vertebrae;

sympathetic fibers reach most of the cervical spinal nerves via the vertebral nerve.

The caudal continuations of right and left sympathetic trunks (Fig. 28.7), consisting of sympathetic trunk ganglia (1) and **INTERGANGLIONIC RAMI** (2), are situated along the dorsal surface of the thoracic, abdominal, and pelvic cavities.

The sympathetic trunks are situated on each side of the vertebral column external or superficial to the parietal pleura (thoracic cavity) or parietal peritoneum (abdominal and pelvic cavities).

At the approximate level of the 13th thoracic spinal nerve, a relatively large nerve arises from a sympathetic trunk ganglion and passes caudoventrally into the abdominal cavity past the lateral surface of the crus of the diaphragm. This **MAJOR SPLANCHNIC NERVE** (3) is adjacent and ventromedial to the lumbar continuation of the small sympathetic trunk, which also is situated lateral to the crus of the thoracic diaphragm.

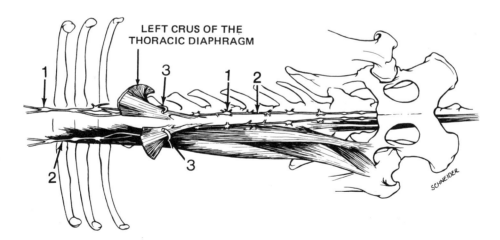

Fig.28.7. Abdominal and pelvic portions of the sympathetic trunk, ventral view.

The major splanchnic nerve (1, Fig. 28.8) supplies fibers to the aorta, adrenal gland, and the plexuses of fibers over the proximal portion of two of the major arteries to the abdominal viscera.

These plexuses are named the **CELIAC** (2) and **CRANIAL MESENTERIC** (3) **PLEXUSES** according to the artery they are situated around.

Sympathetic ganglia, **CELIAC** and **CRANIAL MESENTERIC**, are present in the plexus of sympathetic and parasympathetic fibers. Postganglionic sympathetic fibers course along with branches of these two arteries to the visceral structures they supply.

The sympathetic trunk is larger in the lumbar region than at the level of the caudal portion of the thorax.

LUMBAR SPLANCHNIC NERVES (4) arise from a number of sympathetic trunk ganglia and course ventromedially to any of several ganglia or visceral structures.

Lumbar splanchnics arising from ganglia at the 5th to 7th lumbar spinal nerve levels pass ventromedially to the **CAUDAL MESENTERIC PLEXUS** and **GANGLION** (5). Fibers belonging to the **INTERMESENTERIC PLEXUS** (6) may be observed spanning the distance between the cranial and caudal mesenteric plexuses. Some postganglionic fibers are distributed with the femoral artery to the pelvic limb.

RIGHT and **LEFT HYPOGASTRIC NERVES** (7) are composed of predominantly postganglionic sympathetic neurons coursing from the caudal mesenteric ganglion (where

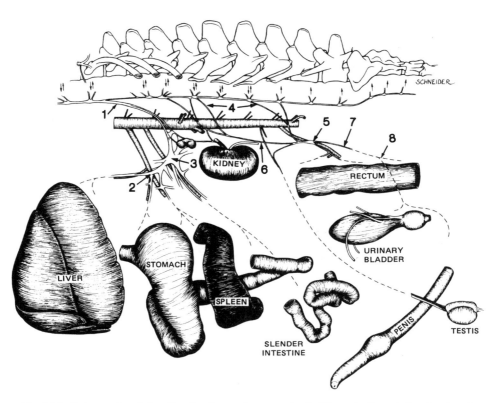

Fig.28.8. Schematic of the distributions of sympathetic fibers in the abdominal and pelvic cavities, lateral view.

their nerve cell bodies are located) to the pelvic plexus (8) on the lateral surface of the pelvic portion of the rectum. The sympathetic fibers course through the pelvic plexus to reach the various pelvic visceral structures; some postganglionic fibers pass out to the pelvic limb with the ischiatic and femoral nerves.

The right and left sympathetic trunks (1, Fig. 28.9) are more slender in the sacral region and tend to converge toward the median plane. Postganglionic sympathetic fibers pass from sympathetic trunk ganglia through communicating rami to sacral spinal nerves. The sympathetic trunks extend into the caudal region.

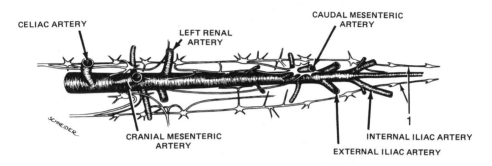

Fig.28.9. Schematic of the relative positions of right and left sympathetic trunks and abdominal aorta, ventral view.

A

M

Q

R